THE SINGLE SOURCE CANCER COURSE

Volume 1:
Prevention

By

S. Wilking Horan

ISBN: 1439273847
ISBN-13: 9781439273845

Praise for

The Single Source Cancer Course

DR. MICHAEL ENGELBERG,
Medical Oncology, Comprehensive Cancer Center, Cedars-Sinai Medical Center, Los Angeles, California:

"Includes the best analysis of breast cancer I've read. I have no doubt this book will prove to be of great value to many people."

PHYLLIS DILLER,
Legendary comedienne, actor and author:

"Susan's Layering Effect is brilliant!"

MARY BUFFETT,
Bestselling author of *Buffettology* and *The Tao of Warren Buffett*, Simon and Schuster:

"This is by far one of the best books I've read on diagnosis, recovery and positive spirit because it so deftly packages Susan's ideas in a form that anyone can identify with. A great read that you will want to keep by your side, to refer to over and over."

JAMES CROMWELL,
Academy Award nominated actor and activist:

"*The Single Source Cancer Course* is a thoroughly researched, comprehensive encyclopedia of cancer facts - an essential and invaluable resource for anyone."

GREG MOODY,
Author and thirty year veteran of radio, newspaper, television and online reporting, *Critic At Large*, KCNC-TV, Denver, Colorado:

"I come from a family of cancer survivors. And, the greatest difficulty in dealing with cancer is simply finding information. Where do you look? Who do you listen to? What information is nonsense, what is anecdotal, what is hard fact? The truth is, we search thousands of places to bring together the information we need to comfort ourselves, our friends, our families. Until now. Susan Wilking Horan has created the ultimate reference guide for all of us. Thousands of facts, contacts and information sources are suddenly at your fingertips in a highly readable, easily referenced format. You're not alone. You're no longer in the dark. Information is at hand and you can find it right here."

Thanks

Thanks to the following people for their patience, input and answers to my numerous questions, many of which were posed completely out of context:
Dr. Michael Engelberg, Oncology, Los Angeles, California; Dr. Edward Share, Gastroenterology, Los Angeles, California; Dr. Steve Horan, Orthopedics, Denver, Colorado; Dr. Lisa Becker, Obstetrics & Gynecology, Littleton, Colorado; Kate Horan, Ultrasonography, Denver, Colorado; Peg Horan, Speech and Language Pathologist, Insurance Referrals; Toborcia Bedgood, Radiological Therapist, Los Angeles, California.

With additional thanks to the following people for additional reasons:
Dr. Joseph Yadagar, Dr. Mitchell Karlin, Dr. Kristi Funk, Dr. C. Michelle Burnison, Terry Magnatta, Erin Rogers, Jim Agee, Michael Garrett, Kristi Blicharski, Mark Fleischer and my computer guru Evan Leonard who kept all my computers and printers running throughout the long writing and re-writing process.

DISCLAIMER

The information contained within this book and all related materials is intended only as an educational aid. This information is not intended as medical advice for individual treatments or conditions, nor is it intended as a substitute for advice by a physician or any other health care practitioner. Readers should consult their personal medical professionals to properly evaluate the comprehensiveness and utility of the information within this book. Readers who suspect they may have a specific medical problem should consult their physician to secure a proper diagnosis and determine a safe and effective course of treatment. And, of course, in the event the information or advice within this book differs from information or advice provided by a health care professional, readers should always follow the recommendation of the health care professional.

Who Should Read This Book?

I will begin by stating that I am not a medical doctor. I have never been to medical school nor did I study pre-med courses in my undergraduate years. Rather, I studied Psychology in college and graduated in 1988 with a Bachelor of Arts Degree from the University of California, Northridge. I then went to law school and graduated in 1993 with a Juris Doctor Degree from Loyola Law School, Los Angeles.

I believe this is important because this book is not a textbook. It is not designed by a doctor to be read by other doctors. It is not written in dense medical terms that only those with a specialized education can understand. It is not a publication or treatise written to gain promotion or tenure. And it is not associated with, nor does it promote, any particular medical organization, community or business over another.

Quite simply, this is a "how-to" book written by one ordinary person for the benefit of other ordinary people. I have survived three different cancers over the last fifteen years. I have spent more time in hospitals, doctors' offices and medical facilities during that time than I care to remember. My expertise on the subject comes primarily from personal experience. And I have taken this experience, combined it with my research and writing skills as an attorney and my knowledge of psychology to produce this one-stop-shopping guide to a better understanding of cancer and its many related issues.

Just as important is the fact that I do not advocate anything in this book. I do not advocate one cancer treatment over another or one scientific study over another or one course of action over another. I do not present information that reflects one school of thought over another. While I do present that information upon which the most respected medical organizations and publications the world over appear to agree, I also present information that is in controversy and scientific findings that are contradictory. For information is not static, but fluid and ever-changing. There are many experts on cancer and not all of them are in agreement, and findings that state one thing today will often state something completely different tomorrow.

To that end, I have done my best to present a comprehensive layperson's guide to preventing, treating and surviving cancer as we understand it today. I have utilized the most reliable and up-to-date sources available and have distilled their vast oceans of information into the pages before you. I simply present information and ask the reader to reach her or his own conclusions. For if I advocate anything in this book it is that each individual take full responsibility for her or his personal life and health. I advocate that each individual be as fully informed as possible. I advocate that each individual become pro-active rather than re-active. I advocate that each individual make her or his own decisions based upon thorough research, consultation and analysis. And, I hope this book will make that task a little easier.

Cancer is common. Eventually, it will affect everyone in one way or another. Everyone will either wage her or his own personal battle against the disease or be drafted into the personal battle of another. Accordingly, the person who should read this book is one who:

1) Desires concise information on cancer-related issues in an accessible, user-friendly format;
2) Is at present engaged in a battle with the disease;
3) Knows someone who is engaged in battle with the disease;
4) Requires clear information regarding cancer treatments;
5) Has survived cancer and requires guidance in navigating the health care and legal systems, and;
6) Seeks a better understanding of the nature of the disease and common-sense steps to help in its prevention.

How to Read This Book

When it comes to cancer we are surrounded by a world of information. Literally, truck loads exist. Indeed, I have an entire guestroom filled to the ceiling with research materials that attests to that fact. Yet, too much information is just as confusing as too little. Perhaps, it's even more confusing. The trick is to understand what information is essential to the cancer process. This information must be separated from the excess and the facts must be distinguished from the fiction. It must then be reduced to its essence and presented in a user-friendly source that is comprehensive without being unnecessarily cumbersome.

This is what I hope my book has accomplished–at least, to some small degree. It's the result of years of personal research, years of personal experience and years of listening to and counseling others. In the interest of accessibility, it has been divided into two Volumes. The first is entitled "Prevention" and the second is "Treatment and Survival." Clearly, readers who have never had cancer may wish only to read Volume 1, while readers who now have or have had cancer in the past may wish to read both. And, although each volume contains approximately 300 pages, please trust me when I say that each is written in simple language that's easy to understand.

So, let's discuss the progression of this book in the same manner in which it was written. We'll start with the first volume and proceed to the second, with each chapter laying the foundation for the next. We'll move slowly and logically through the information one small step at a time.

Volume 1

"Prevention" begins with a short history of cancer and a thorough discussion of what we believe cancer to be. This is important because we need to understand the basics of what cancer is and how it begins if we ever hope to prevent it. I believe one of the biggest obstacles my readers will face will be overcoming unfounded fears and outdated misconceptions of the disease. It's necessary to replace fear with knowledge, for knowledge truly is power. And, it's crucial for you – the reader - to remove the paralyzing blinders often associated with cancer, and to arm yourself with the latest information and universally accepted facts and figures.

Once we've broken the ice, Volume 1 moves on to a discussion of statistics. That's right, statistics. Now, this has nothing to do with mathematics so please don't panic. Rather, this section discusses the way in which scientific studies are conducted and findings are presented. This is important to understand because new information on cancer is always emerging.

New studies are always being published and quite often, the results of one will contradict the results of another. This section will help train us to ask the right questions about such studies and to reach our own conclusions by applying common sense and logic.

Next, we will dive into an exploration of those things that are believed to cause cancer. Now, it's very difficult to establish a direct link between many commonly accepted causes of cancer and the disease itself. Accordingly, this book will present the terms "cause" or "causes" in quotes. I do this simply to remind the reader that it's hard to "prove" something causes cancer. Rather, it is more accurate to say that certain things have been associated with or linked to the development of cancer. These are the things we will explore in this book.

Indeed, I have organized this particular material into thirteen different areas of exploration. These include:

1) Heredity

2) Solar Radiation
3) Air Pollution
4) Water Pollution
5) Pesticides and Chemicals
6) Viruses

7) Drugs
8) Ionizing Radiation
9) Hormones

10) Occupation
11) Diet
12) Alcohol
13) Tobacco

As you can see the first area, **Heredity**, is in a category of its own. The second area includes the five major **Environmental** "causes" of cancer. The third includes those "causes" associated with **Medical Conditions and Treatments**. The last includes those "causes" associated with **Lifestyle**.

Indeed, these "causes" are those that have been studied extensively and have been generally accepted as those most associated with the development of cancer. Of course, new agents are always coming under suspicion within the cancer research community, but those listed here will give the reader a solid understanding of the usual suspects. And, once this is established, we will thoroughly discuss the major cancers that are implicated by these thirteen areas of concern.

Now, having this foundation of knowledge is essential. Understanding the connection between the most commonly accepted "causes" of cancer and the cancers related to them will allow us to evaluate our own lives and bodies and our own possible risk for some cancers. In fact, this is so important that it is presented twice in this book; first in a short, superficial way and then in an in depth, detailed way beginning with many of the ground-breaking cancer studies of the 1980s and the 1990s.

This leads us to a section of the book I call "The Layering Effect" which, in my opinion, may be the most important section. The Layering Effect is an exercise which allows us to assess the **possible** cancer risks for an individual. It's presented in the same way as our previous section on "causes" and related major cancers. First, we profile five hypothetical individuals and their lifestyles. We apply our "Layering Effect" in an effort to identify known cancer risks each individual may face. We add the "layers" of risk together and then list the possible cancers for which the individual may be at risk. Based upon this, we make suggestions as to how each individual may decrease or mitigate his or her potential risk.

Now, the first two profiles will be simple. The second three, however, will be much more detailed. And once we've done this, we'll evaluate our own risk by applying "The Layering Effect" to ourselves with a personal worksheet included in the chapter. Of course, this exercise isn't perfect and it's not infallible. For as we will say many times, we cannot predict with certainty what cancers may or may not affect us. But, this exercise is an effective tool that will help us understand our **potential** risk for different cancers and the ways in which we may decrease or mitigate that risk.

Of course, Volume 1 would not be complete without a thorough discussion of the most common screening and detection procedures for the most common cancers. Prevention is pro-active. It is not re-active. It's vital to monitor our own health and well-being by utilizing all the tools available to us. Yearly exams, regular visits to our physicians and age and risk-related tests must become a part of our regular healthcare routine. For fighting cancer is very much like certain sporting events. The best defense is a strong offense. Let's not live in fear but, rather, act confidently with the benefit of knowledge.

Finally, both volumes of this book are dotted with several personal notes from my own experience and several synopses of scientific studies. The former notes help to illustrate specific points in our discussion and the latter studies help to test our knowledge and teach us to think for ourselves and come to our own conclusions.

Volume 2

Congratulations! If you've finished Volume 1 you now have a better understanding of cancer and its "causes" than probably ninety percent of the general population. You're learning to evaluate information and to reach conclusions based upon your own knowledge and common sense. And, you're aware of the importance of screening procedures and regular medical check-ups according to your personal risk profile. Yet, having a firm knowledge of cancer and incorporating preventive measures into everyday life does not guarantee any individual will remain cancer-free.

Volume 2 addresses this very issue. Suppose you've taken advantage of every applicable screening procedure **and** you've undergone regular and necessary medical exams **and** you still develop some form of cancer. What do you do now?

To begin, it's important to understand that developing cancer even when you've been careful and responsible **does not mean your preventive measures have failed**. Rather, it means that if a cancer does develop, your preventive measures in all likelihood will have detected it early when the cancer is highly treatable. It also means that because of your good health practices, you are probably in fairly good physical condition at the time of diagnosis. And this, of course, means that you'll be better able to withstand any treatment that might be required. All of these things are extremely important if and when your battle with cancer becomes personal.

Volume 2 discusses cancer treatment and cancer survival. Now, most cancers will require treatment that involves some form of surgery. In the first section of Volume 2 we'll discuss several of the most common cancers and the surgical procedures typically recommended. After surgery, many cancers will require chemotherapy, radiation or both.

As these two latter treatments are the most common, we discuss each in great detail. We'll explain what they are, how they work and how they're administered. We'll also examine the possible side effects and discuss the potential dangers of each treatment. We'll discuss the short-term and long-term conditions you might face from undergoing these treatments including the ways in which each impacts reproduction. This is an honest and frank discussion that I refer to as "all the things you need to know that no one wants to tell you." For I believe one must be fully informed before one can make responsible choices and decisions. Then we'll finish this section by discussing some additional therapies also commonly used in treating cancer.

Next, we'll move on to a section entitled, "Basic Medical Know-How." For if you or a loved one has cancer, knowing the ins and outs of your medical community and how it functions is a necessity. We'll begin by discussing the role of the technician. The technicians, by the way, will be responsible for most of your day-to-day care. It is they who will monitor your regular check-ups, conduct your necessary procedures and interface with your doctors. You need to understand what their job is, what you should expect from them and how far their responsibility extends.

Then, we'll discuss the role of the doctor. After all, your life is in the hands of this professional. So I caution you, never take anything for granted. Never just hand your well-being over to another individual without careful consideration. Accordingly, the importance of this section is to instill in you the need to think for yourself. Its purpose is to make you aware that no one should be allowed to make decisions about your life without your input. You must work in concert with your physician. You must question her or his actions. And, you must take responsibility for your own well-being. In so doing, one of the most important relationships of your life, in one of the most crucial times of your life, will be successful and rewarding.

And of course, this leads us to our next discussion of your role as the patient. So far we've examined the responsibilities your technicians and doctors have toward you. Now we'll examine the responsibilities you have toward them. We'll also discuss in great detail your legal and privacy rights as you move through the medical network.

Now that we have the basic nuts and bolts of your treatment out of the way, we'll spend a little time on pain management. While this may not be an issue with cancer itself, it's often an issue that results from the treatments of cancer. We start by clearing up the confusion that exists on the subject of narcotics. We'll discuss the various drugs that are available and why some are legally sanctioned and others are not. Apart from these drugs, we'll also examine additional procedures and techniques for treating pain or discomfort. Then we'll finish this section up with a discussion of several alternative and complementary medical techniques.

At this point, we'll move our discussion from cancer patient to cancer survivor. This is a big transition, and this new role encompasses issues quite different from those we've already investigated. First, we'll discuss the physical concerns. The focus here, of course, is to maintain health and monitor for any future occurrence or a recurrence, for as a survivor, you must be vigilantly aware. You must engage in strict post-cancer check-ups, blood tests and screening procedures. You must adhere to a positive, healthy lifestyle. And, you must be dedicated to simple, yet essential, good health practices in your daily routine for the rest of your life

Second, we'll discuss the emotional concerns associated with cancer survival, of which there are many. We'll examine the anger, anxiety, grief and depression that can result from a battle with cancer. We'll examine how your personal relationships with family, friends and lovers may be affected. We'll also examine how your relationships in the workplace may change, what your legal rights within your workplace are and how you can protect those rights.

Third, we'll discuss the financial concerns of a cancer diagnosis. This is a most important issue, for a battle with cancer can devastate the life savings of an entire family. In this section you will learn how to make the system work for you. You'll become an expert on medical insurance issues and how they may apply to your case. You'll become familiar with federal and state sponsored insurance programs as well as private plans. You'll learn how to extend your insurance, change your insurance and protect your insurance. For those who don't have insurance, you'll learn how to help yourself by utilizing other available programs, funds, foundations and clinical trials.

We'll also discuss disability benefit programs and survivor benefit programs. We'll discuss your medical rights and the procedures in which you can appeal a negative decision from your insurance carrier. Then, we'll discuss medical facilities, how they differ from one another and how you can protect yourself from treatment and billing mistakes.

Of course, the United States passed new health care reform in March of 2010. I don't profess for a second to fully understand it, nor have I spoken to one other person who believes they fully understand it. Indeed, it may be years before the full impact of this reform becomes clear. Nevertheless, I have included a small section in this volume that attempts to clarify some of the aspects of this reform and how they may relate to the issues we have discussed. Finally, Volume 2 ends with a list of organizations that can help you through every step of your cancer experience as well as a synopsis of cancer research and its future.

Now, I've included a list of sources for the information found within these pages in the reference section of each Volume. It's just not possible, however, for me to list *every* source that may apply. If I were to do so, the reference section of this book might be longer than the text. Accordingly, I typically list one or two sources. When discussing scientific studies, I sometimes cite the initial work that laid the foundation for the area of study. Sometimes I cite a few of the ground-breaking studies, many of which were conducted in the 1980s and the 1990s. And, sometimes when there are far too many studies and researchers to list, I simply cite the pages of a comprehensive source.

Moreover, readers will notice the term "Id." appears often in the reference section. Id. is an abbreviation of the Latin term "ibid." It simply means that a citation is identical to the previous citation of "the immediate past one." Typically, in legal documents Id. is only used when the previous citation contains one source. This book, however, is not a legal document. As a result, and in the interest of brevity, I have used Id. even when the previous citation contains two or more sources. This means that the text being referenced comes from all the same sources as the previously referenced text.

Similarly, other citations within this book may not always conform to the rules of the legal profession. The rules and opinions for citing information continue to change as does the technology for gaining information. And, sometimes certain information is just not available. As a result, some citations may lack a page or section number, or an author's name or full date. Other citations may appear as they were cited in a previous publication, correct or not. In any event, they remain sufficient enough to point those readers who wish to conduct their own research on a topic in the right direction.

Much of the basic cancer information within this book can be found in the literature of many organizations including the American Cancer Society, the National Cancer Institute and the World Health Organization. For readers who want more information on specific subjects, one internet search will probably yield several pages of additional references. And for readers who wish to know more about scientific studies, there are a few websites in particular that contain data on nearly every cancer study that's been conducted. These are wonderful reference tools and two of my favorites are:

PubMed

(http://www.ncbi.nlm.nih.gov/pubmed/) and;

Journal of the American Medical Association Archives

(http://pubs.ama-assn.org/).

Finally, direct quotes found within the text of this book have been credited, of course, to the specific source in which they were found.

I want to end this section by once again offering my heartfelt congratulations to each and every one of you who has the courage and the determination to read this book. It's not easy to face our fears. And, it's not easy to tackle this particular subject. But in reading this book, you are arming yourself with the most powerful weapon on earth– knowledge. And as you continue to expand your knowledge, you continue to expand your ability to protect yourself and your loved ones. Remember, we are engaged in a war. And the best way to win any war is to learn everything you can about the enemy. Let's not stand helpless on the sidelines. Let's not stick our heads in the sand and hope the enemy passes us by. Let's not ignore its presence and convince ourselves we are immune. Let's not allow it to surprise us and catch us off guard. Rather, let's be prepared! Let's meet this enemy head-on with confidence and power! Let's be pro-active! Let's go after it before it comes after us! Together we can save lives. And, together we can halt the march of this enemy and turn the tide in our favor! For this, I applaud you all!

Introduction

To know the road ahead, ask those coming back.
Chinese Proverb

I've been through colon cancer, skin cancer and breast cancer. And I'm still here. I was a healthy, young, athletic, slim, non-smoking vegetarian when I was diagnosed with colon cancer over ten years ago. During the next decade, while recuperating not only from that disease but from the treatments I received, including chemotherapy and radiation, I also developed skin cancer. And to top it all off, I was diagnosed with breast cancer in 2007. I was ill prepared for my first cancer, better prepared for my second and firmly prepared for my third, for I did my homework. I studied. I researched. I know what it takes to survive. And the full benefit of my knowledge lies within the pages of this book.

As anyone who has experienced the same can tell you, the road from cancer prevention to recovery and survival is difficult, filled with unexpected turns, detours and a multitude of pitfalls and obstacles. And not knowing my way the first time, I took every wrong turn, got lost with every detour, fell into every pitfall and stumbled over every obstacle. For the great problem with cancer is that when one or a loved one is diagnosed with the disease, time becomes a critical issue. One must gather information quickly. One must make decisions quickly. One must act quickly. And to further compound this unavoidable reality, cancer is a subject that doesn't lend well to simple phrases, immediate comprehension or easy choices. Rather, cancer is a complicated subject that must be dissected carefully to be understood. It's a disease that raises enormously important questions for which clear answers are not always evident. And, it's a disease the existing information for which is far too vast to be adequately collected, sorted and digested in a limited period of time.

In addition, a diagnosis of cancer often leaves one in a state of emotional turmoil in which one's ability to make objective and logical decisions becomes clouded and compromised. And, of course, the diagnosis is only the beginning, for the road that leads one from diagnosis to survival and recovery can be long and arduous. Each step requires one to be fully aware and informed, regardless of the fear, doubt or confusion one may encounter along the way.

Accordingly, this brings us to the purpose for this book. It's a handbook, really. It's one source that contains just enough of the essential information necessary to guide one from cancer prevention to cancer survival. In Volume 1 of this book, we'll discuss the history of cancer; describe what it is, how it begins and why. We'll discuss our deep-rooted fear of the disease and many of the misconceptions that surround it. We'll discuss the field of statistics, how statistical information applies to cancer, and the ways in which we can analyze that information to separate fact from fiction. We'll discuss the known risk factors associated with cancer, first from the perspective of the risks themselves, then from the perspective of the major cancers they implicate. We'll supply tools that will enable one to objectively determine her or his potential cancer risks and provide examples to illustrate the usefulness of these tools. We'll outline the ways in which one can protect oneself from cancer through lifestyle choices, screening procedures and early detection.

In Volume 2, we'll move on to discuss a diagnosis of cancer and a variety of the cancer surgeries and treatments that may follow. Not only will we describe these surgeries and treatments, we'll be extremely frank in discussing the problems they may create and the ways in which one may prepare for, avoid or mitigate such problems. We'll explore the roles of both patient and medical personnel, the importance of these relationships, as well as the patient's legal protections and privacy rights. Moreover, we'll discuss the many issues one will face as she or he makes the transition from cancer patient to cancer survivor. We'll discuss the necessary follow-up programs that one must adhere to, and the physical and emotional issues that may surface. And, of course, we'll discuss the financial aspects of cancer including insurance, disability, employment rights and other legalities. We'll discuss the differences among treatment facilities, hospital billing practices, clinical trials and the resources through which one may find additional help. We'll punctuate each section with personal notes and a variety of news headlines to drive our points home and hone our analytical skills. And we'll emphasize the importance of personal responsibility and the necessity of thinking for oneself throughout.

In essence, this book is a compilation of cancer basics. It provides a solid starting point, sure footing and a useful map for the road ahead for those who wish to protect themselves from cancer, as well as those fighting cancer. And while this book is an essential source, it's not an exhaustive source, for it simply isn't possible to include all of the world's information on cancer and all its aspects within one source. Furthermore, some of this information is constantly changing. Accordingly, I apologize in advance to those whose questions may not be answered in this book. I apologize to those whose specific cancers may not be discussed in this book. And I apologize to those who seek information that may be beyond the scope of this book.

I also apologize for the fact that much of the information within this book pertains primarily to the developed and industrialized countries of the world. This is in no way a statement about the relative importance of one country or population compared to another. Rather, this is a practical reflection of reality in that cancer information and cancer statistics typically are more current and available in the developed and industrialized countries of the world. It's within these regions of the world that most of the populations generally know how to read and have access to the luxury of books through their homes, schools or libraries. As a result, these are the populations that may most benefit from the information within this particular book.

Moreover, as a citizen of the United States, some of the statistics and information relating to certain matters such as insurance and finances will be unique to the United States.

Finally, as a resident of California, some of the examples within this book will be limited to that particular state, only because the information needed to make the point may have been, in some cases, more accessible.

Having said this, I nevertheless hope that most readers will find the answers and information they seek within these pages. I hope that some of the fear associated with this disease will be dispelled. I hope that the many ways in which one can protect oneself from this disease will be incorporated into one's life. And I hope that those who strive to prevent cancer, have been diagnosed with cancer, are currently fighting cancer or have survived cancer will themselves find hope, knowledge and inspiration within these pages. For, this is the book that I wish I had had when I was diagnosed with my first cancer.

I've been down this road before. Indeed, I've been down this road three times. I know the way. I can help shed light on the path and illuminate the darkness. I can help one navigate the terrain, avoid the wrong turns, negotiate the detours, anticipate the pitfalls and sail over the obstacles. I've already jumped through all the hoops, and if just one reader can benefit from my mistakes, or learn from my experience, the purpose of this book will be served.

S. Wilking Horan

TABLE OF CONTENTS
Volume 1: Prevention

Part 4: The Layering Effect Revisited

Part 5: Screening and Detection

Part 6: A Quick Review

Volume 1: Prevention

Part 1:
Cancer: An Overview

Chapter 1:
Well Begun Is Half Done

"Come to the edge," He said. They said, "We are afraid."
"Come to the edge," He said. They came. He pushed them . . . and they flew.
Guillaume Apollinaire

Cancer. Few words have the power to intimidate, frighten and chill to the bone as this one simple utterance. It's the one word that no one wants to hear, and everyone fears they will. It's the word that stops time in its tracks and changes the lives of all who hear it. It's a word that establishes a moment of truth by which all future events will be measured. It's a word that shakes the very foundation of who we are, what we think and how we feel. It's a word that threatens all one holds dear, all one lives for and all one hopes for. It's a word that forces an acknowledgment of mortality now rather than at some vague time in the future.

Cancer is not a delicate subject, and as such we won't discuss it here in a delicate manner. Cancer is a harsh reality that must be faced squarely if it is to be fought effectively. And while the waters in this pool are intimidating, we won't test them timidly with our big toe and wade in slowly. Rather, we'll plunge right in, squarely in the middle of the deep end, and confront them directly with courage and confidence. So, let's hold on tight, brace ourselves, take a deep breath and jump!

Not surprisingly, a diagnosis of cancer, the prospect of cancer, the mere mention of the word "cancer" is for many people the most frightening thing imaginable. The thought of cancer entering our lives or those of our loved ones in any way creates confusion and panic. It paralyzes us with fear and replaces the reality of our everyday lives with feelings of hopelessness and impotence. We must ask ourselves, "Why?" Why is there so much fear associated with this disease?

This is the most important of questions, because such desperate reactions and emotions are largely misguided and unwarranted and are based primarily on an outdated and inaccurate image of this complicated disease. First, cancer is not the death sentence that it used to be. It's true that cancer historically has been a brutal and highly lethal enemy of humankind, but its power has been greatly reduced thanks to the ever-increasing advances in medicine and technology. And although it remains a strong adversary that must be faced and fought, its reputation as a "killer" has greatly diminished.

So we must begin by removing the shroud of mystery that has so long enveloped this disease in darkness, ignorance and fear. For similar to the monsters we fear hiding under our beds and in our closets by night, when exposed to the light of day this "monster" becomes much less frightening than the culprit of our imagination. And in this case knowledge, the great equalizer, will be our light. It will illuminate our path and empower us with the ability to understand our foe, for we cannot fight an enemy we don't understand.

And make no mistake about it, cancer is our enemy, and we are in for the fight of our life. It's a personal fight in which we must take responsibility for our own life, our own health and our own recovery. It's a fight that will require determination, sheer guts and the ability to make difficult decisions. And it's a fight in which we must make a commitment to not only arm ourselves with all the weapons and tools modern society has to offer, but to educate ourselves as to their proper application, for all the tools in the world won't help us if we don't know how to use them.

Surviving cancer isn't easy and it may take several years to recover. But, we're all much stronger than we think, for when the wonders of medical science team up with the power of the human will, great things can happen. We must begin by developing an understanding of what cancer is and what it is not. It's imperative to separate information from misinformation, fact from fiction and the present from the past. And as we do so, cancer will become a mere fact of life, a challenge that can be faced and fought as any other we may encounter.

Chapter 2:
A Short History[1]

There is an old adage that states, "Nothing is new under the sun." Cancer is certainly not a "new" disease, and although we have no idea as to when it first appeared in human beings, we do have some idea as to when its presence was first acknowledged. The earliest evidence we have of cancer comes from seven Egyptian papyri that were discovered in the late nineteenth century. Known as the *Ebers Papyrus*, these records appear to have been written in about 1600 B.C., although it's believed the sources of their information may date back to 2500 B.C. These papyri provide us with the first direct knowledge of Egyptian medicine and the first descriptions of cancer.

Indeed two of them, the *Edwin Smith* papyri and the *George Ebers* papyri, not only describe the surgeries for cancer, but outline the numerous mechanical, pharmacological and, of course, magical treatments for cancer as well. The field of medicine was raised out of the realms of magic and superstition, however, as medical and scientific history advanced through the combined Greek theories of disease and the Roman practices of surgery. Disease was re-defined as a natural process the treatment of which was based upon objective observation and experience.

As centuries rolled by, the search to discover the causes of cancer and its proper treatments continued. The Medievals believed that cancer was the result of an excess of "black bile" and that it was only curable in the earliest stages. In the second century A.D., human illness was thought to be the result of Satan, sin, astrology or the ancient Greek theory of the four bodily humors, which referred to blood, phlegm, yellow bile and black bile. Indeed, this "black bile" theory continued throughout the sixteenth century as the medical community began to treat cancer with a variety of pastes laden with arsenic.

It wasn't until the seventeenth century, however, that scientists began to ask "how" rather than "why" and in the process laid the foundation for modern medicine. This was the age of great scientific discovery when Newton's laws of gravity and Galileo's invention of the telescope advanced the world's understanding of its physical universe. Science was aided by exciting new instruments, including the microscope which was discovered by Dutch eyeglass maker Johannes Jansen and his son Zacharias. Robert Hooke's observations of plant structure as "little boxes of cells" led to the nineteenth century theory that the "cell" was the basic unit of living organisms. William Harvey observed and proved the continuous circulation of the human blood system and with the cancer theory of "black bile" discarded, researchers began in earnest to look for answers elsewhere.

It was during this time that a scientist named Gaspare Aselli discovered the vessels of the lymphatic system and suggested that abnormalities of the lymph may be the primary cause of cancer. Medical attention now began to focus on the lymph nodes, the removal of which now became a more common procedure when located near a tumor site. Indeed, it also was during this time that the first mastectomies were performed in conjunction with the removal of the enlarged lymph nodes near the breast. And in addition to the numerous medical and scientific advances, Englishman John Graunt provided the first example of scientific quantification, which led to the improvement of health care through the gathering of statistics.

The eighteenth century was the "Age of Reason," with revolutionary political and intellectual ideals consuming both sides of the Atlantic. The arts soared with the openings of new national museums around the world, and proliferating magazines and newspapers spread information to an ever widening public. In science, the study of the origin of disease or "pathology" and physical diagnoses were becoming more common. The first systematic experiments in cancer were conducted and **oncology** or "the study of cancer" was established as a medical discipline. During this century, Dutch scholar Hermann Boerhaave first theorized that chronic inflammation of body tissues could result in tumors that might become cancerous. The relationship between the development of cancer in workers, such as English chimney sweeps, and the conditions in which they worked were investigated for the first time, as were the carcinogenic effects of tobacco use. The inescapable correlation between many environmental hazards and cancer was made clear and the first hospitals specializing in cancer care were opened.

Similarly, the nineteenth century overflowed with spectacular advances in technology and industry, as well as science and medicine. During this century Louis Pasteur began the study of bacteria and the battle against infectious diseases. Charles Darwin published his theory of evolution, Joseph Lister conducted his experiments with disinfectants and Crawford Long introduced the use of ether and the term "anesthesia" was coined. Indeed, it was the combination of Lister's and Long's work that greatly lowered surgical mortality rates and allowed the science of surgery to quickly advance.

Cancer research also quickly advanced with William Conrad Rontgen, the recipient of the first Nobel Prize in medicine, and his discovery of x-rays, the isolation of radium by Pierre and Marie Curie, and the first observations of cancer cell anomalies by Johannes Muller, an observation that pushed researchers to study the link between disease and cell growth and behavior.

In addition, the first cancer statistics were compiled in France and Italy where researchers found that the cancer death rate was rising and that women died more frequently than men. Using further analyses by sex, age and occupation, Domenico Rigoni-Stern also surmised that cancer was more common in cities than in the country; that the rates of cancer increased with age; and even that unmarried individuals were more likely to develop cancer than those who were married.

Yet, as incredible as all of the world's advances were throughout these past centuries, the amount of knowledge gained in the twentieth century alone was greater than the entire prior history of the world combined. From the early 1900s to the years of World War II, huge strides were made in comprehending the functions of organisms as well as their chemistry and structure.

Based upon the accomplishments of their predecessors, scientists began to battle infectious diseases with newly developed drugs. Through the science of chemotherapy, natural and synthetically produced drugs were used to treat a variety of diseases and the pursuit to control cancer through chemical means began. For the first time x-rays were used to diagnose and treat illness, and in conjunction with radium they were used to combat cancer.

The "causes" of cancer began to be documented and conclusively identified. The carcinogenic effect of viruses was established as was the role of hereditary and the link between cancer and chromosomal anomalies. Long suspected physical factors such as the sun and solar radiation were positively identified as carcinogens. The eighteenth century theory regarding the chimney sweeps of England and the possible carcinogenic effect of chemicals became fact in 1915 when experiments supported the connection. In the United States, the first nationwide organization dedicated to cancer public education was begun, the first modern statistics on cancer rates and deaths were published and the first article on cancer's warning signs appeared in a popular women's magazine.

In the years following World War II and throughout the second half of the twentieth century, the boundaries of scientific research exploded and reached deep into the frontiers of both outer and inner space. Information could now be processed with astonishing speed and molecular biology revealed the inner workings of cells as well as their fundamental makeup. A virtual scientific revolution began when James Watson and Francis Crick presented their model of deoxyribonucleic acid, or DNA, the cellular material that carries the genetic information for all living organisms. It was found that segments of DNA combine to form individual genes, which in turn form the chromosomes that are found in the nucleus of a cell. Based upon this model, the genetic code was broken and a multitude of new discoveries followed regarding the structure and functioning of DNA and the basic building block of all life – the cell.

Armed with this important information, science continued its efforts to solve the most basic issue of all, the origin of cancer. Great strides were made in the areas of cancer causation and the suspicions of earlier ages regarding the dangers of chemicals, viruses, chromosomal anomalies and the environment were confirmed one by one. Epidemiologist Richard Doll pioneered the first studies linking lung cancer to smoking. The role of chemical carcinogens was scrutinized and important research conducted by James and Elizabeth Miller demonstrated that many carcinogens are actually "pre-carcinogens" which means they do not cause cancer in and of themselves, but rather cause errors in the genetic code of the DNA which in turn may cause cancer.

Building upon this research, Howard Temin and David Baltimore isolated an enzyme called reverse transcriptase, which explained how viruses that contain ribonucleic acid, or RNA, convert their genetic makeup into DNA–research that made modern day genetic engineering possible. It was genetic engineering that in turn provided researchers the means to study the process by which a normal cell turns into a cancerous one. Two such researchers, George Todaro and Robert Heubner, theorized that cancer was caused by a particular class of genes known as the oncogenes, meaning that no matter what the "cause" of the cancer was, be it chemical, viral, genetic or other, some essential mechanism remained the same.

And while conducting further genetic studies, Peter Duesberg and Hidesaburo Hanafusa discovered that the RNA virus that caused cancer in animals contained a gene that, in turn, produced a protein necessary for cancer development. Indeed, when the gene was removed and the protein was not produced, the RNA virus was rendered incapable of inducing cancer. Miraculously, Duesberg and Hanafusa had discovered the first oncogene, a gene directly responsible for transforming a normal cell into a cancerous one.

Furthermore, the relationship between viruses and cancer continued to be explored as researchers linked the Epstein-Barr virus to cancer for the first time. Directly on these scientific heels came proof that RNA viruses are linked to human cancer when Robert Gallo demonstrated that human T-cell leukemia was "caused" by the human lymphotropic virus type 1 or HTLV-1. A related virus known as HTLV-11 was soon isolated from patients affected by another leukemia, and based on the work of Gallo and French scientist Luc Montagnier, a third virus called HTLV-111, later known as human immunodeficiency virus or HIV, was identified and isolated. It is, of course, HIV, which can develop into the human autoimmune disease known as AIDS, and from the time of this discovery research regarding AIDS and cancer has been intricately intertwined.

The charge into the world of molecular biology and genetic engineering pushed forward during the latter part of the century, and scientists made great strides in establishing the relationship between chromosomes, their genes and cancer. Just as the oncogenes that cause cancer had been isolated in the 1970s, genes that suppress the growth of cancer were later discovered in the 1980s. Known as "tumor suppressor genes," research found that cell growth becomes restrained when these genes are present. Yet in the absence of these genes if, for example, these natural suppressors are damaged or missing the complete DNA that forms the gene, cancer can develop. Indeed, cancer usually develops when a series of damaged genes that lack these natural suppressors accumulates in a cell.

The 1990s also produced evidence that linked known environmental carcinogens to specific DNA damage. For instance, it was found that solar radiation changes the character of tumor suppressor genes in the skin, thus creating a vulnerability to cancer in the tissue. It also was found that specific chemicals in cigarette smoke "activate" certain genes in cells of the lung that make them more susceptible to the harmful effects of the chemical carcinogens. Ultimately, it was this evidence and the new era of gene research that laid the foundation for several bold new programs such as the Cancer Genome Anatomy Project and the Human Genome Project. It was the goal of these programs to assemble a full index of cancer causing genes and to pinpoint the location and function of each gene in the inherited set of "instructions" that govern the functioning and behavior of human beings.

As inroads into the origins and "causes" of cancer were forged, so too were those that advanced the methods of detecting and treating the disease. Surgery began to be used in conjunction with radiation therapy, and as new chemotherapies joined their ranks a strong alliance in the war against cancer was created. As early as the 1970s, approximately forty-five new chemicals had been found effective in fighting twenty-nine different forms of cancer. And researchers found that as effective as these individual chemicals were, they were even more effective when used in certain combinations. Indeed, it was one of these combinations that succeeded in curing certain forms of childhood leukemia, and it was another four drug combination that raised the cure rate of Hodgkin's disease from nearly zero to eighty percent.

Chemotherapy, however, is a treatment that lacks the ability to discern between cancer cells and normal cells. As a result, a basic course of treatment will poison and destroy many normal cells as well as the cancerous ones. In an effort to reduce this "overkill," the 1980s and 1990s oversaw the development of new treatments that actually fought cancer by enhancing the body's own immune system rather than utilizing lethal chemicals. One such treatment known as the "biologicals" has the ability to identify the antibody producing antigens of specific cancer cells and stimulate these antigens into producing the antibodies necessary to fight the cancer in question.

In addition, the great innovations in genetic engineering over the last decade not only shed light on the mechanisms by which a cell becomes cancerous, they also enabled researchers to chart the extremely complicated immune system of the human body. This feat, combined with the new biotechnology known as "hybridoma technology," has allowed science the means to manipulate and strengthen the human immune system.

It's this combined knowledge of the nature of cancer, the human immune system and the power of antibody-producing antigens that for the first time gives researchers hope that the quest for a cancer vaccine may someday become a reality. Work is already underway to develop cancer vaccines that prevent the recurrence of cancer and vaccines that protect high-risk individuals from developing certain cancers. Research into other vaccines that mark tumor cells for destruction or work as immune system stimulants also are being investigated. This idea of "immunizing" individuals against cancer has intrigued scientists for the last century, and it's this brave and enlightened experimental research that keeps this dream alive.

As the new century and, indeed, the new millennium begins, the world is blessed with an arsenal of weapons focused solely upon the treatment and potential elimination of cancer. Yet, the most important aspect in the war against cancer is early detection and diagnosis, a fact that cannot be emphasized enough. Earlier decades could only study the organs and soft tissues of the human body through anatomical dissections. Through the great advances in computer technology over the last decade, however, diagnostic imaging has been transformed into a precise and powerful life-saving device.

It's now possible to visualize the inner structure of the body and to "see" areas that haven't been accessible before through physical exams or x-rays. Imaging techniques such as ultrasonography, computed tomography or CT scans and magnetic resonance imaging shed light on anomalies and tumors allowing them to be detected at extremely early stages of development. New testing procedures for evaluating the existence of cancer cells such as the Papanicolaou or PAP smear for cervical cancer and the Prostate Specific Antigen or PSA test for prostate cancer warn of problems before they become insurmountable. And this new information concerning routine testing, warning signs, self exams and diagnostic procedures all combine to offer the most comprehensive cancer protection program ever known to humankind.

We find ourselves now on the threshold of the twenty-first century. We live in a time when medical miracles are becoming everyday occurrences. We live in a time when dreams are becoming realities. The last few decades have ushered in a new era of knowledge and progress that have greatly diminished the stranglehold that cancer once had upon women and men the world over. More individuals are surviving cancer today than ever before, and with all the information and all the tools medical research has provided, we're winning the war. So, again we must ask ourselves . . .

Chapter 3:
Why Are We So Afraid of Cancer?

We fear things in proportion to our ignorance of them.
Titus Livy

The reasons for our fear exist for many reasons, yet the most significant one may be the simple fact that old attitudes die hard. Cancer has had over five thousand years to build its notoriously negative and frightening reputation. It's difficult to dispense with ideas and fears that are centuries old in the span of a few short decades. Let's face it; cancer is a disease with a past that is hard to overcome. There's an eighteenth century story about Dr. Oliver Wendell Holmes and his great friend, noted author Nathaniel Hawthorne. When Dr. Holmes discovered that Hawthorne had been diagnosed with cancer, Dr. Holmes shook his head in resignation and replied, ". . . the shark's tooth is upon him . . ."[2]

Indeed, in those days having cancer was just like falling victim to a shark. Both were attacks by lethal, overpowering forces that rose from mysterious depths to overtake and consume. There was little chance of escape, few survived and most simply accepted defeat and surrendered to the demise that was certain to follow.

More recently, and throughout the first half of the twentieth century in fact, cancer retained its reputation as a "death sentence." Most of those diagnosed with the disease didn't survive. Yet this was so because surgical procedures were still developing, treatment programs remained for the most part experimental and our knowledge of the disease was limited and often inconclusive. In addition to the dire statistics and the lacking technology, cancer was and is a disease that can strike anyone. It knows no boundaries and will attack regardless of age, sex, race, nationality or a multitude of other factors that vary significantly from one individual to another. It also can occur in any part of the body, and as a result, no one at any time can feel completely safe or protected from a possible invasion.

In decades past, with limited technology, it wasn't often possible to detect cancer in its early stages when the disease is easier to fight and defeat. The symptoms and warning signs of specific cancers were largely unknown, and little of this information was dispensed and made available to general populations. People didn't understand that self-awareness and vigilant observation were instrumental elements in the war against cancer. They didn't know how to conduct self exams or that such procedures were even necessary.

Unlike the urinalysis for diabetes or the blood test for syphilis, there was no test an individual could undergo to detect the presence of a cancerous or pre-cancerous condition. There were few diagnostic procedures available that could detect cancer in its early stages, and those that did exist lacked the refined technology to render their findings conclusive. And in spite of the advances that medical research was making, the overall knowledge of the nature of cancer and its "causes" was still preliminary and often speculative.

Yet, we're no longer living in the early twentieth century - or the late twentieth century of the 1980s and the 1990s. We're now living in a time when we can reap the bounty of the incredible advances made during the latter part of the twentieth century when knowledge was doubling every ten years. We now live in a time when the past shortcomings of knowledge and research are quickly disappearing and are being replaced with tremendous and powerful insights and information. Confusion is becoming clarity. Speculation is becoming fact. And fear is becoming hope.

Strangely, as dangerous a foe as cancer may be it's not the most dangerous. Cancer hasn't been in the past nor is it now our greatest enemy. Indeed, cancer claims less lives each year than heart disease, yet cancer remains the disease we fear most.[3] Perhaps it's because we believe that heart disease is easier to understand. Perhaps we find heart disease less threatening because it's limited to one part of the body. Perhaps we believe heart disease is easier to prevent with proper diet and lifestyle changes, or that it's easier to detect and treat. Whatever our reasons may be, the fact remains that heart disease is a much greater threat to us and our loved ones than cancer.

The fear we have of cancer, therefore, isn't wholly logical or substantiated. It's exaggerated. It's a fear that exceeds the actual threat the disease presents. To gain a proper perspective, cancer claimed the lives of approximately 7.9 million individuals worldwide in the year 2007. Heart disease, however, is responsible for approximately 16.6 million worldwide deaths each year or one third of all global deaths. In the United States, cancer strikes approximately one and a half million people annually and is responsible for approximately one out of every four or about 500,000 deaths nationwide. Heart disease in the United States claims approximately 600,000 lives each year.[4]

Clearly, therefore, misconceptions prevail. Cancer is serious, but it can be curable. More and more individuals survive the disease with each passing year. We're winning the war against this enemy, and although we haven't completely destroyed it, we have it on the run. Modern medicine and research have provided us the means to reduce its negative impact on society and the individual. And as the technological march to victory continues, we can become active participants in the battle by employing the forces of knowledge and information. For as both of these elements increase in our awareness, the misconceptions about cancer and the fear surrounding it will decrease.

The choice will become ours to make. We can live in fear, or we can just live. To begin, therefore, it will be helpful to have an elementary understanding of the foundation upon which all cancer information and analysis is based. For an understanding of this foundation will not only enable us to analyze information on our own, it will enable us to recognize the flaws and inaccuracies in the analyses of others. It will enable us to think for ourselves. So let us put aside any preconceived notions we may have about the subject and begin anew.

Chapter 4:
Introduction to Statistics

In 1936 the two candidates in the United States presidential election were Alfred M. Landon and Franklin D. Roosevelt. Prior to the election, a magazine called the *Literary Digest* sponsored a telephone survey to determine which candidate would win the election. Of the more than two million people who were polled it appeared that Landon would defeat Roosevelt by fifty-seven to forty-three percent. When the election was over and the votes were counted, however, it was Roosevelt who won by a margin of sixty-two percent to Landon's thirty-eight percent.[5] So, naturally we must ask, "If such studies can be so misleading, are the numbers they indicate of any real value and do we need to pay any attention to them at all?"

Strangely, perhaps, the answer to this question remains unequivocally, "Yes," as the information to be gained from such numbers is potentially tremendous even when, and sometimes because, they are inaccurate. The use of statistics and the theories behind the science find application in a variety of areas, many of which often result in sustained and positive changes that greatly benefit humanity.

Statistics can be used to further our understanding of chemistry, medicine, sociology, agriculture, education and economics. Statistical analyses can be used to initiate much needed social reforms in the areas of crime prevention, poverty awareness or city and population planning. Endangered wildlife can be better protected through revised regulations and more efficient laws governing air pollution, resource distribution and privacy issues may be enacted. Educators may discern the most effective teaching methods and disease and epidemics can be better controlled by applying standard statistical techniques.

In our case, it's imperative to filter the information we receive about cancer to separate that which is accurate from that which is not. It's important to think for ourselves and evaluate data from our own perspective. We must not simply accept information without investigation and we must not allow ourselves to be bullied or intimidated by data with which we're confronted or by the source of that data. We must learn to question information, and when faced with statistics that claim one thing or another about the disease, we must be critical and careful.

We must selectively build our own warehouse of knowledge, for it's in this way that our individual understanding of the disease will be enhanced and unproductive fear and anxiety will be eliminated. For while it's one thing to recognize the serious nature of cancer, it's quite another to react with unfounded emotion or panic. The ability to be discerning will enable us to make clear choices and informed decisions about our personal situation and the course of action we wish to pursue.

Indeed, the potential of statistics to help society and enhance our daily lives is enormous, yet this beneficial potential is not automatic. Potential is something that must be carefully nurtured and critically assessed to become a reality. Numbers can be manipulated and statistical analyses are only as accurate as the data upon which they are based. As a result, therefore, the answer to our initial question remains "yes." It's imperative we pay attention to statistical data not only to gain an accurate perspective of the world in which we live, but to train ourselves to recognize numbers and data that are flawed – those that are designed not to illuminate, but to deceive and distort our perception of the world in which we live.

Although the study of statistics can be difficult and dense, the discussion within these pages will make every effort to keep the subject simple and clear. We'll begin, therefore, with a definition of "statistic" which is a numerical measurement that describes a characteristic of a group.[6] For example, if five women in a group of ten women are over thirty, then we can say that half of the women, or fifty percent of the women, are over thirty. The figure "fifty percent" is a statistic. It's a number that measures and describes the characteristic of age within the group of women. The "fifty percent" in this example is a single statistic, whereas the term "statistics" refers to the complete science by which characteristics are measured with numbers.

Indeed, the science of statistics began with the previously mentioned John Graunt, the seventeenth century storeowner whose ample spare time and curiosity prompted him to study and analyze a weekly church publication called the "Bills of Mortality."[7] This publication listed the christenings, births, and deaths, as well as their causes, among the group, or population, of the church. Graunt analyzed this information and in 1662 published his observations and conclusions in a small work not surprisingly entitled "Natural and Political Observations Made upon the Bills of Mortality."

Although perhaps lacking in literary excitement, Graunt's publication was nevertheless the first printed interpretation of social and biological information taken from raw data. Graunt noted the differences between the birth and death rates of men and women, and documented the existence of a surprising consistency among events that to date were considered chance occurrences. It was this initial work that allowed people to evaluate, expect, plan and understand some small part of the world in which they lived. It was this work that scientists and researchers the world over, past and present, consider to be the birth of the science we call statistics.

This science of numbers, like any science, however, has its strengths and weaknesses. While statistics can be extremely useful in understanding current conditions and in determining future trends, it isn't a tool that enables us to predict with certainty what will or will not occur. In this way, statistics is different from the science of mathematics. Mathematics is a scientific tool that is "deductive" in nature. This means that mathematics uses previous conclusions to predict or "deduce" new conclusions with certainty.[8]

For example, we know from mathematics that three times two equals six. We know that three times three is nine. With these conclusions we can predict that three times four will be twelve, and that three times four million will be twelve million. This latter conclusion is one we can predict with certainty, even though we cannot actually see or demonstrate the conclusion by counting it out in tangible objects. Yet, we "know" that the figure of twelve million is, and will be, correct based upon our prior conclusions.

Statistics, on the other hand, is more "inductive" in nature. This means that we cannot predict future conclusions with the same certainty afforded us by mathematics. Rather, we can only infer that events or conditions will occur. We can only make generalizations about information that may or may not correspond to reality.[9]

Let's say, for example, we have numbers that indicate 1) more men smoke cigarettes than women and that, 2) the number of men who smoke has increased each year for ten years and that, 3) the number of women who smoke has decreased each year for ten years. Based upon these three statements we can reasonably predict that in next year male smokers will outnumber female smokers. This, however, is not a certainty.

Our presidential election is another example of inductive reasoning. A particular outcome may appear "likely" to occur, but many factors may change that would render our prediction completely inaccurate. And the ways in which statistics and the predictions garnered from them can go wrong are numerous and far more common than one might expect. For statistics, like any tool used properly, can be extremely valuable. Like any tool, however, statistics also can be misused in ways that render the end result of an analysis suspicious, unreliable and undependable.

There are three kinds of lies:
lies, damned lies, and statistics.
Benjamin Disraeli

Since this statement was uttered over a hundred years ago, it also has been said that, "Figures don't lie; liars figure" and that statistics are used "more for support than for illumination" much like, as one author noted, "a drunk uses a lamppost."[10] Each of these quotes is a statement of protest against the many ways in which the use of statistics can be abused, both unintentionally and intentionally. Indeed, a statistic may be wrong as a result of the information obtained, the analysis of the information or the conclusion based upon the information.

First, a numerical analysis may be inaccurate because the data was simply wrong or incomplete, or the method of gathering the data was compromised in some manner. Or, the case may be that the data was accurate and properly gathered, but that the analysis of the data was flawed or that the conclusion of the analysis was inaccurate. It also is possible, however, that an analysis may be inaccurate because the individual or group responsible for the study has suppressed certain data, emphasized other data and mislabeled the final results of the data in a concentrated effort to support personal objectives.

For example, many statistical analyses strive to find the "average" figure or value in a large sample group. Now, to most people the average is the figure we get when we add all of the values of a group together, and then divide that figure by the number of values involved. In other words, if five people were ages fifteen, twenty-nine, forty-five, sixty-two and eighty-one, we would find their average age by adding them all together to get 232, then by dividing by five to get 46.2. As a result, we could say that the average age of this group of people was 46.2 years old.

This figure, however, is only one type of average, which is called the "arithmetic mean."[11] There are also other types of "averages" known as the median, the mode and the midrange, among others. And for each of these different averages, the method of calculation is different and the results can vary significantly even though all of them can claim to be the "average."[12] If we were to calculate the median average, for example, we would arrange the above ages in increasing order, as they already are, and using the number in the exact middle as our median, we would report the average age as being 45 not 46.2. And, although this discrepancy may not strike us as being enormous, larger figures can yield larger discrepancies that indeed may be enormous.

To make things more difficult, there is no objective criterion that demands one figure be used over another in determining the average that most represents the group. As a result, the researcher is free to select the "average" figure that best supports the position she or he is trying to put forth.

To further illustrate this point let's examine the following statistics compiled from one class of students to determine their average I.Q. score. The mean was calculated to be 110, the median was 120, the mode was ninety-five and the midrange was one hundred. If the school conducted this study in an effort to show that more teachers were needed to enhance the student potential, the mode of ninety-five would probably be used to measure the average I.Q. If, however, the study was conducted to demonstrate the outstanding teaching techniques of the school, the median of 120 would most likely be used.

In another example, employees of a certain company may believe that they're underpaid and that all salaries should be raised. To support their argument they would choose the lowest average in an effort to illustrate the need for a salary increase. On the other hand, negotiations may find the company's management team choosing the highest average to negate the need for salary increases. Whenever confronted by an "average," therefore, it's advisable to find out which average is represented in the data.

As is often the case, however, if additional information isn't available, we need to understand that the figure stated as "average" may be misleading. When we refer to an average within these pages, it generally will refer to the average age human beings typically develop a particular cancer or the average risk an individual faces for developing a particular cancer. In the first instance, average will not be a specific number, but an age group such as children under the age of fifteen, women in their twenties and early thirties, or men over the age of fifty. In the second instance, average risk will refer to individuals who don't possess a specific risk for developing a particular cancer, an issue we'll discuss further in the next section.

Indeed, while the averages mentioned within these pages reflect a consensus of research, they also should be considered responsibly calculated estimates rather than absolutes.

There are numerous other ways in which statistical information may be erroneous. For instance, the numbers themselves can be somewhat deceptive. If, for example, the average median base annual salary for a registered nurse in the United States in 2004 was determined to be approximately $41,000, the reported figure may be stated as $41,243. It's reported in this way because the detailed precision of exact dollars and cents makes the figure appear more reliable and creates a sense of confidence in the observer regarding the accuracy of the figure.[13]

Similarly, many statistical figures are merely guesses based upon related prior guesses, such as the amount of money placed in secret Swiss bank accounts, or the number of trees growing in the national forests of a particular country. The verbal way in which results are reported also can be manipulated to give erroneous impressions.[14] This may be especially true in the area of advertising where a consumer may hear that ninety-five percent of consumers who bought a particular make of washing machine in the last fifteen years still own the machine and are happy with their choice. This claim sounds as if the washing machine itself is well made, lasts a long time and is an exceptional buy. It may not say, however, that ninety-five percent of the consumers questioned still have their washing machines because they all bought their machines within the last six months.

The true nature of data also can be misrepresented through a variety of visual devices such as charts and bar graphs.[15] While the numbers and figures of an analysis may, therefore, be accurate in and of themselves, their end result may "appear" to say something else. For example, a statistical analysis may be used to calculate the amount of money that an industry has spent on pollution abatement over a ten year period. The study may indicate that with each passing year the industry did indeed increase the funds allotted to the protection of the environment. This increase from year to year, however, may only have been a small increase of perhaps one percent.

Yet, this result may be illustrated by a bar graph in which the small increase appears to be much larger simply because of the way the graph is drawn. Visually, the one percent may be represented by an additional inch in height in each graph for each year rather than allotting one eight of an inch for each one percent. As a result, while the numbers remain accurate, the overall study is manipulated in a way that visually "tricks" the observer into thinking the increased spending is much greater than it actually is. The intent of the graph is to trigger an "intuitive impression" in the observer based upon a visual pattern. By doing this, the true nature of the statistic may be lost as the observer is more influenced by the erroneous impression she or he "sees" than by the facts.[16]

There are other visual techniques that can "trick" the eye as well. For example, the result of a study may accurately indicate that one person's salary is twice as large as that of another person. This result may be illustrated by depicting two three dimensional pictures of a gold bar with one being twice as large as the other. Although this sounds logical, if one gold bar is drawn twice as tall, twice as deep and twice as wide as the other, it actually will appear to be eight times larger than the other, not twice as large. As a result, even though the data is accurate, the analysis is accurate and the conclusion is accurate, the result of this study is represented in a manner that deceives the eye and – consciously or subconsciously – "tricks" the observer into thinking that the difference in the two salaries is much greater than it actually is.[17]

Similarly, when the dimensions of a simple two dimensional object such as a flat square, not a cube, are doubled, the area of the new square is actually four times the size of the original rather than two times the size. As consumers, students and observers, therefore, it's important to always analyze the data and the numerical information contained in a visual aid rather than allowing ourselves to be swayed or impressed by its general shape or pattern.

In addition to these manipulations, it also is important to know that the size of the sample from which the information is obtained may be subject to criticism as well.[18] If, for example, eight out of ten consumers prefer brand A over brand B, the result of the survey should not claim that "eight out of ten consumers" recommend brand A. It's deceptive to make such a statement because the sample size is too small to support a generalized claim. Even if the sample size is large, it must be representative of the overall group or population being surveyed or studied to avoid biased conclusions. This brings us to our opening example.

As mentioned, an extensive telephone survey was conducted in 1936 to assess the winner of that year's United States presidential election, a survey that indicated Alfred M. Landon would soundly defeat Franklin D. Roosevelt. Of course, Landon did not defeat Roosevelt by a landslide and, in fact, Roosevelt defeated Landon by a landslide. Although the survey was a complete failure, it's a wonderful example of what is called a "biased sampling."[19] First, it's important to note that in 1936 few American households owned telephones. Indeed, telephones at that time were quite a luxury, and most of the households that had telephones at that time were affluent. Moreover, the affluent households in 1936 were largely comprised of business and corporate individuals most of whom belonged to the Republican political party. Landon, of course, was a Republican candidate.

As a result, most of the two million individuals interviewed by the telephone survey were Republicans, who resoundedly supported their candidate Landon. In other words, the sample used in the survey was not representative of the entire population of the United States. Many individuals who comprised the country's other political parties were never contacted, which rendered the entire survey "biased" and the conclusion completely inaccurate.

Clearly, as the data to be analyzed becomes more complicated and comprehensive, the possibility of flaws entering the analysis also increases. While many flaws are unintended, it's the intentional manipulation of statistics that remains most troublesome. The few examples found in these pages are hopefully helpful, yet they barely touch the field of deceptive statistical practice which is so vast that entire books have been devoted to the subject. It's not surprising that this phenomenon is quite common in the areas of society where statistics are used to advertise and sell and where industries and livelihoods depend upon promoting a particular point of view.

Unfortunately, deceptive statistical practices can flourish in any area of society, including those that exist primarily for altruistic purposes. It's human nature to desire personal success, attention and recognition from and among one's peers. In every discipline, foundation and industry it's possible to find individuals who may compromise and manipulate statistics to gain importance for themselves, further a cause, change public opinion or secure financial funding. Even within the best intentioned statistical analyses the data can be inconsistent, argumentative and full of contradiction from one source to another.

For these reasons, the statistical information reported in this book has been accumulated from only the most respected cancer research and medical institutions in the world, and no statistic has been used without collaboration from at least two additional sources using the most current information available. Yet, by its very nature, information is constantly changing and evolving, and as a result, the statistics found in these pages as well may be somewhat less accurate when read than when written.

The lesson to be learned from this discussion, however, is to acknowledge that information of every sort permeates the world in which we live. While the beginning of the twentieth century was known as the "Industrial Age," the beginning of the twenty-first century has been dubbed the "Information Age." It's an age of great technology, high speed communication and around the clock media and news coverage. We're surrounded by and bombarded with information of every conceivable nature, and it's important to realize that much of that information is misleading, biased and deceptive. Accordingly, we must learn to question the information we receive and the reliability of the source of that information. We must analyze headlines and news reports carefully in the light of knowledge and common sense before arriving at our own informed and logical conclusions.

For the ability to understand the use and abuse of statistics, even to a small degree, will not only enhance our accurate understanding of cancer, it will allow us to become more responsible and educated members of society in general. Further, as we become less susceptible to the deceptions that permeate our world, we'll become more capable individuals who make intelligent decisions and opinions that benefit others as well as ourselves.

Chapter 5:
This Disease We Call Cancer

Compiling statistical information on any subject is a daunting task. Yet, this task becomes especially difficult when the subject at hand is one that encompasses the entire world population. With great appreciation, however, for several sources including the **American Cancer Society**, the **National Cancer Institute's Surveillance, Epidemiology, and End Results (SEER)**, the **World Health Organization** and the **International Agency for Research on Cancer,** we're able to paint a fairly clear statistical picture of this disease.

To create this picture, however, it's necessary to understand and combine three different elements or statistical "rates."[20] The first element is called the "incidence rate." This rate refers to the number of new cases of cancer reported each year in every 100,000 members of a given population. In most countries, this rate is monitored by local and regional "tumor registries," which are organizations that collect the data and then, in most cases, transfer the data to a country's department of vital statistics. It is this incidence rate that gives us information about the types of cancer that occur, how often each occurs and who and where they strike.

Indeed, the only cancers that are not included in the incidence rates for any population are basel cell and squamous cell skin cancers, and it's the incidence rate that will appear most often throughout our discussion of this disease. The second element is called the "mortality rate," which refers to the number of deaths each year from cancer for every 100,000 members of a population. The third element is called the "relative survival rate." This element, of course, refers to the number of people who are still alive after being diagnosed with any form of cancer.[21]

This last element, however, requires clarification to fully understand its significance and limitations. To begin, the survival rate is a study based upon those individuals living five years after being diagnosed with cancer. This five year figure will include all individuals, whether they're cancer free, in remission or in the process of being treated for a still existing cancer. In addition, it's a "relative" study, which means that the statistical information has been adjusted for normal life expectancy factors affecting cancer survivors, such as the possibility of death from heart and other diseases or accidents. This rate appears to be helpful when determining the odds of cancer survival in a given general population; however, it's far less helpful when used to predict individual prognosis.

First, the relative survival rate is based upon individuals who were diagnosed and treated for cancer at least eight years prior to the analysis. As a result, this rate doesn't reflect the significant yearly advances in medical treatment that today's cancer patients are afforded.

Second, the rate doesn't take into account many factors that influence individual survival such as the existence of additional illnesses or personal lifestyle habits and behaviors.

Another term we discuss throughout this book is the "risk" associated with certain cancers and the individuals most likely to develop those cancers. There are two ways in which cancer researchers use this term, and the first is known as "lifetime risk."[22] This risk refers to the probability, or chance, that any individual has for developing or dying from cancer over her or his lifetime. In the United States, for example, men have a little less than a one in two lifetime risk, or chance, of developing some form of cancer. This means that not quite one out of every two American men will be diagnosed with cancer at some point in their life. For women in the United States, the lifetime risk is a little more than one in three, which means that at least one out of every three American women will develop cancer during their lifetime.

The second use of this term is known as the "relative risk,"[23] which refers to the strength of the relationship between specific risk factors and a particular cancer. This term examines the risk of individuals who share certain traits or harmful exposures when compared to individuals without the trait or exposure. For example, it's estimated that males who smoke have a twenty-fold relative risk for developing lung cancer when compared to males who don't smoke. This means that these smokers are twenty times more likely to develop lung cancer at some point in their life than nonsmokers. It's the relative risk that we'll see again and again throughout our discussions of the most common cancers, the factors related to their development and the individuals who appear most likely to develop those cancers.

In the year 2000, of the nearly fifty-six million deaths worldwide from all causes approximately twelve percent were attributed to cancer. In that year, the incidence rate indicated that approximately ten million individuals were diagnosed with cancer and the mortality rate indicated that approximately 6.2 million individuals died from the disease. In the year 2007, approximately 11.3 million individuals were diagnosed with cancer, and approximately 7.9 million of these individuals died as a result.[24]

Indeed, in many countries cancer is responsible for more than twenty five percent of the country's recorded deaths. This is certainly true in the United States, where one of every four deaths each year is directly attributed to cancer.[25] The risk of cancer, of course, varies from region to region, suggesting that geographic, environmental and cultural factors influence what type and to what extent cancers exist. Yet, while cancer incidence rates historically have been greater in industrialized countries, cancer is now emerging as a major threat in developing countries as well.

If current predictions hold true, the worldwide incidence rate for cancer will steadily continue to rise and increase fifty percent by the year 2020.[26] By comparison, this means that by the year 2020, fifteen million new cases of cancer will be diagnosed each year compared to the ten million cases of cancer diagnosed around the world in the year 2000. Additional predictions estimate that the number of cancer deaths that occurred worldwide in 2008 will double by the year 2030 to over thirteen million deaths per year.[27]

Clearly, these statistics are staggering. It's important, however, to gain perspective by examining these numbers a little more closely. First, more individuals are surviving cancer today than at any time in history. For example, in many of the world's industrialized countries, including the United States, nearly half of those individuals diagnosed with cancer will survive the disease. Second, the increase in the incidence rate and the decrease in the mortality rate are due in large part to important early cancer detection methods and procedures.

Furthermore, when examining mortality rates, it's important to realize that many cancer deaths occur as the result of late diagnoses. In fact, in developing countries it has been reported that eighty percent of those affected by cancer are already in a late and incurable stage of the disease at the time of their diagnosis.[28] Finally, medical and scientific evidence indicates that of all the cancers that plague the world, literally one third can be prevented and another third can be cured.[29]

To reach this goal of prevention and cure, however, education, personal awareness and diligence become essential. For, clearly, a fundamental understanding of this disease will be not only helpful to many individuals in the years to come, but perhaps necessary as well. And even if this disease doesn't directly affect our life, the chances of having a loved one whose life is directly affected are significant. To begin, therefore, it's important to understand a little more about the basic building block of the human body, the cell. For it is within the cell–in fact, within one solitary cell–that every cancer has its beginning.

The atom, being for all practical purposes the stable unit of the physical plane, is a constantly changing vortex of reactions.
The Kabbalah

Simply defined, a cell is a small microscopic structure that contains a center part known as the nucleus. The nucleus is enclosed by a thin layer of tissue called a membrane. It's within the nucleus of a human cell that deoxyribonucleic acid, or DNA, is found. And it's the DNA, or segments of DNA, that form individual genes which in turn combine to form forty-six chromosomes.[30] It is, of course, within these cells that all individual characteristics such as eye color and height are determined, and that all of the body's functions including metabolism, reproduction and locomotion are programmed and carried out.

The human body is a living mechanism that grows to maturity through a process known as cell division or "mitosis."[31] Mitosis is simply the process by which one cell divides into two, two divide into four and so on. When a cell divides, it produces two new cells that are exactly like the parent cell in every way except for size. The new cells, of course, are smaller and do not reach the size of the parent cell until they mature. An additional process known as cell differentiation allows new cells to develop into different types of cells that have specialized functions. Cell differentiation, for example, accounts for the differences between cells found in the lining of the stomach, cells within a hair follicle or cells of the lung tissue and respiratory system.[32]

Most normal cells continue to divide until the human body reaches maturity, and then they stop. Other cells, however, such as those responsible for the growth of hair and nails, continue to divide throughout the human lifetime. Similarly, cells that promote tissue growth to replace or repair damaged tissues such as those of the skin also continue to divide, multiplying themselves as many as seventy times throughout a human life span.

The end result of this division, of course, is a fully grown, mature human body capable of limited regeneration and containing approximately sixty trillion cells, give or take a few.[33] And through it all, the processes of cell division and differentiation promote orderly growth and development, turning on when necessary and turning off when their work is complete.

Telomeres and Free Radicals

It's possible, however, for these two processes to be disrupted or altered in such a way that normal cell division is compromised. In the case of cancer, the alteration to the processes results in the uncontrolled division of cells and an excess of tissue growth. In other words, the cells don't know when to stop multiplying. They continue to divide and create new tissue, an abnormal process that will not cease and that can be controlled only by destroying or removing the cells in question. And any living organism composed of and sustained by the division of cells, be it plant, animal or human, is at risk for developing this complication.

In human beings the cycles of cell division appear to be regulated, at least in part, by certain segments of the DNA known as "telomeres." Once again, our DNA forms genes, which in turn form chromosomes. Telomeres are the segments of DNA found on the ends of each chromosome. They actually have been described as being similar to the little "plastic caps on the ends of shoelaces."[34] Each time a cell divides, the telomeres become shorter, and when they become too short, the cell stops dividing, a phenomenon of normal, non-specialized cells that should coincide with human maturity.

It appears reasonable, therefore, that in human cancers a cell may simply stop responding to the signals of the telomeres or of the normal growth processes and continue to divide without control. This would indicate that the segment of the DNA that forms the telomeres might perhaps be damaged in some way. As a result, the telomeres may lose their ability to properly instruct the cell to stop dividing, creating a situation of uncontrolled growth.

Another factor in uncontrolled cell division, however, appears to be influenced by another organism known as a "free radical." A free radical is a damaged molecule missing an electron.[35] They're found in the environment in sources such as ultraviolet radiation and in air pollutants such as cigarette smoke. Yet, they also are found in and produced by the human body. In fact, free radicals within the human body are normal by-products of human metabolism created as the body converts food into energy.

While the name sounds strange, we can think of it in this way. Free radicals roam freely throughout the body and the environment, and express themselves in an extreme manner. Indeed, because a free radical needs and wants its missing electron, it will attack any other molecule from which it can steal an electron to complete itself. Free radicals have the ability to break through the membrane of a cell, enter its nucleus and take an electron from key components of the cell such as its fat, protein and DNA. When this occurs, the cellular DNA may be damaged and, of course, DNA that's damaged or incomplete is believed to be the origin of cancer. For when the integrity of the DNA becomes compromised, the instructions held within the DNA become altered and the communication between the DNA and the cell breaks down.

The human body, however, also possesses built-in defenses that protect cells from the potentially harmful effect of free radicals. For instance, the body manufactures enzymes, organisms that are protein-filled molecules. Some of these enzymes actually have the ability to convert free radicals into water thereby completely neutralizing the threat. In addition, antioxidants may help neutralize the effect of free radicals. It's believed that oxygen damage, or oxidation, to human cells is responsible in part for the aging process and the onset of certain diseases, including cancer. Known antioxidants such as vitamins E and C, selenium and beta-carotene are thought to prevent this process of oxidation and, in turn, also aid in the neutralization of free radicals.[36]

Knowing this, it has been theorized that if one's food consumption is decreased, one's metabolic rate will decrease, the production of free radicals within the body will decrease and the risk of cell damage from free radicals will decrease. While such a theory appears to be reasonable, the production of free radicals remains an ongoing process as long as the human body is alive and taking some form of nourishment. And, of course, free radicals are always in the environment. There's always the chance, therefore, that one of these molecules, because it only takes one, will penetrate the membrane of a cell, damage the instructions of the cell's DNA and create the foundation for uncontrolled cell division and growth.

When this occurs, be it the result of telomeres, free radicals or other complex processes, what begins as one misguided cell can uncontrollably multiply itself into millions of misguided cells. This production of too much tissue results in a lump or mass commonly referred to as a tumor, which can be either benign or malignant.[37] Benign is defined as being favorable or having a kind disposition, and clearly a benign tumor is usually not harmful and is certainly not cancerous. A benign tumor may be small or large; it may be felt in the tissue, seen on the skin or detected by an x-ray. In any case, it's a tumor that stopped growing before any surrounding tissue was harmed or damaged. And while it may reach a size that's troublesome because it occupies too much space, a benign tumor doesn't invade normal tissue or spread to other parts of the body.

In contrast, malignant is defined as a harmful influence or effect, and tumors classified as such are cancerous. Unlike a benign tumor, a malignant tumor is composed of cells that continue to divide without restraint. They grow until they begin to displace and crowd normal cells and compete with them for necessary nutrients. At this point, these tumors also can begin to invade and destroy normal tissue. Such tumors may prevent the body's organs from functioning properly or they may obstruct important blood vessels or air passages.

Pieces of these tumors also can break off and travel to other parts of the body through the blood and lymph systems, the body's main avenues of circulation. It's the bloodstream, of course, that carries nutrients to the tissues and it's the lymph channels that return water and proteins from the tissues back to the blood. When malignant cells enter either system, they can be deposited in any other part of the body where they'll continue to grow and invade other organs, a process called "metastasis."[38]   Some malignant tumors, or cancers, grow slowly while others grow rapidly. Yet, none of them stop growing, and none of them will remain confined to a small area without eventually harming nearby healthy tissue. This is the difference between tumors that are either benign or malignant, and this is why the latter are so dangerous.

Not all cancers, however, are characterized by the existence of malignant tumors. For example, leukemias, which are cancers that affect the blood, are not characterized by tumors. Rather, they're characterized by the uncontrolled growth of abnormal white blood cells.

Leukemias target the blood-forming tissues of the body, which include the bone marrow and the lymph system.[39] As the production of abnormal white blood cells increases, they begin to compete with healthy cells for available nutrients and interfere with the normal functioning of the body's vital organs. These abnormal white cells also begin to outnumber and overwhelm the normal white cells of the body's immune system and decrease their ability to fight bacteria and infection. A more accurate statement in describing cancers, therefore, might be to say that while all cancers are not characterized by the existence of malignant tumors, they are characterized by the uncontrolled and unlimited growth of abnormal cells.

Clearly, the human body contains many different types of cells. Because cancers begin within the cells there are, accordingly, many different types of cancers. It was reported in 1978 that over one hundred cancers already had been identified.[40] Today, it's estimated there are at least two hundred different kinds of cancer.[41] Yet, because new ones are constantly being discovered, it simply isn't possible to determine how many exist. And each cancer varies depending upon the part of the body, and the type of cell, in which it begins.

While different types of cancers can occur within one body part, most cancers are given the general name of the body part in which they begin, such as breast cancer, colon cancer or lung cancer. Cancers that originate in the bone and muscle tissue are known as sarcomas, and because they occur in tissues that may lie deep within the body, these cancers are often more difficult to diagnose and treat.

In contrast, cancers that develop in the skin or in the "skin" or lining of the internal organs are known as carcinomas. Understandably, these cancers are often easier to diagnose and treat because they're located in body parts more obvious to the eye or medical instruments and are more accessible. Those that affect the human blood system are leukemias, and those that target the lymphatic system are called lymphomas.[42]

Cancers may differ from one another in many ways, including size, texture, rate of growth and susceptibility to treatment. Some are more common in children while others are more common in seniors. Some occur more frequently in developing countries whereas others are predominant in nations that are already industrialized. Yet, all are alike in that they constitute a serious threat that when left unchecked, may prove deadly.

The Big Os—Old Age and Opportunity

One of the few things we know about cancer that we can state with complete confidence and without refute is that it is, in part, a disease of "old age." Although the cancer rates for individuals of all ages are rising, the occurrences of cancer in children and young adults remain relatively rare when compared to the occurrences of cancer in older individuals. In fact, less than half of all cancer cases are diagnosed in individuals under the age of sixty-five.[43] To fully understand this phenomenon, therefore, it will be helpful to examine "old age" and the underlying factors that contribute to this natural process.

Simply defined, aging refers to the physical and mental changes that occur in an individual over time.[44] Typically, most humans find that as they age certain aspects of their lives begin to change. It's quite common, for example, for physical strength and agility to decline. It also is common for one's mental capabilities to decline in ways that may be evidenced by various degrees of memory loss or forgetfulness. The body itself may experience more difficulty in healing and repairing damaged tissues and may become more susceptible to disease and infection.

On the other hand, many individuals who remain physically and mentally active throughout their lives may continue to enjoy exceptional physical and mental prowess. Indeed, a sixty-year-old individual who has always exercised regularly can expect to retain about eighty percent of the physical stamina she or he possessed at age twenty-five. Clearly, it's not possible to predict what will happen to any individual, as each of us is unique. We each possess our own particular genetic makeup, our own health histories and our own stress patterns and habits of personal nutrition and exercise. And while some older, athletic individuals may retain organs and muscles as healthy or healthier than those of younger individuals, it's inevitable that some decline in the body's ability to function properly will occur as we age, regardless of any and all attempts to the contrary.

The reasons for this inevitability are numerous. And while doctors who specialize in the health of older individuals known as "gerontologists" have yet to agree upon the precise biological processes that permit aging to occur, several theories abound.[45] Among them is the **worn template** theory that speculates that each time a cell divides it produces new cells that are slightly less perfect than the original.[46] This concept can be likened to the "Xerox" process of duplication. In this process, we start with one original image of which a copy is made. The copy is then used to make another copy, that copy is used to make another and so on.

Each time this occurs, the copying mechanism becomes more and more likely to introduce and produce errors—errors that may result in an image that lacks the precision and accuracy of the original. In the case of dividing cells, therefore, this would mean that the entire process of mitosis is one, which creates slightly inferior cells with each division. It follows that when the process ceases at human maturity, cells created later in the process are more and more inferior, and as a result, create tissues that are increasingly inferior. In theory, the tissues degenerate according to their level of inferiority, with the most compromised of them breaking down first and beginning the aging process. The less compromised break down later and the least compromised, those closest to the original image, break down in the last stages of the aging process.

Another long standing school of thought is known as the **accumulated toxins** theory.[47] Proponents of this concept believe that the human body is continually exposed to chemicals and other harmful elements that literally poison the body's tissues. As time passes, the amount of harmful elements in the body reaches a saturation point at which time the accumulation of toxins is so great the body can no longer neutralize or expel them. The toxins remain in the tissues and organs of the body where they eventually compromise the healthy functioning of both. And, of course, when the body no longer functions properly it becomes more susceptible to disease, infection and the inevitable process of degeneration.

A third theory concerning the aging process is known as **immune surveillance**.[48] Here, it's believed that as the body grows older, it experiences a progressive decline in its ability to detect and destroy harmful foreign elements. This ability to protect the body tissues lies within the domain of the immune system, which is a collection of cells and proteins. It's these cells and proteins that work together to target and attack human disease and infection. Theorists believe that the passage of time hinders the human immune system and gradually erodes its ability to differentiate healthy cells and tissues from damaged ones. With this control mechanism compromised, harmful elements are allowed to proliferate throughout the body. They threaten and eventually overtake healthy tissues, weakening the body, hindering its ability to function properly and prompting the degenerative process we call aging.

Regardless of the theory one supports, however, the bottom line in each of the above and numerous others is that aging is the result of simple wear and tear on the body tissues. As years go by, each area of the body, each muscle and fiber, each tendon, vessel and organ is used over and over again. And as this use continues, the point is eventually reached where the body part can no longer perform its corresponding job as effectively as it once could. The point is reached where it takes more energy, more effort and more time to accomplish the same result, and eventually the desired result may not be accomplished at all.

It isn't a difficult concept to understand and differs little from the ways in which other mechanisms fall victim to ordinary wear and tear. When any product, for example, is new and without defect it should operate smoothly and efficiently perform its function. As it ages, however, and the product is used over and over again, certain aspects of it may become weak and begin to interfere with proper performance. Whether we're speaking of automobiles, carpet or kitchen pans, if used regularly over long periods of time all will eventually weaken and lose their ability to provide the result for which they were originally designed. Repetitive motion, metal fatigue, bumps and jolts and excessive heat eventually weaken the components of an automobile. Carpet wears thin from continuous friction, weight and dirt. And the sturdy kitchen pan will eventually fall victim to heat and flame, constant handling, washing and abrasion.

Similarly, the fibers and tissues of the human body will gradually degenerate, be it from less than perfect copies of cellular material, growing amounts of poisons and toxins or the breakdown of its immune system, the body is susceptible to the same inevitable end result of longevity. Every inanimate structure, and every living organism, is constantly being bombarded by a variety of factors that compromise the innate strength and durability of its components and tissues.

This mechanical wear and tear upon the human body takes its toll in a number of ways. Among them, the elasticity of the skin and blood vessels gradually decreases, allowing the skin to become loose, more wrinkled and more easily bruised due to the weakened capillaries. Certain organs experience a decline in performance, including the heart whose eventual inefficiency at pumping results in a reduced tolerance to exercise and the liver, which becomes less effective in filtering toxins from the blood. The bones, of course, may become brittle as a result of lost calcium, and the loss of nerve cells in the brain may result in a loss of acuity and clarity in one or all of the senses.

The joints and muscles may lose their flexibility and strength and the arteries of the circulatory system may harden resulting in high blood pressure and poor circulation. The lungs, which unlike some of the body's other organs, cannot be "exercised" or saved from deterioration, will over time lose their elasticity resulting in less efficient breathing. As if this were not enough, when these tissues reach this state of advanced age and weakness they become susceptible to invading disease and infection.

It also is important to realize that as the body and the living tissues of the body age, so too does each individual cell. In fact, once the body reaches maturity and the process of mitosis or cell division stops, the cells themselves begin to age rapidly. The same things we associate with physical aging in general, including decreased strength, flexibility and elasticity characterize this aging process of the human cell. Actually, when observed through a microscope, the difference between young and old cells is quite obvious to the eye. While young cells have an elongated oval shape and are compact and tightly aligned, old cells begin to lose their shape, becoming raggedy, less oval, irregular around the edges and loosely aligned with one another.[49] Unfortunately, when a cell ages and becomes weak, it too becomes extremely susceptible to invading disease and infection.

It's when this advanced stage of cellular aging is reached that cancers typically make their appearance. The body cells lack their original strength. They become tired, unable to perform their functions properly or efficiently, unable perhaps to repair damaged DNA, and unable to protect themselves from harmful elements. These harmful elements, both internal and external, that are responsible for the aging and degeneration of our body cells are numerous. The free radicals that roam throughout the body bombarding our cells now stand a much better chance of penetrating these cells that over time have become more vulnerable to an invasion. Carcinogens that have been consumed over a lifetime may begin to accumulate and overpower cells of the digestive tissues and organs, the respiratory tract and the reproductive system. Cells also become more vulnerable to the environment and the harmful effects of ultraviolet radiation, air and water pollution and chemical products.

It's a simple fact of life that organisms of any size become weaker, more susceptible and more vulnerable to invasion and takeover by harmful, stronger elements as they age. This is true of the human body, its tissues and its cells. This is why cancer becomes increasingly common as individuals age, and this is why cancer is called a disease of "old age."[50]

Yet, it's important to realize that cancers may not be detected for years or even several decades after their inception. Known as the **time bomb effect**[51], a cancer may have begun in one single cell of body tissue thirty or forty years before invading enough cells to make its presence known. In the beginning, the host tissue to a cancer cell may be healthy enough to fight the invader and prevent it from growing and spreading quickly. With age, however, this same tissue will lose its "edge." It will weaken in the ways we've already discussed and will provide the foundation for the accelerated growth of abnormal cancer cells.

Indeed, one of the reasons cancer rates are rising steadily is because people are living longer, a new longevity that's the result of modern medicine and technological advances. At the beginning of the twentieth century, for example, many lives were claimed by diseases such as tuberculosis, influenza, smallpox and polio. Add to this existence of rampant disease the facts that basic good nutrition was lacking and medical diagnoses and procedures were primitive. As a result, many individuals died relatively young and the "average" age of most of the world's populations was much younger than the average age of populations today. Because cancer is a disease of old age, many individuals were spared from its harm only because they died from other diseases at younger ages.

This doesn't mean that these individuals didn't have cancer – it merely means that many of them died from other causes before their cancer was discovered. Today, however, many of these diseases have been eliminated as deadly threats to humanity, as have many other contributing factors. As a result, more individuals are living to be older. The irony, of course, is that while research and technology have succeeded in wiping out these past threats and prolonging our lives, they also have increased our risk for developing cancer as we continue to age.

As we all know, however, cancer isn't limited to older individuals. Not all cancers take decades to develop, as many children and young adults are diagnosed with various forms of the disease every year. Indeed, some cancers are found primarily in these age groups. Clearly, the role played by advanced age in the development of this disease doesn't stand in the spotlight alone–it shares the stage with another player known as simple opportunity. The basic formula that underlies cancer development, however, remains the same regardless of an individual's age. For whether one is eighty or eight, body cells that are weak, vulnerable and unable to fight off a harmful invasion become likely hosts for future cancers.

In the case of aging, we already understand that older individuals possess body cells that have become weakened due to this natural process. In a younger individual, however, body tissues and cells become weak as the result of numerous other factors. In some, heredity is responsible for this weakness. One's parents determine one's DNA and genetic makeup. If, therefore, one or both parents possess an inherent weakness in certain body parts and the cells that comprise them, this characteristic may unavoidably be passed on to their offspring. As a result, such offspring may be "predisposed" to certain diseases and run a greater risk for developing cancer as children or young adults. In this case, it's this predisposition that creates the opportunity for the invasion and growth of cancer. Similarly, other individuals suffer particular weaknesses because their mother was exposed to certain chemicals, drugs or medical procedures while pregnant with the individual. Others experience cellular weakness due to their own exposure to harmful elements in the environment, toxic foods or water, chemicals, radiation, drugs and medical procedures. There are, unfortunately, many additional elements of the modern world that contribute to the breakdown of human tissues and cells. These are the things that in spite of age create the additional opportunities for cancer to develop and thrive early in an individual's life. And with this understanding, we come to the most important aspect of the nature of this disease, a concept we will refer to as . . .

The Cancer Blueprint

This is an important concept, and one we'll refer to again and again throughout our discussion of this disease. For regardless of the factors that appear to be responsible for the onset of cancer, be they age related, chemically induced, genetically determined or any other, the underlying basis of any cancer remains the same. This concept simply stated is:

> **Cancer begins in body cells that have been damaged or weakened to the point they are no longer capable of repairing themselves or defending themselves from the invasion and negative effects of harmful elements.**

Having said this, let's now consider a few examples to drive the point home. First, let's examine one of the most common and potentially harmful elements of our environment, ordinary sunlight. Medical experts the world over have warned us of the potential danger of excessive and unprotected exposure to the sun. This is because sunlight produces ultraviolet radiation, which is comprised of particles that act much like the free radicals found within the human body.

As mentioned, it's these particles that damage the tumor suppressor genes found in the skin and, like free radicals, these particles have the ability to penetrate the skin cells and damage cellular DNA. Medical professionals continue to urge individuals to use sunscreens, wear sensible clothing and avoid outdoor activities during certain hours of the day to avoid the damage caused by ultraviolet radiation–damage commonly known as sunburn. And while most individuals, especially those with lighter skin, have experienced sunburns at one time or another, it's a routine occurrence rarely considered serious.

It's important to realize, however, that sunburn indicates the surface cells of the skin have literally been burned by the sun's ultraviolet radiation. Repeated sunburns, minor though they may seem, result in an accumulation of burned tissue and damage to the surface cells of the skin. One intense sunburn may damage not only the surface skin cells, but deeper tissues as well. In either case, as the damage continues and the skin cells are bombarded and burned by ultraviolet radiation again and again, they become weakened, eventually losing their ability to protect themselves. In this weakened state, these cells become more vulnerable to penetration by the harmful particles of ultraviolet radiation. Once inside the cell, these harmful particles can now damage the DNA contained within each cell. If this occurs, the cellular genetic coding itself will become compromised and the information and instructions contained within the DNA will become altered.

We already know that through the process of mitosis, when a healthy cell divides, it creates two identical healthy cells. In the case of a damaged cell, however, the process of mitosis results in two identical damaged cells. In addition, we also know that the cells of the skin, as well as the cells of the hair and nails, divide quickly and continue to do so throughout the course of one's life. This means that skin cells whose DNA has become damaged from sunburn have ample opportunity to divide and create a multitude of cancerous tissues. This combination of facts may be, in part, one reason why skin cancers, including basel cell, squamous cell and melanoma, are the most common cancers in the world.

Our second example also concerns the skin, as this large breathing organ is exposed to harmful external factors perhaps more than any other organ of the human body. We often hear that moles on the skin should be monitored and periodically inspected for any unusual changes. This is because a mole indicates that these skin cells are already functioning differently from the majority of our skin cells. The tissue is different in many ways, including color and texture. And while some moles may eventually grow, change color and become cancerous, many remain harmless. Even these harmless moles may present an opportunity for cancer to develop.

For instance, let's consider a mole located on an area of the skin where it is constantly being irritated. This might be a mole on the back of one's neck repeatedly hit or scraped when one uses a brush or a comb. It might be a mole located on one's waistline where it's exposed to continual rubbing or scratching from the elastic or fabric in one's clothing. In each of these situations the tissues of the mole are being subjected to repeated irritation and friction by the simple movements and tasks of one's daily routine. As the years go by, however, this constant irritation can result in damage to the tissues and cells of the mole.

Moreover, as this damage accumulates, the cells of the mole become weakened and more susceptible to disease and infection. They also become more vulnerable to harmful elements, including the free radicals of the body or the ultraviolet radiation of the earth's atmosphere—elements that can damage the DNA contained within the cells. And this series of events, this Cancer Blueprint, lays the foundation for the potential development and growth of the disease.

Similarly, the tissues of the throat may have an increased risk for cancer if one suffers from chronic and long-term heartburn referred to as "acid reflux disease" or gastrointestinal esophageal reflux disease also called GERD. Under normal circumstances, digestion involves a process in which food enters the mouth, passes through the throat or "esophagus" and enters the stomach. A structure known as the "esophageal sphincter" is located at the point where the esophagus connects to the stomach. Once food passes into the stomach this sphincter closes tight and prevents food from traveling back into and up the esophagus.[52]

For a variety of reasons, however, this sphincter sometimes fails to close properly allowing food and stomach acids to move backward into the esophagus. When this occurs, one may experience a burning sensation in the chest and a regurgitation of food and digestive acids. This condition, known as heartburn, isn't considered particularly serious and is fairly common with one in ten adults experiencing it at least once a week.

Some individuals, however, experience severe heartburn symptoms of chronic and even nightly regurgitation and vomiting of stomach contents. When the condition becomes this severe it's called acid reflux disease rather than ordinary heartburn. This is a difficult condition that's not only extremely uncomfortable to live with, but one that constantly exposes the tissues of the esophagus to the harsh digestive acids from the stomach. Each time this occurs, the tissue of the esophagus, which isn't designed to digest or pass harsh acids, becomes irritated. This irritation, when continued for a period of years or even decades, will have a cumulative effect that may eventually damage the esophageal tissue.

If the tissue becomes damaged, the cells of the tissue also become damaged and weakened as a result. This brings us back to our Cancer Blueprint whereas 1) cells that have become weakened 2) become vulnerable to harmful invasions of infection and disease 3) that may damage the integrity of each cell's DNA and, 4) lay the foundation for the development and growth of cancer.

Hopefully, these few examples help illustrate the way in which cancer begins its march and establishes its occupation within the human body. This basic understanding is only half of the equation. For once we understand this Cancer Blueprint and the role played by cellular weakness, it's important to understand the factors that create the weakness in the first place. It's this combination of concepts, cellular weakness and its causes, that will enable us to evaluate our own risk for developing cancer and allow us to take the necessary steps to protect ourselves. This brings us to the second half of the equation and to another concept we'll refer to as . . .

The Layering Effect

As we continue in our efforts to keep a dense subject as simple as possible, this concept refers to the risk factors associated with cancer. Although there are no doubt many unknown factors that contribute to the development of cancer, we'll focus on those known or at the very least, those suspected of having links to cancer. If old age isn't the underlying factor in a diagnosis of cancer, opportunity is. And there are thirteen major factors that provide this opportunity including:

1) Heredity	**8) Ionizing Radiation**
2) Solar Radiation	**9) Hormones**
3) Air Pollution	**10) Occupation**
4) Water Pollution	**11) Diet**
5) Pesticides/Chemicals	**12) Alcohol**
6) Viruses	**13) Tobacco**
7) Medical Treatments/Conditions	

Of course, this list is by no means complete as new information about cancer and its "causes" surfaces every day. It does, however, provide a good foundation from which to begin our discussion of cancer and its risks, a discussion this book will begin now and re-examine in greater detail later.

Simply put, the Layering Effect is an exercise that forces one to objectively evaluate each risk factor on our list and the ways in which each impacts her or his life. As already mentioned, it's difficult to state unequivocally that one thing or another "causes" cancer, for cancer is an extremely complicated disease the initial origin of which still eludes the research and medical communities of the world. If it were understood completely, we already would have vaccines, shots and pills that would magically destroy existing cancers and protect us all from future cancers.

We do, however, understand enough about cancer to see trends and links and patterns, and recognize that certain elements of our lives and our lifestyles appear to increase our risk for developing certain forms of the disease. Although this understanding is limited, when it's combined with ordinary common sense, we can create a powerful defense that goes a long way in reducing our individual risk for the disease. For similar to basic sports theory, when it comes to fighting cancer, the best defense is a good offense.

Our list doesn't appear in alphabetical order, but rather is organized according to the amount of control we as individuals have over each risk. We'll examine each one individually beginning with those over which we have the least control, moving on to those over which we have limited control and concluding with those over which we have almost complete control. For, clearly, those factors over which we have little or no control are potentially more harmful and, therefore, may intrinsically be more important for us to understand.

Additionally, we'll refer to each factor as a "layer of risk" either adding layers or removing layers as we discuss each. Having established that, we are going to start this exercise by discussing factor number one–heredity. Of all the possible layers of risk associated with cancer, heredity remains the most inescapable one, the one that remains constant regardless of any conscious choice on our part or any lifestyle alteration we may attempt. As a result, it's the most crucial layer of risk for every individual, and as such we'll discuss it in greater detail than the others.

Heredity

Heredity is defined as the transmission of genetic characteristics from parents to their off-spring.[53] Indeed, every trait we possess from the color of our hair, eyes and skin, to our talents and athletic abilities, to our particular physical strengths and weaknesses have been largely pre-ordained by nature and the law of genetics. To a certain degree, so too has our ability to protect ourselves from disease and infection and our susceptibility to specific ailments and anomalies. It's well known that certain physical conditions such as Tay-Sachs disease, Sickle Cell Anemia and Cystic Fibrosis are inherited conditions passed to an individual from one or both parents. It's also becoming increasingly clear that the risk of developing cancer, especially certain forms of cancer such as those of the breast and colon, also is determined at least in part by our genetic makeup.

To protect ourselves from this possibility, therefore, it's necessary for each of us to know as much as possible about our family medical history. This is a project that will take energy and time, yet its value cannot be emphasized enough as this knowledge for many of us will make the difference between life and death. To begin, one must start by contacting one's living family members and relatives. It's vital for families to conference with one another and to communicate and share all relevant medical information. It's important for each family member to know what conditions and diseases have affected other family members, and it's important to know which family members have been so affected.

It also may be necessary to research available hospital and physician medical records that may document the presence of disease or the cause of death of relatives now deceased. One should go back, if possible, to great grandparents, as well as grandparents and aunts and uncles on both sides of the family. Most importantly, one must make every effort to know the medical history of parents, siblings and children. For these family members are referred to as "first-degree" relatives[54] and it's their genetic makeup that will most closely reflect our own and any predisposition we may have to developing a variety of diseases, including cancer.

If research of our family relatives indicates that a particular cancer appears more than once in a single generation, or if the same cancer appears from one generation to another, that particular form of cancer may be genetic. If a cancer known to be genetically influenced, such as breast or colon cancer, appears even once in any generation that particular cancer may have a genetic etiology. In addition, if an individual developed a cancer early in life while in their twenties, thirties or forties, that cancer may be genetically influenced.[55] Once we have this information, we can take the appropriate steps necessary to protect ourselves from the cancer in question and avail ourselves of all procedures that may detect the disease at the earliest stage of its development.

It's important, however, to remember that even with this familial information we still may not have the whole story. True, medical records of a deceased relative may indicate if they had cancer or if their death resulted from cancer. Yet, if death was the result of something else, a likely scenario for those who lived several decades ago, the person in question may still have had cancer. Their disease simply may have been undetected and undiagnosed at the time of death.

Moreover, many of us may not have access to information about our grandparents, uncles and aunts, or parents. Some of us don't know who our relatives are and some of us don't even know the identity of our biological parents. In such cases, although our proactive ability to defend ourselves against some specific cancers may be somewhat limited, many protective tools remain. For those who suspect a family history of cancer, there are genetic counselors and genetic screening programs that can determine a predisposition for some cancers, such as breast and colorectal cancers. There are numerous tests, exams and medical procedures designed to detect many additional cancers early in their development. And, we have our own intelligence and common sense to guide us, inform us and warn us of possible harm.

In any case, it's essential that we take every possible step to secure this information for heredity remains the one layer of risk that as yet, we cannot escape. A genetic predisposition for cancer means that our DNA may already be altered or damaged at the time of our birth. If this is the case, it may not be necessary for a harmful agent to invade a weakened cell before cancer is expressed, for the DNA is already compromised. Our Cancer Blueprint essentially has been sidestepped. The harm has already been done and the damaged cell is free to multiply and create additional cells that are identically damaged.

Further, such genetically influenced cancers are believed to be more virulent and possibly more aggressive than other cancers.[56] It becomes clear, therefore, why heredity remains the most important layer when determining our own personal risk for specific cancers. As such it's in a class of its own while the remaining layers of risk, with a few exceptions, can be divided basically into three additional categories of environmental, medical and lifestyle issues.

Environmental

In the first group we have **solar radiation**, **air pollution**, **water pollution, pesticides** and **chemicals** and **viruses**. Beginning with solar radiation, we once again have a factor that cannot be eliminated. It can, however, be avoided and controlled to a certain extent. The use of sunscreens, the wearing of proper clothing and the practice of minimizing our time in the sun are simple tools that afford us a great deal of protection.

Similarly, air and water pollution are hazards that exist in our environment. Yet, these risks are more difficult to control as it's not clear what conditions actually constitute "pollution" of these resources. We're not certain of all the agents that might be harmful to us, of the level at which these agents become harmful, or in many cases, if these agents exist in our water or air in the first place. Once we're aware of possible danger, of course, we can then take steps to correct the situation, minimize our exposure to the situation or avoid the situation.

Yet, our roles as dictated by family, business and community responsibility demand we function in a world where our awareness of air and water pollution may remain elusive. Even if we're aware of potential harm, it may not always be possible for us to breathe fresh clean air or drink purified water. The amount of control we exercise over these layers of risk, therefore, remains limited and often inconsistent.

The same is true of pesticides and chemicals believed to be possible carcinogens, although the link between many of these products and cancer is not conclusive. We can always determine for ourselves if or to what extent we utilize such products in our own lives and around our own homes. We cannot, however, control the actions of others in our neighborhoods and communities. Nor can we control the government guidelines that allow or forbid the use of such products. We can use natural products instead of harsh pesticides or chemicals, we can purchase foods raised without pesticides or chemicals, and we can influence our legislatures to examine additional data and adopt more appropriate measures for the production and use of pesticides and chemicals. Even with these abilities we don't have complete control over this suspected risk and as a result we remain vulnerable to its potential harm.

The last risk in this group are the viruses, microscopic infectious agents that live in the environment and multiply only after invading living cells. A virus contains its own genetic material, and when it invades a cell, it takes over by instructing the host cell to manufacture whatever the virus needs to reproduce.[57] In some cases, this alteration predisposes the host cell to the development of certain cancers including cervical cancer, Kaposi's sarcoma and Burkitt's lymphoma.[58] Viruses are contagious and can be transmitted through bodily fluids such as saliva, blood and by sexual intercourse. This is a layer of risk, therefore, that we can control to a large degree by changing or adopting certain lifestyle habits. By following the guidelines for safe and protected sex, for example, and by avoiding shared needles for tattoos or intravenous drugs, our risk to the viruses associated with cancer will be greatly reduced.

Medical Conditions/Treatments

The layers of risk associated with this second group include specific **medical conditions** or **treatments, ionizing radiation** and **hormones**. First, there are several physical conditions with which we may be born that may contribute to the development of future cancers. Technically, anything with which we're born could be classified as a hereditary factor. Some physical conditions, therefore, may implicate two areas of risk: medical conditions and heredity. We'll refer to this as a cross-over risk. Yet, because we're writing about obvious physical body conditions that are known to be linked to specific cancers, we'll place this factor within the medical risks. Second, there also are many medical treatments that have been used to combat a variety of ailments in the past that appear to contribute to one's cancer risk in the present.

Various drugs, including some anticancer drugs and drugs used in certain forms of chemotherapy, also have the unfortunate potential to "cause" future cancers while treating current cancers. Similarly, immunosuppressive drugs have been linked to the development of cancers.[59] Immunosuppressives are drugs used widely in treating a variety of autoimmune diseases and in preparing patients for organ transplants. These drugs work by inhibiting one's immune system to prevent the body from identifying necessary medical agents or donor organs as foreign material. This allows the body to benefit from the medicines or accept the new organ rather than rejecting either as a harmful invader. When the immune system is inhibited, however, its ability to recognize and fight true harmful invaders is compromised. As a result, numerous infections and diseases including certain cancers, have ample opportunity to develop and grow.

The next two layers of risk, ionizing radiation and hormones, also are cross-over risks that technically could be included in more than one layer of risk. The first, ionizing radiation, can come from environmental sources such as cosmic rays and radioactive materials within the earth's crust such as radon and radium. In that case, our control over this risk will vary depending upon the circumstances. It's also true that exposure to this radiation can be produced by nuclear material and devices within our environment, another situation that allows most individuals even less control. For our purposes, however, we'll put this layer of risk in the category of "medical" for a number of reasons.

Radiation is a known "cause" of cancer and one of the most extensively studied human carcinogens.[60] Similar to the ultraviolet rays of solar radiation, ionizing radiation has the ability to enter and alter the molecular structure of a cell. It's believed that this alteration results in damage to the cell's DNA, which as we know can lay the foundation for cancer to develop. Yet, ionizing radiation is used in a variety of medical treatments for the very reason that it can alter the molecular structure of a cell. Radiation has been used in therapy to treat spinal disorders, ringworm, cancer and atypical conditions of the thyroid and tonsils–and, of course, in routine x-rays. As it alters and destroys damaged cells, radiation also damages healthy cells that may once again subject an individual to future cancers.[61]

The third cross-over layer of risk, hormones, could be categorized as a component of heredity as well as a medical factor. After all, we're all born with a predominance of either male or female hormones. Further, the naturally occurring intrinsic hormones of testosterone and estrogen have been implicated in some cancers, including those of the prostate in the former and breast, cervical and endometrial in the latter. Our discussion, however, will focus more upon exogenous hormones added as supplements rather than upon naturally occurring endogenous hormones.

For example, the female hormone estrogen is used to combat menopausal symptoms through Hormone Replacement Therapy or HRT. Drugs with estrogenic properties also have been used to treat a variety of reproductive conditions in women. Similarly, male androgens have been used in the treatment of renal conditions and various types of anemias. The use of estrogen in some situations, however, has been linked to breast, cervical and endometrial cancer in females as well as to testicular cancer in males, while the use of androgens has been linked to liver cancer in males.[62]

Clearly, all three risks in this group, medical conditions and treatments, ionizing radiation and hormones, involve difficult situations in which difficult decisions must be made. On the one hand, the use of these treatments may provide the means necessary to fight, detect or manipulate uncomfortable, harmful or life-threatening medical conditions. On the other, many of these treatments may prove beneficial in one area of our health only to prove damaging in another. This becomes a situation of medical trade-offs that demands our decisions be cautious and well informed. As the decision maker, the individual maintains control over these layers of risk, although it's control that must be tempered with caution and balanced with common sense.

Lifestyle

This last category includes the four layers of risk over which we have perhaps the greatest amount of control. **Occupation**, **dietary habits** and **alcohol** and **tobacco use** are all lifestyle risks that can be reduced or completely eliminated. Of the four, occupation may be the most difficult to change or control. An individual must first have a choice of opportunities before she or he can leave an existing job to begin a new one. And, of course, one must be able to adapt one's skills to a new position that may offer a healthier workplace environment. The remaining three risks, however, are among the easiest to control. For example, our diets. There's a wealth of information today that outlines the steps necessary to insure proper nutrition, health and longevity. And, while some of the world's populations have limited resources and, therefore, limited control over this risk, much of the world can control it to a large degree.

The final two layers of risk, alcohol and tobacco use, can be completely controlled by every individual in every part of the world. Alcoholic beverages have been associated with certain cancers, but only to a limited degree. The harm induced by such beverages depends entirely upon the strength of the drink and the amount consumed.[63] Both of these factors are determined by each individual's personal choice.

Similarly, the use of tobacco is a personal choice, a risk that can be eliminated completely by a simple change in lifestyle. This lifestyle change is perhaps the most important decision any individual can make as tobacco use, especially in the form of cigarette smoking, is the single most preventable cause of excess mortality in many of the world's countries, including the United States.[64] Indeed, one third of all cancer deaths in the United States are directly linked to cigarette smoking, yet the simple choice to avoid cigarette smoking and the smoke of another's cigarette gives us total or near total control over this extremely dangerous layer of risk.

Risk Analysis

Now that we have a basic knowledge of the risks, a subject that will be discussed in greater detail in the next section, we can determine our own "risk profile," or in other words, our possible potential for developing certain cancers. To do so, we'll begin at the top of the list with heredity, the layer of risk over which we have the least control, and continue down the list to tobacco use, the layer of risk over which we have the most control. We'll examine each risk carefully and determine if that risk applies to our personal life. If it does, the risk will be added to our list. We'll then move on to the next risk and the next, examining each independently and either adding it to our list or omitting it. Adding one layer at a time, we'll end up with a personal profile that will help us assess our own personal cancer risk. Once our list is compiled, we'll re-evaluate it and remove or modify the layers where elimination or alteration is possible. Let's use a few simple examples to help clarify this exercise.

Profile #1:

Our first individual is a fifty-five-year-old female whose maternal grandmother developed breast cancer at the age of sixty. Our individual also underwent childhood radiation treatments for a skin disorder on her back and chest and began Hormone Replacement Therapy (HRT) for menopausal symptoms at the age of forty-five.

Beginning at the top of our list, heredity clearly is a layer of risk that must be included in this profile. Breast cancer is known to be a genetic disease, and our individual has a close blood relative who has had the disease. Moving down our list, two medical treatments are implicated in our individual's profile, including the radiation therapy she received as a child and the HRT she's receiving as an adult.

The first, ionizing radiation, has been linked to the development of certain types of cancers and as such must be added as the second layer of risk in our profile. It also is noteworthy that this therapy was applied to our individual's chest area, which may further contribute to a vulnerability of these tissues. The second, the use of extrinsic estrogen through HRT, may increase a woman's risk for breast cancer, especially if the use is long-term and the dose is relatively high. Such estrogen exposure also has been linked to the development of cancers of the uterus. This fact adds a third layer of risk for our individual and creates a risk profile that includes **1) heredity, 2) ionizing radiation** and **3) hormones.**

Now it's our job to examine this list again and determine which layers of risk can be either removed or modified. Again, starting at the top with heredity we have a layer that at this point in time, based upon current medical technology, we cannot remove. Our individual cannot eliminate this layer of risk, as she cannot change the fact that a close blood relative experienced breast cancer. Nor can she undo her past treatment with radiation. Accordingly, these two layers of risk will remain in her profile. The third layer of risk, however, can be reduced or removed by substituting natural products or medications in place of her current HRT, which has been ongoing for ten years. Such products do not contain estrogen, yet help reduce the discomfort of many symptoms associated with peri-menopause, menopause and post-menopause.

Furthermore, it appears our individual already carries an increased risk for developing breast cancer based upon heredity, and possibly, her radiation exposure as well. Since these are layers over which she has no control, it may be advisable for her to take the necessary steps to remove or reduce this third layer of risk. In doing so, even though her risk profile indicates a possible predisposition for breast cancer, she may decrease her overall risk for developing the disease. By removing or reducing this layer she also may reduce her risk for developing related cancers of the uterus. As a result, her risk profile has changed in the following way:

Heredity	Heredity
Ionizing Radiation	Ionizing Radiation
Hormones	{Controlled}

In review, our individual remains vulnerable to breast cancer through her possible genetic predisposition for the disease. She also remains vulnerable to those cancers that have been linked to radiation therapy. She can, however, reduce her risk for breast cancer and possibly uterine cancer by reducing or eliminating her use of extrinsic estrogen through HRT. We need to remember, of course, that our adjusted profile does not mean our individual will never develop breast or uterine cancer. It does indicate, however, that her apparent risk for these specific cancers has been acknowledged and dealt with in a positive and pro-active manner.

Profile #2:

Our second individual is a male with fair hair and blue eyes. He's a commercial fisherman who smokes a pack of cigarettes daily and whose father suffers from respiratory disease.

Again, starting at the top of the list with heredity, we know of no family history of cancer. There is, however, a history of lung disease that may or may not indicate a genetic predisposition, not necessarily for cancer, but for a generalized weakness of the lung tissues. Knowing that vulnerable tissue is susceptible to many diseases including cancer, just to be safe, heredity should be listed on this individual's risk profile. Furthermore, heredity is once again implicated as our individual's genetic light coloring increases his risk for developing cancers of the skin.

In addition, our individual spends a great deal of time outdoors in the sun and, accordingly, solar radiation must be included as an additional layer of risk in the profile. Moving down our list, the next layer of risk that pertains to our individual is occupation, for it's our individual's job as a commercial fisherman that exposes him to excessive solar radiation. Finally, a fourth layer of risk, tobacco use, is added to create a risk profile that includes: **1) heredity, 2) solar radiation, 3) occupation** and **4) tobacco use**.

Once again, we will now examine each layer of risk in the profile with the intent of altering or eliminating those we can. Heredity remains in the profile as the one layer over which we have the least control. Our individual cannot change the fact that his father suffered from a lung disease that may indicate a genetic weakness of these particular tissues. Nor can he change his inherited light coloring. Solar radiation, on the other hand, is a layer of risk we can reduce, if not eliminate completely. The use of sunscreens and protective clothing can help tremendously in averting the harmful effects of ultraviolet radiation even in an individual with fair hair and eyes.

Occupation, on the other hand, may not be a risk that lends itself easily to alteration in this case. But by practicing good "sun sense" as mentioned above, the cancer risk posed by this layer is greatly reduced. Finally, the fourth layer of risk, tobacco use, is entirely within our individual's control and therefore can be completely eliminated. Not only is cigarette smoking associated with a number of different cancers, it's directly linked to lung cancer. In light of the possible genetic predisposition to diseases of the lung our individual may face, the decision to eliminate this fourth layer of risk would be highly advisable. As a result, this individual's risk profile has changed in the following way:

Heredity	Heredity
Solar Radiation	{Controlled}
Occupation	{Controlled}
Tobacco Use	{Eliminated}

Once again, this individual began with several layers of risk that indicated a possible genetic predisposition for lung disease and, therefore, possibly lung cancer. His genetic coloring and exposure to the sun through his occupation also indicated a risk for skin cancers. Through a process of examination, however, he can control or remove the three remaining layers of risk and create an adjusted profile that indicates less risk for both lung and skin cancer.

Again, the initial profile doesn't mean that the individual would definitely have developed either cancer, nor does the adjusted profile guarantee that either cancer, or other cancers, will ever develop. The profiles do indicate, however, that the individual has an apparent risk for cancers of the lung and skin that can be reduced first, through acknowledgment and second, through action.

In essence, therefore, the Layering Effect is a tool that allows us to create a personal profile of the cancer risks that most apply to us. It's a tool that helps us gain the proper perspective of our cancer risks, enables us to make conscious choices about those risks and take deliberate proactive steps to reduce those risks. We cannot fight an enemy until we recognize it as such. And, we're in a far better position to fight that enemy when it is recognized from a distance than when it's storming the castle wall.

We've briefly discussed the risks for cancer and, as a result, the above examples are rather simplified. Regardless of their simplicity, however, each example is sufficient to illustrate the important concept of a cancer risk analysis. This analysis, the Layering Effect, combined with our Cancer Blueprint, will give us a solid foundation upon which we can build an extremely useful understanding of this disease we call cancer. As we continue through the next two sections of this book we'll discuss in greater detail these layers of risk and the most common cancers associated with these risks. And, when armed with this additional information we'll examine a few more risk profiles in greater detail.

Part 2:
Cancer: "Causes" And Effects

Once again, this book will continue to refer to the term "cause" or "causes" of cancer in quotes simply because it's so difficult to say exactly what the "cause" or "causes" of cancer may be. There's an enormous amount of information about cancer and the factors that contribute to its development. Such information, however, may be incomplete, for many unknown factors that work in combination with these known factors may exist as well. Keeping that in mind, this book will do its best to explain the phenomenon of cancer growth and the risks that science has shown are associated with that growth. Our discussion will begin again with the risks over which we have the least control and continue through those over which we have the most. This time, however, our discussion will be more complex as we move through each section again, beginning with heredity and continuing through the environmental, medical and lifestyle risks.

Chapter 6:
Heredity

All human cancers involve the malfunction of genetic material that controls the growth and division of body cells. While most human cancers are caused by a combination of heredity and environmental factors, five to ten percent of many cancers such as that of the breast, are considered primarily hereditary.[65] When a cancer is hereditary, it means that the cancer is "caused" by a defective gene that may be passed on from one generation to the next. This phenomenon predisposes the members of a family in whom this defect is present to an excessively high risk for developing that particular type of cancer. Unlike many other factors, heredity is one risk that cannot be eliminated or avoided simply by altering one's lifestyle. As such, one's genetic makeup may be the most significant layer of risk regarding the development of certain forms of cancer and quite frankly, according to some theorists, the development of every form of cancer.

When a particular cancer, due to hereditary traits, strikes several blood relatives, it's referred to as a "family cluster." Indeed, such clusters have been reported for virtually every form of cancer. It's been estimated that close relatives of a cancer patient share twice the normal risk for developing the same type of cancer.[66]

In addition to those cancers whose etiology is known to be hereditary, other important signals that may indicate a family predisposition to a specific cancer include two or more members who are affected by the same cancer. This is especially important if the members are "first-degree" relatives, a term that refers to one's parents, one's siblings or one's children.[67] The age at which the cancer is diagnosed also is important in that clusters usually strike predisposed individuals at a younger than average age. While such familial cancer clusters are often due to inherited factors they are, however, also influenced by chance associations as well as environmental factors.[68]

The "chance" factor[69] plays a considerable role when determining the etiology or origin of any cancer. For example, it's estimated that in the United States alone each person faces a forty-five to fifty percent risk for developing some form of cancer during her or his lifetime. This means that approximately one out of every two people will eventually develop cancer. Additionally, cancer is considered in part to be a disease of "old age." In other words, the longer a person lives, the greater the chance for developing cancer. And in today's world of advanced medical technology, people are living longer than ever. As a result, more people are developing cancer, and it's more and more common for many families to have at least one or multiple members with a cancer history.

The role of this "chance" factor, however, may be reduced or eliminated if a number of specific conditions exist. As mentioned, if the cancer occurs in the same body site or organ in multiple blood relatives, and if it occurs at an early age, genetic factors take precedence over chance. Similarly, cancers that appear in more than one place within the particular site or organ once again are often linked to hereditary factors rather than chance. For example, women with a familial history of breast cancer may not only develop the cancer at a relatively early age, they also may develop two primary breast cancers in the same breast, or one primary breast cancer in each breast.

Environmental factors, on the other hand, are more difficult to identify and separate from the possible hereditary factors. The relationship between the two is complex and requires careful analysis. While a cancer may be genetically induced, the age at which the cancer develops may depend, at least in part, upon environmental triggers. One who may be genetically predisposed for developing colorectal cancer, for example, may be able to delay or possibly even avoid the disease by making proper dietary habits and physical exercise lifestyle priorities.[70]

Similarly, cancers that appear to be linked primarily to external factors are still influenced by heredity and the gene pool of an individual. For instance, lung cancer is strongly associated with cigarette smoking, airborne pollutants and one's workplace environment. Yet, an individual's risk for developing lung cancer also depends upon whether or not one is genetically susceptible to diseases of the lung and respiratory tract. It's always possible for one individual to live in an urban area, smoke heavily, work around hazardous materials and never develop lung cancer. It's also possible for another individual to live in a rural area, never smoke, work in a hazard free environment and develop lung cancer. Each case involves a tangled combination of factors the outcome of which is impossible to predict with certainty.

In spite of these complications, however, it remains vitally important to have knowledge of one's family medical history and exercise common sense based upon that knowledge. Familial cancers triggered by environmental factors can be reduced through education and the avoidance of related harmful carcinogens. If one suspects a family history of lung ailments, for instance, it would be wise to refrain from cigarette smoking. In melanoma- prone families or in families where the members have light skin, fair hair and blue or green eyes, a program of reduced sun exposure combined with proper sun protection similarly may substantially reduce their risk for skin cancers.

In recent years the amount of research investigating hereditary factors and their relationship to specific cancers has increased greatly. The inherited susceptibility to cancer was first discovered in the genes that are responsible for a childhood malignant eye tumor known as retinoblastoma or RBI.[71] Following this important discovery, breast cancer was identified as a hereditary disease when the genes BRCA-1 and BRCA-2 were isolated. New techniques in molecular biology continued to identify several additional human cancer genes that have been implicated in the development of cancer.

Furthermore, these new and advanced techniques also revealed a new class of cancer genes called **tumor suppressor genes** or **antioncogenes.**[72] In fact, it was research conducted among families with known hereditary cancers that led science to the discovery of the antioncogenes. These are genes that have the ability to inhibit the development of cancer when they're functioning normally. When these genes are damaged, however, they lose their protective effect and cancer develops with greater frequency. It's these damaged genes that may be inherited and passed on to future generations increasing the risk for developing certain forms of cancer among family members.

On the other hand, it appears that the protective power of tumor suppressor genes is enhanced in some individuals, a quality also inherited and passed on to future generations. For example, there are certain ethnic groups whose incidence rates for specific cancers are far below the average rate. Acute lymphocytic leukemia, for one, is the most common childhood cancer in most of the world's Western countries, yet it's rare among Arab, Indian and black children in the United States and Africa.[73] Similarly, Ewing's sarcoma, which is a skin cancer, melanomas, nonmelanomas and testicular cancer are rare among the world's black populations.[74]

In 2003, the **Human Genome Project**[75] succeeded in its goal to map every gene within the human body and detail the function and importance of each. In so doing, the Project made it possible to not only identify each human gene, but to determine if those genes are damaged in a way that may promote the development of specific diseases including cancer. The purpose of identifying such gene factors, of course, is to promote early cancer detection to increase an individual's overall chance of survival. However, this technology, known as "gene mapping," comes with a price. As is often the case with new technology, it comes with new psychological, ethical and legal issues that must be considered as well. Every individual who discovers through the process of gene mapping that she or he has damaged genes associated with the development of disease also must consider the consequences of this knowledge.[76]

For example, will an individual who discovers predispositions for certain cancers through gene mapping also be faced with overwhelming emotional stress or social stigmatization? Will the individual be able to obtain health insurance? As a result of the mapping, will the individual be at risk for losing her or his current insurance? If insurance is available, will the cost increase for those whose cancer risk appears to be hereditary? Will other members of the family be able to obtain affordable insurance? Will future generations be able to obtain insurance at all? If the individual is able to obtain affordable insurance and a cancer develops will the treatment be covered by the policy or will the cancer be considered a preexisting condition? Will insurance companies pay for procedures that a genetically fragile individual needs early in life in order to detect possible cancers? Will employers be reluctant to hire an individual with a predisposition for certain cancers?

And although new laws prohibiting discrimination based upon genetic information are increasing, are those laws being enforced? In the United States, for example, forty-six states had enacted such laws as of 2009.[77] More states have joined these ranks in the past few years, however, state laws differ dramatically. Some are very narrowly drawn and some are quite broad. And, while the federal government enacted the Genetic Information Non-Discrimination Act of 2008 (GINA), this Act only provides a minimum of protection.[78] One must understand the rights to which she or he may be entitled in one's state or country of residence.

To use an old adage, these questions raise issues that merely form the tip of the iceberg. For the information gleaned from gene mapping will not only expose the possibility of future cancers, it also will isolate the genes associated with every hereditary condition within the entire spectrum of human frailty. While gene mapping, and the goals behind it, remains a tremendous breakthrough from a scientific viewpoint, it may have serious, unintended consequences from a different perspective. The promise of early cancer and disease detection and the possible prevention of each is enormous, yet the potential for harm exists as well.

We'd like to think that with each new scientific breakthrough we also possess the wisdom with which to use the knowledge properly and humanely. This is not always the case, however, as different elements of our societies have different goals. Those elements that exist to conduct business and make profits may not view this particular breakthrough in the same altruistic light as the elements of science and medicine. Such information, therefore, may create a quagmire of sticky societal issues that may prove extremely difficult to isolate and solve. As a result, it's clear that before gene mapping becomes commonplace, its use and the information it yields must be protected through the responsible and careful evaluations of society. For the highest goal of knowledge must be to promote maximum benefit for all humanity while minimizing potential harm.

Personal Note

When I was diagnosed with colon cancer, it was a tremendous shock for all who knew me. I displayed no obvious risk factors for the disease. My diet was low in fat, void in meats and high in fruits and vegetables. I didn't smoke and drank alcohol rarely. I was active and athletic, I had always been lean and I was half the age of the typical colon cancer patient. Unknown to me at the time, however, was the fact that colon cancer ran in my family. Indeed, I didn't research my family medical history until my surgeon told me that my disease, in his opinion, could only be the result of genetic factors. Both my maternal and paternal grandparents were deceased at the time of my diagnosis. I was aware that my maternal grandmother had undergone a mastectomy and survived breast cancer, but no additional information regarding my other grandparents and additional cancers was available.

One of my maternal uncles, however, had been diagnosed with and treated for colon cancer when he was in his fifties. Further, following my diagnosis, another maternal uncle was diagnosed with the disease, and my mother was diagnosed with colon polyps. This indicates that one or both of my maternal grandparents in all likelihood had a predisposition for colon cancer, even though cancer wasn't the cause of their deaths and was not mentioned in their medical records. All of this information, of course, is not only vital to me, but also to my siblings and cousins, as well as their children.

Chapter 7:
Environmental

Solar Radiation

This type of radiation exposure is, of course, that which is produced by the earth's sun. It's this type of radiation exposure that's the primary cause of all cancers of the skin including basal cell cancer, squamous cell cancer and melanoma. The first two, known as the non-melanomas, were responsible for many deaths in the United States during the 1950s and the 1960s. Fortunately, the mortality rate from these skin cancers declined in the 1970s, and today both are considered to be more than ninety percent curable. Melanoma, on the other hand, is far more lethal, with mortality rates that have increased in recent years. Indeed, when the new cases of melanoma are combined with those of the nonmelanomas, skin cancer becomes the most common cancer in the world.[79]

The harmful relationship between the sun and human skin appears to have been documented first in the late 1800s when sailors exposed to the sun developed a skin condition called "Seemannshaut" or "sailor's skin."[80] A report published in 1894 by German researcher P.G. Unna documented the apparent relationship between sunlight and skin cancer, and the early 1900s produced additional evidence of this relationship through studies conducted among farmers and Caucasians in particular. It was not until the 1930s, however, that scientific evidence forged the theory that sunlight contained ultraviolet-B radiation, and when the sunlight was strong enough to burn human skin as in a typical sunburn, the ultraviolet-B light produced a carcinogenic effect.

To clarify this subject, let's first establish that solar radiation includes light that's visible to the human eye. It also includes other wavelengths, such as ultraviolet light that are invisible to the human eye. As we know, this ultraviolet light is composed of two types of light known as ultraviolet A, or UV-A, and ultraviolet B, or UV-B. When scientifically measured with a device known as a nanometer, UV-A is radiation that falls within the 320 to 400 range, and UV-B radiation falls within the 290 to 320 range.[81]

Both cause aging and wrinkling of the skin, and both have the ability to damage DNA directly or indirectly by activating oxygen molecules that in turn damage the DNA. It's UV-B radiation, however, that's responsible for most of the tanning and redness of the skin associated with sun exposure. It is this tanning and redness that's most associated with the future development of skin cancers.[82] Furthermore, UV-B light is the greater contributor to localized immunosuppression of the skin, which in itself will inhibit the body's natural cancer-fighting abilities.

The strength of UV-B light in any location is determined primarily by the latitude of the location, which is its distance from the equator, the altitude and the sky cover. For example, in the United States, Atlanta, Georgia and El Paso, Texas have the same general latitude, which measures 32 to 33 degrees north of the equator. El Paso, however, has a drier climate and a higher altitude than Atlanta. These two factors increase the amount of solar radiation, and as a result, El Paso has an annual UV-B count approximately thirty-eight percent higher than Atlanta. In addition, the time of year and time of day also determine the amount of UV-B radiation, although to a lesser degree.[83]

For example, the greatest amount of UV-B exposure occurs during the summer months, with sixty percent of each day's total occurring between the hours of 10:00 A.M. and 2:00 P.M. A good rule to remember when the time of day is unknown, therefore, is that when one's shadow is longer than one's height, the sun is less than forty-five degrees above the horizon and UV-B radiation is at its lowest intensity. And while latitude, altitude and climate all impact the amount of UV-B in the atmosphere, latitude remains the most critical of the three. Indeed, there's a direct inverse relationship between nonmelanoma skin cancer and latitude. This means locations of lower latitudes, or those closer to the equator, have the highest incidence rates of nonmelanoma skin cancer, including both basel and squamous cell cancer.[84]

There's another factor, however, that's even more important than latitude when determining the amount of UV-B exposure, and that factor is the amount of ozone in the atmosphere. Ozone is a type of oxygen commonly produced from an electrical discharge such as that which occurs during a lightning storm. The "ozone shield" is a layer of ozone that hangs in the atmosphere about thirty to forty feet above the earth's surface. This shield protects the earth from excessive ultraviolet radiation in that ozone gas has the ability to actually absorb most of the UV-B light in the upper atmosphere. Indeed, it's because of this ozone layer that only small amounts of UV-B light, perhaps one percent, actually reach the earth's surface.[85]

Unfortunately, in the 1970s researchers discovered that ozone molecules in the stratosphere over parts of Antarctica were being destroyed. This "Ozone Hole" was thought to be caused by man-made substances known as chlorofluorocarbons.[86] Called "CFSs" for short, chlorofluorocarbons are substances found in many products, including refrigerants, aerosol propellants, computer chip solvents and styrofoam insulation. Today's research estimates that the ozone layer could be reduced by another six percent or more over the next several decades if the world's production of CFSs continues at its current rate.[87] Clearly, as this reduction continues, greater amounts of ultraviolet radiation will penetrate the earth's atmosphere. As UV-B exposure increases on earth, the risk of developing skin cancers among humans also will increase.

To put this in perspective, for every one percent decrease in the ozone layer, the earth could experience a two percent increase in UV-B radiation. In response, many nations the world over have begun to implement environmental guidelines which call for a reduction in and a possible elimination of CFS production over the next several years. Further, on an individual level, solar radiation is an environmental factor that can be altered through lifestyle to reduce one's risk for developing skin cancers.[88]

As a result, any increased risk from UV-B exposure may be balanced by taking preventative measures, such as limiting sun exposure and using sunscreens and protective clothing. Hopefully, this combination of societal safeguards and individual responsibility together will help mitigate any harmful effect created by this recognized decrease in the ozone layer.

Headline:

Airline Pilots and Attendants Get More Breast Cancer[89]

Apparently true, at least for female airline pilots and attendants. This increase in breast cancer appears to be related to their increased exposure to ultraviolet radiation. Radiation exposure is a known risk factor in the development of breast cancer. This particular sample group spends a great deal of time flying at high altitudes where the intensity of radiation from ultraviolet light is greater than that found on the surface of the earth. And, it's this increased intensity, combined with repeated exposure, which appears to contribute to the higher than average incidence rate of breast cancer among women in these particular professions.

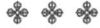

Air Pollution

Pollutants in urban air have long been suspected as contributing to the development of certain cancers and in particular to the development of lung cancer. Yet, it's difficult to substantiate this suspicion because it's hard to define and measure what we mean by "air pollution." In recent years, most of this suspicion has focused on the combustion of fossil fuels. Fossil fuels, of course, are found primarily in motor vehicle exhausts, especially diesel engines, as well as residential and commercial space heating, oil and coal-fired power plants and industrial emissions.

While some studies have found a link between some of these combustion factors in urban air and lung cancer rates the evidence is not clear. Apparently, one reason for this confusion is that cigarette smoking and occupational hazards also may contribute to the higher lung cancer rates in urban areas, and it's difficult to separate the effects of each factor.[90]

In an attempt to do so, however, specific research was conducted among a number of male individuals with average smoking habits. The result of this research suggests that the causative effect of urban air pollution on lung cancer among men is much less evident than the effect of smoking on lung cancer among men. Yet, it appears that the carcinogenic effects of smoking on the lung are enhanced in urban areas, which indicates that pollutants in the urban atmosphere, while they may not be as harmful in and of themselves, may increase the carcinogenic potency of tobacco smoke. It appears, therefore, that while evidence linking airborne pollutants directly to the risk for lung cancer is inconclusive, such pollutants appear to be possible co-factors that become significant when combined with known carcinogens.[91]

Interestingly, some of the strongest evidence that supports the link between specific air pollutants and the risk for lung cancer comes from China where the lung cancer rates in certain regions is unusually high.[92] In these regions it was discovered that many of the men and women lived in houses without chimneys and whose only source of heat came from burning a locally produced soft coal. It's believed that the smoke and fumes released into each home's indoor environment by the coal-burning devices were contributing to the country's high rates of lung cancer. In addition, cooking oil vapors released into the home environment by high temperature wok cooking is also believed to increase the risk for lung cancer, especially among Chinese women primarily responsible for the preparation of meals.[93]

Similarly, lung cancer rates are excessively high in neighborhoods around the world that are adjacent to arsenic – emitting smelters.[94] Arsenic is an element that occurs naturally throughout the earth's crust and can be used as either a therapeutic agent or as a poison. In the latter case, arsenic poisoning can be caused by the ingestion or inhalation of arsenic itself or by substances containing arsenic. When arsenic is used in the production of pesticides, herbicides or dye, it can be released into the air as an industrial waste byproduct. Of course, once it's released into the air it becomes a component of the oxygen one breathes and, as a result, directly affects the lungs and respiratory system.[95]

More evidence of the harmful effects of exposure to certain airborne substances comes from several studies that have focused on radon. Radon is an inert radioactive gas produced through the natural decay of radium and uranium. It's found everywhere in the earth's crust yet certain conditions appear to pose special problems. For example, studies conducted among uranium miners have found that these individuals share an incidence rate for lung cancer that's higher than average. In these studies, it's believed that the exposure to the radioactive emissions from radon in the uranium mines is directly linked to this apparent increased risk.[96]

Concern also has focused on radon exposures that occur in the home. In particular, there is special concern about those homes that have been made airtight by the new efficiency of insulation. In these cases, the insulation definitely keeps the home warm in the winter and cool in the summer. Unfortunately, it also can lock radon, which can enter the home through cracks in its foundation, the water or specific building materials, in the home's atmosphere where it may accumulate undetected.[97]

Indeed, both the National Cancer Institute and the Environmental Protection Agency estimate that about 13,000 lung cancers a year in the United States may be the result of exposure to radon in the home environment.[98] Although a certain amount of radon is commonly found in many homes it's important that the amount not exceed a certain level. Radon is measured fairly easily in units called "picocuries." The amount can be determined by a number of companies that specialize in radon testing and according to the EPA, indoor radon levels above four picocuries per liter of air should be modified to reduce the risk for lung cancer. It's true that some organizations believe that the indoor radon level in a home can rise as high as ten picocuries per liter of air before it becomes dangerous. The EPA, however, stands by its suggestion that levels above four picocuries should be modified to ensure maximum protection.[99]

Additional airborne pollutants believed to contribute to the risk for cancer include asbestos (a word which comes from the Greek root meaning "inextinguishable")[100] and, of course, tobacco smoke. In fact, asbestos in the workplace has become a significant factor when determining one's risk for lung cancer. Similarly, tobacco smoke, especially when produced by cigarettes, is a well established risk factor in a number of cancers. Cigarette smoke in the home environment is believed to be linked not only to an increased lung cancer risk for the smoker, but to a small yet measurable risk increase among non-smoking family members of smokers.[101]

This phenomenon, known as secondary or passive exposure, environmental tobacco smoke or simply ETS, is significant and helps confirm the suspected link that exists between specific air pollutants and the risk for cancer. This is distinguished from a second phenomenon, known as third-hand smoke, which refers to contamination that remains in the environment for hours or days after a cigarette is extinguished. While not directly linked to cancer, third-hand smoke is believed nevertheless to be a health hazard for infants and children as it lingers in materials such as furniture, carpet and clothing.[102]

So while the relationship between air pollutants in general and cancer is difficult to establish, the relationship between tobacco smoke and cancer is not. Indeed, the harm presented by all forms of tobacco use creates its own layer of risk. As a result, risk presented by other air pollutants typically won't be a substantial issue unless an individual is employed in an occupation or industry where the risk has been clearly documented.**[103]**

Water Pollution

Many of the harmful elements that account for water pollution are the same harmful elements we discussed in the prior section on air pollution. In industrialized countries, drinking water comes to us from two sources: 1) the city and county reservoirs and water treatment plants in urban areas and, 2) the groundwater that supplies spring and well water in rural areas. In each case, the water may contain a complex mixture of known and suspected carcinogens, including asbestos, trace metals, radioactive substances and a variety of chemicals. Some of these elements are found naturally in water while others may be the result of industrial waste or the water treating process itself, which may create small quantities of harmful chemicals. For example, drinking water in urban areas is often treated with chlorine in an effort to purify the water and neutralize any harmful bacteria.[104]

Unfortunately, this process of chlorination can produce byproducts known as trihalomethanes or "THMs" that are potential cancer-causing chemical compounds. These compounds include substances such as chloroform and are formed when the chlorine reacts with organic compounds in the water. In some city water supplies where the level of organic material is high there's suspicion that such byproducts may increase the risk of gastrointestinal and urinary tract cancers among the population. To reduce this risk, therefore, water is often filtered first so that the amount of chlorine needed for purification is reduced and the resulting amount of harmful byproducts is decreased as well.[105]

Yet, the greatest threat to drinking water remains the environmental pollutants created by industrial societies. Asbestos has already been implicated in cancer risk as an airborne pollutant. Unfortunately, asbestos fibers also can be found in the water supplies of many countries, including the United States. The highest levels are often found near cities and industrial centers because asbestos was used extensively in building construction until 1975 when it was replaced by other materials.[106]

Primarily used as a form of insulation, asbestos also was used to line cement water pipes in many industrialized regions. Over the years as the water pipes age, asbestos fibers become dislodged, seep into the water and are transported throughout the supply area. Although research indicates the danger from asbestos is greater when the fibers are airborne, asbestos in drinking water is considered harmful and may increase one's risk for certain cancers.[107]

In addition to asbestos, there are several trace metals found in drinking water, including arsenic, chromium and nickel. These substances may enter the water supply from industrial plants and mines or by seepage from soil or water piping. They also may be the result of water treatment processes or the natural breakdown of rocks and minerals. Of these metals, arsenic may be the most harmful. While the levels of arsenic in most drinking waters of many countries, including the United States, are fairly low and aren't considered a public health threat, the high levels of arsenic in drinking water in other countries such as Taiwan have been linked with several types of cancer, including that of the bladder, kidney, lung and liver in both sexes, as well as the prostate in males.[108]

Another metal that has come under close scrutiny recently is chromium. This element doesn't occur in pure form on its own but rather is derived from a mineral known as chromite. Traces of chromium can be found in plants and animals, and it's believed to play an important role in human nutrition. Because it's highly resistant to rust, chromium also is used extensively in industrial settings where it's used to plate other metals and harden steel.

While chromium in itself is not usually considered harmful, derivatives of this metal, including chromium 3 and chromium 6, may be harmful when elevated levels are found in drinking water. When these two derivatives seep from their intended location into nearby water sources, alarming "clusters" of cancers appear in the nearby populations. Cluster, again, refers to a large number of individuals in a relatively small area who exhibit cancer levels far above the average. Both chromium 3 and chromium 6 in drinking water have been linked to a number of cancers and rare leukemias, but due to increased awareness and publicity their levels are now much more closely monitored.[109]

Additional metals in drinking water, such as nickel, also may be harmful if found in large amounts. The combination of agents also may produce harmful results as in the case of nitrates. Nitrates themselves don't cause cancer, but when they combine in the body with certain amines they form nitrosamines, many of which are powerful carcinogens in animals and potential carcinogens in humans. Ingested nitrate comes primarily from food, but water can be the primary source of consumed nitrate in the United States, for example, where nitrate in drinking water is close to or above the level set by the Environmental Protection Agency. Nitrates are seldom eliminated by the water treatment process and while the evidence linking nitrates to human cancer is weak, it requires close and sustained investigation.[110]

In addition, radioactive substances may be found in a water supply depending on a number of circumstances. First, the local rock type in any given area may contribute to a contaminated water supply. Radium, of course, is the radioactive material produced by the disintegration of uranium and also exists in the uranium minerals of carnotite and pitchblende. Any water supply affected by such geology, therefore, is at risk for radioactive contamination from radium, which can accumulate in bone tissue and lead to bone cancers. Second, the handling of radioactive compounds by local industries, hospitals and nuclear power plants may greatly influence the safety of local water supplies.[111]

Of course, radon gas remains a key player in the discussion of water pollution as it was in our discussion of air pollution. As previously mentioned, radon is a radioactive material produced from the decay of radium. It's released naturally by the earth's rocks and soil, making it a common source of what is referred to as "background radiation."[112]

Radon also occurs naturally in groundwater and is found dissolved in the water supplies of many countries, including the United States. The ingestion of radon in water usually doesn't pose a serious hazard to human beings because it occurs in low concentrations. Radon in water, however, can become airborne and can be released into household air through showers, washing machines and other water related uses. When waterborne radon is released into the air it can be harmful and may contribute substantially to household airborne levels of this radioactive material. And, airborne radon is considered to be a major contributor to the development of lung cancer.[113]

In contrast to water supplies that come from reservoirs and water treatment plants in urban areas, groundwater is the source of natural spring and well water in rural areas. This is the water that percolates just below the earth's surface, and while it naturally may contain certain materials such as radon, it also may contain a variety of harmful man-made materials. Groundwater becomes contaminated when these materials seep into the rock formations that surround and hold the groundwater supply.[114] Even though natural spring and well water supplies are normally an element of rural areas, this contamination occurs because disposal sites are also commonly found in rural areas.

The most common groundwater contamination occurs as a result of seepage from industrial and hazardous waste disposal sites. The burying of such materials on land has been the most common method of disposal in many countries, including the United States, because it's the cheapest method of disposal.[115] The problem occurs when these disposal sites begin to leak, a condition that unfortunately has been documented in the United States as being quite common near older sites in particular.

Such leakage may result in groundwater contamination from many industrial solvents and chemicals, such as polychlorinated biphenyls or "PCBs" which are toxic and possibly carcinogenic compounds used in plastics, insulation and flame retardants. Similarly, vinyl chloride is a toxic gas produced when vinyl and chlorine are combined to make plastics and adhesives. This gas may be introduced into drinking water from industrial plants as well or in small amounts when the polyvinyl chloride piping used in some water distribution systems begins to seep. In addition, benzene and bis ether, both of which are highly flammable liquids used in solvents, may enter the groundwater at industrial and disposal sites, as may pesticide and herbicide runoff in agricultural regions.[116]

In light of such facts, many industrialized countries have strengthened their regulations and increased their monitoring of industrial and hazardous waste disposal not only in an effort to protect water supplies, but to protect the environment in general. Over the past decade the Environmental Protection Agency in the United States, for example, has adopted rigorous guidelines concerning the disposal of harmful materials and regularly monitors the country's major water supplies for a number of carcinogens.

In addition, there are many organizations that have been studying the possible link between cancer and drinking water for years. As a result of their efforts, with the exception of cluster cancers found in limited areas, the evidence presented appears to indicate that the cancer risk posed by contaminated drinking water remains relatively small.[117]

Pesticides/Chemicals

Pesticides, insecticides and herbicides comprise a group of substances are used to destroy or control pests, insects and weeds in the production of agriculture. To be effective, however, these substances contain a number of chemicals that may prove harmful to humans, animals and the environment, as well as to their intended targets. Indeed, the study of the harmful long-term effects of these chemicals on the human body comprises a major part of cancer research today.

The issue raises extremely important and urgent questions about the use and exposure of these chemicals and their role in the development of human cancers. The potential for exposure is great and extends from voluntary use in one's home and environment as well as involuntary exposure from residues found in food, drinking water, agricultural spraying and military service. Not surprisingly, the political and scientific issues surrounding this topic remain buried in controversy and debate.

The serious study of the harmful effects of pesticides, insecticides and herbicides didn't begin until the 1960s.[118] These studies, however, were limited in that most of this initial research was conducted on a general basis without focusing on specific chemicals. For example, the research indicated that many developed countries in which food supplies were protected by the use of pesticides showed increased rates among farmers for certain cancers including leukemia, non-Hodgkin's lymphoma and cancers of the skin, stomach and prostate.[119] While this was an extremely important beginning, the research failed to identify the specific chemicals responsible for this increase.

It wasn't until the late 1980s that science began to focus on specific chemicals and their possible relationship to the development of cancer. At this time, the International Agency for Research on Cancer concluded that several chemicals used in the production of "target eradicators," such as arsenic and dichlorodiphenyltrichloroethane or DDT may be "probable" carcinogens and, therefore, dangerous to human beings.[120]

This research was extremely important because it was the first to isolate and investigate the potential harm of specific chemical agents such as DDT, one of the most frequently investigated agents. For years, in fact, DDT was the most common chemical agent found in eradicators and was used worldwide as a major agricultural insecticide.

Over time, however, its adverse effect upon the environment became evident, its use was limited and it was replaced with other agents. Indeed, DDT was officially banned as an insecticide in the United States in 1971, a full decade before it was suspected as a possible human carcinogen.[121] The harmful effects of DDT have been validated in several studies since those initial suspicions were documented, validations that include its relationship to human cancers.

Residents of South Carolina in the United States, for example, experience high levels of lung cancer that appear to be associated with high levels of DDT in their blood. Other American studies indicate that high levels of DDT in blood and other tissues appear to be linked with a greater risk for breast cancer among women.[122] Of course, among workers who manufacture DDT, the risk for developing many cancers including that of the pancreas, appears to be higher than average.

In addition to the harmful chemicals found in pesticides and insecticides, those found in herbicides may be implicated in the development of several cancers as well. There are three chemicals in particular that may be particularly harmful, including phenoxy acetic acid, dioxin and triazine. The first, phenoxy acetic acid, has been linked to the development of several cancers, including non-Hodgkin's lymphoma in countries such as Sweden, Canada and the United States. Its use also has been linked with sarcomas in Sweden, Denmark and Italy. And there is evidence that herbicides, which contain phenoxy acetic acid and are used on lawns, are responsible for animal malignancies such as lymphoma that occur in dogs and other pets.[123]

The second chemical, dioxin, also was used extensively in herbicides around the world in forestry and grassland protection, and rice and sugar cane weed control. Interestingly, dioxin was a major component of the much publicized jungle defoliant Agent Orange. It was the job of this "agent" to destroy the vegetation and clear paths for United States military operations in areas of Southeast Asia during the 1960s and 1970s. "Orange" was a code name for the mixture of chemicals found in this herbicide, a name that distinguished it from other widely used herbicides including Agent White and Agent Blue.[124]

Each contained different chemical compounds, yet Agent Orange contained the largest amount of dioxin, a compound that interferes with the normal metabolism of flora. Individuals who have been exposed to dioxin through herbicides appear to be at a high risk for developing a number of cancers, including that of the lung. Individuals exposed to dioxin through Agent Orange or other means may experience a high risk not only for specific cancers, but also for skin disorders such as chloracne and possible genetic anomalies that may be passed to future generations.[125]

The third, triazine, also is a substance contained in a variety of herbicides used for weed control. This chemical is known to be harmful to some animals and has been linked to ovarian cancer among female agricultural workers in Italy where the use of triazine based herbicides is common. And while it's clear that pesticides, insecticides and herbicides are harmful agents by their very nature, it's not clear how far this harm extends.[126]

The evidence appears to link these substances with human cancers, yet none of this evidence is conclusive. The research is too limited and the results are often contradictory. The harm these substances present to the environment and to many of our animals is much clearer than the harm they present to humans. As such, a great deal more time and study is necessary to understand the full implications of their potential harm. Until then, it's of utmost importance to take every precaution to protect not only our environment and our animals, but to protect ourselves by minimizing our exposure to these substances, to use them with caution, to wear protective clothing and wash exposed areas of the skin after every exposure.

Viruses

A virus is a harmful, infectious organism that contains its own genetic material yet cannot multiply on its own.[127] Indeed, the only way a virus can multiply is by invading the cells of living tissue. This invasion takes place when the virus attaches itself to "receptors" located on the surface of a healthy host cell. Once attached, the virus begins to enter the cell wall, and when it's inside the cell the virus "infects" the healthy cell tissue with its own genetic material. This genetic material, either deoxyribonucleic acid (DNA) or ribonucleic acid (RNA) depending upon the type of virus, mixes with the healthy DNA or RNA of the host cell. The virus then begins to "take over" the healthy cell and actually instructs the cell to manufacture whatever the virus needs to multiply.[128]

When these instructions have been completed, the virus has the ability to multiply and the healthy host cell is eventually destroyed. During this process, the host cell becomes altered in a way that makes it more susceptible to certain cancers. It's believed that the virus either induces cancer directly or indirectly when the virus weakens the cell to the point of creating an immunodeficiency condition in the cell. This, of course, makes the cell susceptible to harm from a variety of diseases as well as cancer.

Indeed, it was Francis Peyton Rous who first suspected viruses as possible carcinogens in 1911.[129] His pioneering work laid the foundation for two other scientists, Howard Temin and David Baltimore, who first characterized the molecular biology of a different strain of viruses called the "retroviruses." These retroviruses contain RNA, yet they direct their host cells to produce DNA, a process made possible by an enzyme called "reverse transcriptase."[130]

It was the combined research of these three scientists that earned them the Nobel Prize in 1972 and paved the way for other scientists to further define the role of viruses in the development of human cancer. This research was extremely important for most of the viruses linked to cancer are retroviruses that include the human lymphotropic viruses and the human immunodeficiency viruses as well as the herpes viruses, papilloma viruses, hepadnaviruses or hepatitis B and flavaviruses or hepatitus C. Indeed, it's estimated that approximately five percent of all cancers in the United States alone are virally related while that percentage rises dramatically in less developed countries.

Human Lymphotropic Virus Type 1 (HTLV-1)

Based on the research of Rous, Temin and Baltimore, the first human retrovirus was discovered in 1990 by Robert Gallo of the National Cancer Institute. It's called the human lymphotropic virus type 1 or HTLV-1 and was first recognized in the southern area of Japan. It's believed to be transmitted through contaminated blood products, sexual intercourse and quite often from mother to child through breast feeding and perinatal contact.[131]

This virus, however, may not express itself for several decades. In fact, HTLV-1 is strongly linked with the development of adult T-cell leukemia and lymphoma.[132] These adult cancers occur when the virus attacks the white blood cells derived from the thymus, which is an essential part of the lymph system. These white blood cells are called T-cells because of their relationship to the thymus, and they're a necessary part of the bacteria fighting ability of the human immune system.[133] When the T-cells are attacked by the HTLV-1 virus, however, they lose their ability to destroy harmful agents, the immune system becomes compromised and the body becomes susceptible to specific cancers as well as other diseases.

The autoimmune diseases that HTLV-1 infected adults also may develop include arthritis and polymyositis. Arthritis, of course, is an inflammatory condition of the joints and polymyositis is an inflammation of the muscles, often accompanied by swollen body tissues and insomnia.[134] Forms of polymyositis, such as dermatomyositis, which causes inflammation of the skin and the connective tissues, may develop and are associated with certain malignancies.

HTLV-1 also has been linked to a chronic neurological syndrome similar to multiple sclerosis and causes an immunodeficiency condition in children called infective dermatitis. Because of the way that HTLV-1 affects the human body, it appears to be an example of a virus that may indirectly cause cancer by weakening the body's immune system and thereby allowing cancer to develop.

Human Lymphotropic Virus Type 11 (HTLV-11)

HTLV-11 is related to HTLV-1, but it hasn't yet been linked to the development of cancer in the same way. It is, however, a retrovirus first discovered in a patient who had a rare form of T-lymphocyte leukemia. Surprisingly, HTLV-11 also has been found to occur naturally in certain Native American populations in the United States. As a result, researchers are hopeful that ongoing efforts to support and monitor these populations also will result in promising new research that will enable the scientific community to better understand the virus and its link, if any, to the development of cancer.[135]

Human Immunodeficiency Virus (HIV)

Robert Gallo's initial research on HTLV-1 was not only important in itself, it was instrumental in other research as well. Utilizing his techniques, Gallo and fellow scientist Luc Montagnier of the Institut Pasteur in Paris were able to isolate the human immunodeficiency virus or HIV, as it is known today. Similar to HTLV-1, HIV is a virus that infects and destroys the T-lymphocytes, or T-cells, creating a profound immunodeficiency condition in the human body.[136] Because HIV directly kills T-cells and destroys other mechanisms essential to the health of the body's immune system, one infected with HIV becomes susceptible to a number of disease-producing organisms and cancers. Further, one affected by HIV may eventually be diagnosed with acquired immunodeficiency syndrome or AIDS if 1) the number of T-cells affected by HIV increases to a certain level while the number of healthy T-cells drops to a measurement level less than 200 and, 2) one experiences one or more of a number of symptoms, including fatigue, anorexia, severe diarrhea or depression.[137]

Among the cancers linked to HIV is Kaposi's sarcoma, a cancer of the lining of the blood vessels that occurs on the skin or within the vital organs. Before HIV and AIDS, Kaposi's sarcoma was rare and was found primarily in older males often of Mediterranean ancestry and male residents of central Africa. The occurrence of this cancer now is considered an epidemic form in many countries of the world, including the United States, where it's found primarily among homosexual males.[138]

Other groups at risk for HIV infection include those who share drug paraphernalia or those who have received tainted blood transfusions, although these affectations are much rarer. The other major malignancy that results from HIV infection is non-Hodgkin's lymphoma, a cancer that occurs in all the HIV risk groups and appears to be strongly linked to profound immunodeficiency. Indeed, it has been estimated that eight to twenty-five percent of all future lymphomas in the United States alone will be HIV and AIDS related.[139]

Unfortunately, the risk for developing additional virally associated cancers appears to increase in individuals who are already infected by HIV. For example, data suggests that the human papilloma virus may increase the risk for certain cancers among individuals who are already HIV positive. Similarly, the process of immunosuppression that occurs in individuals living with AIDS may allow other viruses, such as the Epstein-Barr virus and the human herpes virus HHV-6, to express as cancer as well. This research, however, demands further study as it is to date somewhat limited and inconclusive.[140]

Herpes Simplex Virus Type 2 (HSV-2)[141]

Herpes simplex virus type 2 or HSV-2 is a member of the herpes family of viruses and is similar to HSV-1, which is a virus known to attack the mucous membranes of the mouth, creating canker sores. HSV-2, however, is a sexually transmitted virus that primarily affects the male and female genitalia. It also is an infection that may be either symptomatic or asymptomatic. Symptomatic means that the infection becomes obvious with an inflammation of the skin and the appearance of tiny clusters of blisters, although this may not take place for many years after the initial infection. Asymptomatic means that the infection continues to live within the individual, but remains hidden without expressing itself in an obvious manner.

Current research indicates that a large proportion of infections from HSV-2 are asymptomatic although one can be tested for HSV-2 antibodies to determine infection. It also is difficult to determine how prevalent HSV-2 is in a given population because these asymptomatic infections go unnoticed by most individuals and members of the medical community. It's estimated, however, that one in five members of a population may be carriers of the virus.

In the 1960s and 1970s certain studies suggested that women exposed to HSV-2 in adolescence were at a greater risk for developing cervical cancer in adulthood. More recently, however, HSV-2 is not considered to be as important a factor in the development of cervical cancer as it once was. Unfortunately, recent research also indicates that HSV-2 may be a factor in the development of other genital cancers among men and women. Again, this association may be easier to understand if we apply our Cancer Blueprint. As HSV-2 attacks the male and female genitalia, it does so on a repetitive basis that may continue for decades. As the tissues continue to be assaulted they may become increasingly weak and vulnerable, eventually succumbing to additional infections and diseases including cancer.

Human Papilloma Virus (HPV)[142]

Unlike HSV-2, the human papilloma virus is a virus that does play a major role in the development of cervical cancer among women. Known as HPV, this virus is one of a family of viruses that includes more than one hundred viral members. Of the one hundred, approximately twenty types of this virus in addition to HPV have been shown to directly infect the female genital area. The remaining types appear to infect the skin, the rectal area, the oral cavity and the larynx, and create warts on various body sites.[143]

Similar to HSV-2, HPV infections are either symptomatic and obvious, or asymptomatic and hidden. As a result, HPV unfortunately may remain undetected in an individual for many years or even decades. So again, it's difficult to determine what percentage of any given population is host to the virus, although estimates range from ten to forty percent based upon the population studied and the method used in the study.

The relationship between HPV and cervical cancer was first recognized by Harold zur Hausen in 1974 and today's studies continue to support this relationship. Women with HPV not only have an increased risk for developing cervical cancer, they have an increased risk for developing its benign relative, cervical intra epithelial neoplasia. Indeed, it's estimated that women who have been diagnosed with HPV may be ten times more likely to develop cervical cancer than women without HPV. It's important to know, however, that the overall incidence rate of HPV is much higher than the incidence rate of cervical cancer in women who have been diagnosed with HPV. This suggests that it's not HPV alone that induces cervical cancer.

More likely, it's the combination of HPV and other factors, known as co-factors, that determines which HPV infected women eventually will develop cervical cancer. These co-factors might include numerous exposures to the virus, infection with HIV, other sexually transmitted diseases or environmental factors such as smoking, diet and the use of certain oral contraceptives.

Hepadnaviruses–Hepatitis B[144]

Hepatitis B is a virus often acquired when one is exposed to contaminated blood. Individuals who have the greatest risk of exposure are intravenous drug users who share contaminated needles and those who have sexual contact with a person who already has Hepatitis B. Individuals who work in the medical profession and those who receive repeated transfusions also may have an increased risk although donor blood testing has greatly reduced the risk in the latter category. And finally, the virus may be passed to a child by an infected mother.

While many individuals exposed to Hepatitis B experience an uncomplicated infection, the virus is associated with liver damage as well as cancer. The cancer in this case is called hepatocellular carcinoma, a leading cause of death the world over. Hepatocellular carcinoma is a primary malignant tumor of the liver. It's a cancer that appears to be more common in populations where the incidence of Hepatitis B is high and more common still in those individuals who don't have an adequate antibody response to the virus. Scientists today continue their efforts to find a vaccine for Hepatitis B to prevent the primary infection and eliminate its related cancer.

Flavaviruses–Hepatitis C[145]

Hepatitis C is similar to Hepatitis B, although the symptoms it produces often are less severe. Hepatitis C is similar in that it also may be acquired by the sharing of needles among intravenous drug users. Similarly, it may be acquired through contaminated blood transfusions or from needles used in tattooing. The initial source of contact, however, often remains undetected. While the Hepatitis B and Hepatitis C viruses have a different nature, both are associated with liver damage and hepatocellular carcinoma. As each attacks the liver, the tissue is damaged and weakened, which once again opens the door for a variety of medical complications, including this rare form of liver cancer.

Epstein-Barr Virus (EBV)

EBV is another herpes virus commonly associated with infectious mononucleosis. Indeed, mononucleosis is often called Epstein-Barr viral infection because it's the Epstein-Barr virus that causes it. Contracted through the saliva of an infectious individual, mononucleosis also is known as the "kissing disease," yet it can be contracted from exposure to an infectious cough or sneeze as well. Mononucleosis is not usually a serious disease, but it can be an extremely debilitating one, causing prolonged weakness and fatigue.[146]

Unfortunately, EBV is a virus that can lead to an increased risk for specific cancers when it's contracted by one already suffering from immunosuppression. EBV has been linked to certain lymphomas, including Burkitt's lymphoma, which was discovered in the 1960s by Sir Dennis Burkitt. In addition, EBV also has been associated with nasopharyngeal cancer and Hodgkin's disease. [147]

It's important to remember, however, that the relationship between EBV and these cancers appears to be an example of an "immunosuppressive process." This means that the virus only has the potential to express itself as a cancer if the individual is already living with HIV or AIDS and her or his immune system is already severely compromised. While science is in the process of developing an EBV vaccine in the hope of preventing these cancers, this area of cancer research is yet another that requires further investigation.

Headline:

Safe Sex Reduces Cancer Risk[148]

Absolutely. The use of condoms during sexual intercourse dramatically decreases one's exposure to sexually transmitted diseases or STDs. STDs, in turn, have been linked to an increased risk for developing some cancers. For example, the human papillomavirus, or HPV, is an STD that has been linked to the development of cervical cancer in women. The human immunodeficiency virus or HIV is an STD that may result in acquired immunodeficiency syndrome or AIDS, both of which have been linked to cancers, including Kaposi's sarcoma and non-Hodgkin's lymphoma. Herpes simplex virus type 2 or HSV-2 is another STD that appears to be linked to the development of genital cancers among both women and men. The practice of safe sex with condoms can reduce one's risk for contracting STDs and, therefore, can reduce one's risk for developing the cancers associated with those STDs.

Chapter 8:
Medical Treatments/Conditions

Alkylating Agents

While anticancer drugs have proved instrumental in treating and prolonging the lives of thousands of cancer patients throughout the world, some patients have developed additional primary cancers as a consequence of the treatment for their first primary cancer. Chemotherapy, for example, is one of the most commonly and successfully used treatments for cancer, yet it isn't without negative side effects, the most serious of which is the possibility it will set the stage for a future cancer while destroying an existing one.

Chemotherapy is the name given to any treatment that attacks infection and disease with chemical agents. Over the centuries, this term has been applied to a number of different therapies; however, today chemotherapy usually refers to the selective use of certain chemicals to destroy cancer cells. There are a number of different chemicals used in chemotherapy and they will vary depending upon the patient and the type of cancer to be targeted. Unfortunately, there is one class of chemical in particular that has often been associated with the patient's development of future cancers. These chemicals are known as "alkylating agents," the most common of which include cyclophosphamide, melphalan and chlorambucil. And while the risk of bladder cancer appears to elevate after treatment with cyclophosphamide, the overall risk for other additional cancers appears to be the greatest with melphalan and chlorambucil.[149]

The alkylating agents work as any other chemical in chemotherapy by injecting foreign molecules into the genetic material of dividing cancer cells. This infusion of foreign material doesn't kill the cancer cell, but rather disrupts its normal functioning and impairs its ability to grow and multiply. Unfortunately, these agents not only attack the cancer cells, they also damage the growth of normal, healthy cells.

This unintended damage predominantly occurs in cells found in the lining of the gastrointestinal tract, hair, nails, blood and other parts of the body where cells happen to be growing when the drugs are given.[150] These body cells are affected because they also are rapidly growing cells and the alkylating agents which target rapidly growing cells cannot distinguish between fast growing cancer cells and fast growing normal cells. Furthermore, the alkylating agents sometimes produce mutations in healthy cells, and it's these mutations that may lead to future cancers.

For example, the risk of developing bone cancer and solid malignant tumors may increase after childhood treatment with alkylating agents. Within the first ten years after such treatment, however, it's the risk of leukemia that predominates, especially acute myelogenous leukemia or AML (also known as acute nonlymphocytic leukemia or ANL), which is a relatively rare form of cancer.

Unfortunately, many cases of this leukemia have been reported in patients who developed it after being treated with alkylating agents for a previous cancer. This ANL is different from spontaneous ANL in that it appears as early as two years following one's initial cancer therapy, peaks around five years after the initial therapy and is brutally resistant to treatment. In addition, it appears that many instances of this leukemia occur in individuals who received these agents during the treatment of childhood cancers.[151]

Moreover, it's estimated that patients who were treated for Hodgkin's disease with a combination of alkylating agents face a risk for developing AML that is 115 times greater than the risk expected in the general population. In these cases, the risk for developing AML plateaus approximately ten years after the treatment, then decreases. Similarly, women who received alkylating agents in chemotherapy for ovarian cancer appear to have a risk for developing AML much greater than the average woman. The risk in these cases appears to peak at about six years after the treatment. This increased risk also was evidenced when these women were compared to women who were treated for the same cancer with surgery alone. None in the latter group developed AML.[152]

The common thread among this particular leukemia risk, however, is that it increases in each case as the amount of alkylating agents used increases. It's a great irony, as this fact reflects the success of primary cancer treatments that allow patients to survive the initial disease and live longer, only to develop additional primary cancers years later. Yet, it's the accumulation of just such information that's essential to clinical trials and researchers as they struggle to decrease the toxicity of cancer treatments while retaining their positive attributes.

Immunosuppressive Drugs

This class of drugs is used to suppress an individual's immune system for a variety of reasons. Three of the most common drugs in this class include azathioprine, cyclosporin A and adrenal corticosteroid hormones. All three are examples of immunosuppressive drugs used primarily in medical cases involving organ transplant patients and work by reducing the body's ability to reject foreign agents and materials. When a patient receives a donor organ, the organ is identified by the patient's body as an invading and potentially harmful agent. As such, the body's natural immune system will attempt to reject the organ. With the aid of immunosuppressive drugs, however, this natural tendency is inhibited, and the transplant procedure is given more time and opportunity to succeed. While the most common use of these drugs is found among transplant patients, they also are used to treat several autoimmune diseases including rheumatoid arthritis.[153]

Unfortunately, when these drugs suppress the immune system the body's ability to fight genuine harmful agents also is compromised. As a result, an individual becomes susceptible to harm that may increase the person's risk for developing a number of infections and diseases. For example, transplant patients who have been treated aggressively with immunosuppressants share a risk of developing non-Hodgkin's lymphoma fifty times greater than the average individual's risk. This lymphoma usually will develop within one to two years after the transplant operation and is usually found in the brain tissue, a rare site for this particular type of cancer.[154]

Transplant patients also appear to be at greater risk for developing soft tissue skin cancers such as Kaposi's sarcoma as well as melanoma. In fact, about thirty-five to seventy percent of organ transplant patients develop skin cancer within twenty years of the transplant surgery.[155] While several factors contribute to the development of any cancer, the amount and duration of the immunosuppressant treatment in transplant patients appears to be directly linked to the risk for developing future skin cancers. If the transplant patient is treated sparingly with immunosuppressants, the increased risk of developing non-Hodgkin's lymphoma is only about ten times greater than the average.

Apparently, therefore, the risk of developing this cancer also is directly related to the amount and duration of the immunosuppressant treatment. Clearly, ongoing research again is necessary to find a balance in which the beneficial use of such drugs is increased as the potentially harmful effects are decreased.

Radioactive Drugs

The use of radioactive drugs is important when medical professionals want to locate and observe the drug as it travels through a biological, chemical or physical process in a patient's body. This process is made possible because these drugs contain a molecule that has been "tagged" or combined with a radioactive element. Because this element, also called an isotope, is radioactive, it can be seen by various diagnostic tests. These tests measure the amount or level of radioactivity, and the information is then documented by a technician and used to improve treatment.[156]

Indeed, radioactive drugs have been used to treat a number of different cancers, including cancer of the thyroid. They also have been used successfully in the treatment of tuberculosis of the bone which can invade the spinal disks, causing collapse and a rare blood disorder called polycythemia vera. These drugs, however, can become concentrated in the body tissues, causing unintended radiation damage. So, while these drugs are beneficial in many ways, they too have been linked to the development of several diseases, including the bone cancer osteogenic sarcoma, leukemia and a rare form of liver cancer.[157]

Tamoxifen

Similarly, there are individual drugs that provide protection from some forms of cancer only to increase one's risk for others. This appears to be the case with Tamoxifen, a non-steroidal drug used to treat breast cancer in women. Women taking this drug share a greatly reduced risk for developing an additional primary breast cancer when compared to women breast cancer patients who aren't treated with the drug. Unfortunately, women treated with Tamoxifen appear to have an increased risk of developing cancer of the uterine lining or endometrial cancer.[158]

This occurs because Tamoxifen has a different hormonal effect upon different parts of the body. Apparently, in the uterus Tamoxifen acts as an estrogen, which as we know is a hormone, linked to a number of cancers including that of the uterus. In contrast, Tamoxifen acts as an anti-estrogen in the breast, offering protection for these tissues and lessening the chance of future breast cancers.[159]

New drugs called **aromatase inhibitors,** or **third generation aromatase inhibitors**, however, are now being offered as an alternative to Tamoxifen for postmenopausal breast cancer patients as they produce less dangerous side effects.[160] They appear to reduce the recurrence of breast cancer and the cancer's ability to spread. They also carry less risk for the development of future cancers of the uterus.

Unfortunately, these inhibitors increase the risk for bone loss and subsequent fractures as well as possible heart conditions. A third option, however, is an estrogen substitute, which is neither an estrogen nor a hormone and is known as a **selective estrogen receptor modulator** or **SERM**. SERMs are compounds that behave like estrogens in some tissues and like anti-estrogens in other tissues. Among these is a drug known as Raloxifene. Marketed as Evista, this particular product is prescribed primarily to prevent bone loss and osteoporosis in post-menopausal women. Raloxifene, however, also has been found to be as effective as Tamoxifen in preventing invasive breast cancer in high-risk women yet, unlike Tamoxifen, it doesn't appear to negatively affect the uterus.[161]

No drug, however, is without side effects, and the most serious of these associated with the use of Raloxifene is the development of blood clots in the veins. So, while the benefits of Raloxifene balanced against its risks may be preferable to Tamoxifen for many women, choosing the appropriate drug ultimately will be a personal choice that depends entirely upon a woman's personal health, medical history and individualized professional counseling.

Additional Concerns

Chlornaphazine[162]

Chlornaphazine is a drug used in the 1950s and early 1960s in treatments for a variety of medical conditions. It was used, as were the radioactive drugs, to treat the blood disorder polycythemia vera as well as Hodgkin's lymphoma. Unfortunately, chlornaphazine is related to a chemical called beta-naphythlamine, a substance linked to bladder cancer in a number of workplace environments, including the dye industry. When chlornaphazine also was found to cause bladder cancer, its use in medical treatments was discontinued and it was taken off the market.

Coal Tar Ointments[163]

As their name indicates, these ointments are derived from coal tar and, as a result, their use has come under increasing suspicion. These ointments contain polycyclic hydrocarbons, which are the byproducts of fossil fuel combustion and known carcinogens. There is specu-lation, therefore, that the topical use of ointments derived from these hydrocarbons also contains carcinogens that can be linked to an increased risk for skin cancers. The ointments, primarily used to treat chronic skin conditions such as eczema and psoriasis, have always been known as potential skin irritants. New research, however, indicates that psoriasis pa-tients who have been treated with high doses of coal tar ointment do appear to share an increased risk for developing future skin cancers.

This finding is better understood if we apply our Cancer Blueprint, which states that tissue subjected to constant or severe irritation may become more susceptible to infection and disease. In this case, the patient's skin tissue has been affected by the skin disorder psoriasis. The skin is then treated by a substance that appears to contain known carcino-gens. If we then consider additional layers of risk, such as sun exposure, it becomes easier to understand why this skin tissue may be at greater risk for developing future skin cancers. This result would simply reflect an accumulation of conditions that may leave the skin more vulnerable to a number of diseases including cancer.

Inorganic Arsenics[164]

Arsenic has been used for centuries as a therapeutic agent as well as a poison, and it contin-ues to have limited use in treating a number of skin disorders. Inorganic arsenic is a syntheti-cally produced agent that contains the properties of organic or natural arsenic. Although drugs containing these inorganic arsenics have been used in various treatments in the past, their use was discontinued when evidence suggested their use was linked to the develop-ment of skin cancers. These cancers usually appeared on exposed body parts, in unusual locations and in multiple sites. They also were associated with conditions such as arsenical pigmentation, a pigment differentiation caused by arsenic, and hyperkeratosis, a hardening of the skin seen commonly in corns and calluses.

Phenacetin[165]

Phenacetin is an analgesic used to treat pain in a number of medical situations. Analgesics, or "pain killers," relieve pain by acting upon the central nervous system and altering one's perception. While phenacetin was used successfully in this regard for many years, its use was discontinued when it was linked to an increased risk for developing kidney cancer.

Methoxysporalens[166]

Photochemotherapy, or PUVA, is a treatment that combines methoxysporalens with ultra-violet A exposure. First, photochemotherapy, or photodynamic therapy, is a form of chemo-therapy that exposes the patient to ultraviolet A light in an effort to enhance the effect of the chemotherapy drugs being administered. Second, methoxysporalens are substances used topically to treat skin disorders involving irregular pigmentation or lack of pigmentation. When these topical substances are applied in combination with ultraviolet A light exposure, it's believed the chemotherapy drugs have a greater effect. This regimen, which is sometimes used in the treatment of severe psoriasis, unfortunately also has been linked to the development of future skin cancers.

Thiazide Diuretics[167]

The entire field of interpreting drug and cancer relationships, however, remains problematic because it's difficult to show that a cancer is "caused" by the drug and not by the condition for which the drug is prescribed. For example, thiazide diuretics have long been prescribed for high blood pressure. Evidence now suggests that patients using thiazide diuretics for high blood pressure have an increased risk of developing cancers of the kidney. Yet, it isn't clear if the drug is at fault or if the fault lies in the long-term consequences of high blood pressure. Because high blood pressure is one of the most common ailments around the world, and because this condition is often treated with thiazide diuretics, it's essential to conduct more research to reach a clear conclusion.

Protective Drugs[168]

On the other hand, there are some drugs that may actually offer protection from a number of different cancers. Surprisingly, these drugs are commonplace products that include aspirin, ibuprofen and other nonsteroidal anti-inflammatory drugs. Known as NSAIDs, these drugs appear to lower the risk for colon and breast cancer and will be discussed later in greater detail.

Ionizing Radiation

Ionizing radiation is considered a significant risk factor for cancer and is one of the most extensively researched human carcinogens within our layers of risk.[169] Exposure to this type of radiation occurs through a variety of sources, including x-rays and fluoroscopy, radiation therapy, natural sources such as cosmic rays in the atmosphere, radioactive materials in the earth's crust and products that contain radium.

The term "ionization" is defined as the process in which an atom or molecule gains or loses electrons. In therapy, radiation refers to the emission of radioactive energy, rays or waves used in the diagnosis or treatment of disease. Ionizing radiation, therefore, is particularly potent because it, too, like solar radiation, has the ability to actually change the molecular structure of a cell. Accordingly, the cells in living organisms affected by this process may have their growth retarded, their structure mutated or may be destroyed entirely.[170]

Although this effect is desired in certain circumstances, such as medical treatments, it also is these cellular changes that appear to cause cancer. For the most basic building block of living tissue, deoxyribonucleic acid, or DNA, which is contained in the nucleus of every cell, is susceptible to damage from ionizing radiation.

To understand radiation exposure, it's helpful to understand how radiation is measured. First, radiation is measured in units that are called "Grays." This unit, which is abbreviated as "Gy," measures the amount of radiation energy absorbed by a particular body tissue. The danger of radiation exposure depends upon the amount of Gys that are absorbed and the length of time over which the exposure occurs. For example, an exposure that measures in the tens of grays may be fatal if it's received at one time, whereas the same high dose of radiation spread over time may be far less harmful.[171]

Similarly, a single 5Gy dose of radiation received at one time over the entire human body typically would cause death in approximately fifty percent of individuals within thirty days. Yet, patients who receive daily radiation medical treatments of 2Gy to a small part of their body can continue to absorb tens of grays over several weeks without a fatal risk. In comparison, medical x-rays involve a radiation level of less than .25Gy, an exposure so small it's difficult to measure any harmful effect. Radiation from the earth's crust and other natural sources called "background" radiation only measures about 1 to 2 mGy - or 1 to 2 thousandths of a gray per year.[172]

Much of today's knowledge about the dangers of radiation exposure was gained through studies of former patients who were treated with radiation therapy. Before the 1920s, for example, when the dangers of radiation were unknown, radiologists who used x-rays extensively usually did so without protective shielding. As a result, there was an excessively high rate of leukemia among this group of individuals in the early twentieth century. Similarly, prior to 1954 a spinal disorder called "ankylosing spondylitis" was commonly treated with radiation therapy. These patients, however, later developed more cancers, including leukemia, than one would expect in a healthy population.[173]

In addition, an x-ray procedure called "fluoroscopy" was used between 1935 and 1954 to monitor patients with tuberculosis. The female patients who underwent this procedure received an average radiation dose of 1Gy to the breast area, yet they shared a high incidence of breast cancer that occurred between ten and fifteen years after the fluoroscopy was administered.[174]

Similarly, children who were treated with radiation therapy for a number of noncancerous conditions, especially those of the head and neck, experienced a high risk for developing a number of different cancers. For example, prior to the 1950s children treated for enlarged thymus glands with high doses of radiation experienced an elevated risk for developing thyroid cancer and leukemia later in life. During this time, children who were treated for ringworm with radiation therapy appear to share this elevated risk for thyroid cancer and leukemia as well.[175]

Such evidence suggests that exposure to radiation therapy during childhood may be especially damaging because the cells of the body at this stage of development are growing rapidly and appear to be more sensitive and susceptible to harm than the slower growing cells of adulthood. As a precaution, therefore, it's recommended that individuals who underwent radiation therapy for thymus conditions, enlarged tonsils or scalp ringworm while a child consult with their physician to determine their own extent for possible harm.[176]

The study of occupations and historical events throughout the twentieth century also has provided a great deal of information about the harmful effects of radiation. One particularly interesting and classic study was conducted among women employees who painted radium dials during the early part of the century. Radium is a radioactive metallic element often used in the production of durable goods as well as medical devices. It also was used to make clock dials because it provided a shine or an illuminated surface easy to see. Women who were employed in this occupation, however, were found to exhibit high rates of bone sarcomas and head cancers.

During the investigation, it was discovered that these women were unintentionally swallowing large amounts of radioactive radium because it was their practice to lick the ends of their paintbrushes to make fine tips. As a result of this habit, it's believed that each woman received an average dose of 17Gy of radiation in her bone tissue over the course of her employment, an amount exceedingly high even for long-time employees whose exposure occurred over an extended period of time.[177]

In terms of historical events, one of the most crucial in providing information on the effects of radiation was, of course, the use of atomic power during World War II and the effect it had on its Japanese survivors. The lasting harm created by such an exposure is exhibited in many of these survivors who have shown increased rates of leukemia and several other cancers, including those of the breast, thyroid, lung and stomach.

It also was found that women who were exposed to and survived this single blast of radiation run the same risk for breast cancer as the previously mentioned women who were treated with repeated fluoroscopy exposures for tuberculosis. This finding is particularly important because it suggests that in the case of breast cancer, especially in younger women, small doses of radiation repeated over several years may be as harmful as one large, single dose.[178]

Radiation exposure before birth is another issue that raises many questions. While there is some evidence that suggests that low level fetal exposure is linked to the development of childhood cancers, including leukemia, not all researchers agree with this finding. Indeed, studies conducted among the same group of Japanese atomic blast survivors indicated that individuals exposed prenatally while in their mother's wombs don't appear to experience a higher than average rate for cancer. To be safe, however, when diagnosing pregnant women today the standard practice is to use ultrasound in place of x-rays whenever possible.[179]

Of course, other exposures to radiation include the testing of nuclear weapons, which produces radioactive fallout that can create a hazardous environment for all living organisms. This fallout, which is composed of airborne particles of radioactive material, settles to the ground and may remain "active" for many years. Any individual exposed to high levels of such fallout will undoubtedly exhibit an increased risk for several cancers, including that of the thyroid.[180]

In addition, there are many naturally produced radioactive elements that can be harmful to living organisms. Once again, one of these is radon, the gas produced by the natural decay of radioactive uranium. This particular area of study is a good example of research that began as an occupational study and expanded into a broad statement of fact concerning the environment in general. Research began when uranium miners were found to experience unusually high rates of lung and other respiratory cancers. These individuals, of course, worked underground in uranium mines where they inhaled the radioactive radon gas produced by the uranium they were mining.[181]

This connection between occupational radon gas exposure and high cancer levels was the first evidence implicating radon as an environmental hazard in general. Radon remains a great public concern today because of its presence in so many man-made products, such as building materials and so many natural sources such as groundwater. In fact, the danger from radon is so great that some studies estimate ten percent of all lung cancer deaths alone may be the result of exposure to radon gas in the environment. Similar to cigarette smoking, radon remains one of the most universally recognized carcinogens in research today.[182]

Ionizing radiation exposure in humans appears to present the most harm to the breast, thyroid and bone marrow of the human body. Cancers of these areas may not appear until ten to fifteen years after the radiation exposure. Leukemia, however, may develop as early as two years after the initial exposure. Yet, while radiation exists in many harmful forms in our environment, it also exists in many helpful forms in a variety of medical procedures.[183]

One of these procedures, for example, is mammography, which utilizes a low dose x-ray to detect breast cancer in women. While this procedure exposes women to radiation, its benefits, especially in women over the age of fifty, greatly outweigh the small risk of harm resulting from a mammogram. X-rays also are routine in medical exams, dental visits, cancer treatments and a variety of diagnostic procedures. It's important, therefore, to be informed, to exercise common sense and always weigh the small risk of such procedures against the enormous benefit they bestow.

Hormones

Estrogen and Progesterone

The role of hormones and the risk for certain cancers is another extremely complex area, especially for women. Hormones, of course, are naturally produced compounds that help regulate the functions of specific body organs or tissue. For females, the two dominant hormones are estrogen and progesterone, both of which are produced primarily in the ovaries. Estrogen promotes the development of the feminine physical characteristics, while estrogen and progesterone together regulate the menstrual cycle and pregnancy.

Hormones can be either naturally or synthetically produced and are used as drugs in a variety of ways. One of these is a program known as **hormone replacement therapy,** or **HRT**.[184] This therapy usually occurs when a woman's ovarian function decreases and she begins to experience some of the symptoms of menopause, including hot flashes, vaginal discomfort and emotional unrest. HRT also was believed to protect the tissues of the heart in menopausal and post-menopausal women although additional studies on this issue are inconclusive. Finally, HRT is used to combat and prevent bone loss that can result in osteoporosis.[185]

Estrogen, rather than progesterone, is the hormone usually prescribed for women undergoing HRT. Indeed, from 1962 to 1975 the use of estrogens by menopausal and pre-menopausal women in the United States alone increased four times. This "unopposed" estrogen use was, however, followed by an unfortunate increase in the number of American women diagnosed with cancer of the uterine lining or endometrial cancer. Because of this increase, the use of progesterone or its derivatives called progestins gained recognition in the early 1980s as a way of "opposing" or offsetting the increased risk of endometrial cancer due to estrogen use alone.[186]

Today, it's common to prescribe the use of progestins, the most common of which is Provera, for a period of time during the monthly cycle for women who also use estrogen in HRT. And while the addition of progestins to estrogen in HRT is proving to be beneficial in reducing the risk of this cancer, the optimum amount and proper balance of each has yet to be determined.[187]

The risk of developing breast cancer also is a concern among women who have under-gone HRT or whose estrogen exposure has occurred over long periods of time or in high doses. Studies on this subject, however, are contradictory, with some results suggesting breast cancer risk is increased with estrogen use and others suggesting it's not. This research is more con-clusive in that it indicates that menopausal estrogen use doesn't appear to increase a woman's risk for ovarian cancer.[188] Again, research will continue to answer these questions more accu-rately, although past study appears to support the existence of an increased protection from these cancers for women who have used estrogen in combination with progestins.[189]

It's important to note that most of the estrogens used in hormone replacement therapy are natural while the estrogens used in oral contraceptives are pharmaceutically produced syn-thetic estrogens. Further, there are two basic programs of oral contraceptive use. In the first, estrogen is taken alone for the first fourteen to sixteen days of a woman's monthly cycle, then followed by an estrogen-progestin combination during the last five or six days of her cycle. Not surprisingly, this program has been associated with an increased risk of endometrial cancer.[190]

In contrast, the second program, which is the most effective and most commonly used oral contraceptive, is called the "combination" program. This method of birth control in-cludes twenty-one pills, each of which contains a fixed amount of estrogen and progestin. One pill is taken each day for twenty-one days, then a placebo, which has no hormonal value, is taken for seven days. At the end of the twenty-eight days, the cycle is begun again. The use of this combination program has actually been shown to reduce the risk of certain cancers for participating women.[191]

Indeed, research has uniformly indicated that there's a risk reduction of forty to fifty percent for ovarian and endometrial cancers in women who used the combination program at some time in their reproductive history. This same research indicates that the longer a woman uses the combination program, the more her risk is reduced. Moreover, this protective effect ap-pears to last for at least ten to twenty years after a woman discontinues use of the program.[192]

The greatest concern among women who use oral contraceptives is once again the possibility of increasing their chances of developing breast cancer. This concern, however, hasn't been substantiated. This doesn't mean that breast cancer risk is not increased; it just means that the relationship hasn't been conclusively established. On the one hand, some studies have found that oral contraceptive use does not increase the risk of breast cancer in most women. On the other, many studies do indicate that long-term use of oral contraceptives beginning at an early age increases the risk for women under the age of forty-five. There remains the possibility that oral contraceptive use is linked to an increased risk for cervical and liver cancer as well. The evidence supporting this link, however, is difficult to establish and also requires further investigation.[193]

Depot-Medroxyprogesterone Acetate[194]

Depot-medroxyprogesterone acetate, or DMPA, is a long acting progesterone-based contraceptive that's injected rather than taken orally. It's been approved for use in over ninety countries, including the United States, although its approval was delayed in the United States because of concerns that it might increase the risk of breast cancer in women. Limited studies, however, suggest there is no increased risk of breast cancer among women using the drug unless those women already have tumors, in which case the drug may accelerate the growth of those pre-existing tumors.

Granted, research focusing on this hormone-based drug is limited, but to date there appears to be no association with DMPA and a woman's risk for cervical, ovarian or liver cancer. Furthermore, in addition to its apparent benign nature in regard to the above cancers, DMPA may actually provide protection from the development of endometrial cancer.

Diethystilbestrol[195]

Diethylstilbestrol or DES is a synthetic chemical, which possesses properties similar to estrogen. It has been linked to an increased risk for certain cancers in both women and men. During the late 1940s and into the 1950s, women used DES to prevent miscarriage and late complications in pregnancy. When studies in the 1950s, however, failed to report any significant beneficial effect of DES, its use was gradually reduced.

It wasn't until 1971 that young women who where exposed "in utero" to DES while in their mother's womb began to develop a rare form of vaginal cancer called "clear-cell adenocarcinoma." This same group of women also began to develop a rare clear-cell adenocarcinoma of the cervix. In fact, numerous studies have indicated that a woman who has been exposed to DES while in utero has one chance in one thousand of developing either of the above cancers by the age of thirty-four. There is no substantial evidence, however, that DES increases the risk of other types of vaginal or cervical cancers.

In addition, there have been a few studies conducted among women who were treated directly with DES to prevent miscarriage. Although the research among these individuals is limited, it appears at this time that the risk for breast and other types of cancers among DES women is no greater than the risk among women who were not treated with DES. These results, however, aren't based on extensive investigation and it's apparent that further research on this group of women is also necessary to establish clear conclusions.

Unfortunately, the complications of DES are not limited to only women. Evidence shows that males who were exposed to DES in utero may develop more anomalies of the reproductive organs than males who were not exposed. One of these anomalies is the failure of the testes to descend into the scrotum, a condition that appears to increase the risk of testicular cancer. Indeed, many studies indicate that a high proportion of males with testicular cancer were exposed to DES while in utero.

Androgens[196]

Natural male androgens such as testosterone are the hormones responsible for the development of masculine physical characteristics. There is evidence, however, that an imbalance in the level of male hormones due to internal or external factors is related to a man's risk for developing prostate cancer. Indeed, a strong component of prostate cancer treatment involves the manipulation of male hormones to restore proper balance and fight an invading cancer.

There are particular concerns today about **testosterone replacement therapy,** or **TRT,** which is used increasingly in men to treat a variety of symptoms that collectively are being called **andropause** or **male menopause.**[197] These symptoms typically arise in older men and include fatigue, depression, inability to concentrate and a decrease in libido. While some medical specialists believe TRT to be helpful in alleviating such male complaints, others believe the benefit may be slight and worry that the therapy may lead to more severe problems in the future.

Those who have concerns about TRT compare it to Hormone Replacement Therapy for women. We know that HRT was used for years as a way to combat female age-related discomfort and disease before possible harm from its use was suspected. While proponents of TRT agree that its benefit greatly outweighs its risk, others fear that TRT is a risky experiment. Testosterone is related to prostate cancer in that it appears to increase the development of prostate tumors. Critics believe that TRT may stimulate the growth of small existing cancers and may aggravate microscopic prostate tumors in many older men that might otherwise not be harmful.

If this is the case, TRT also may present the possibility of greater harm for men who already have an increased risk for developing prostate cancer. Again, in the absence of long-term study, the use of TRT is a topic that should be discussed carefully with one's physician to evaluate its potential for benefit or harm on an individual basis.

Similarly, synthetically produced androgens function in a variety of ways that may either promote good health or compromise it. For instance, synthetic androgens can be used to treat a number of medical conditions including anemias, endocrine imbalances and general weakness and fatigue. Another class of steroids known as **anabolic-androgenic steroids** also may be used in medical situations to treat a variety of health-related conditions. "Anabolic" refers to muscle building and "androgenic" refers to an increase in masculine characteristics.[198]

As such, these particular steroids are often used with patients who suffer from body wasting and the loss of lean muscle tissue from diseases such as AIDS. This latter class of steroids, however, also is misused by some athletes and body builders to gain strength, enhance performance and develop an improved masculine physique. Unfortunately, when abused in this way, these substances can compromise one's immune system and increase one's risk for developing high blood pressure, jaundice, severe acne, kidney and liver tumors, as well as liver cancer.[199]

Chapter 9:
Lifestyle

Occupation

Clearly, there are numerous environmental hazards that are related to the development of different cancers, many of which are found in the workplace. Individuals are often at greater risk from workplace hazards because the exposure during working hours is usually longer and more intense than other everyday exposures. As a result, the potential harm of certain elements and chemicals often is scrutinized first in workplace environment where data may be easier to obtain. It's this workplace research, therefore, that often spearheads research into the harmful environmental hazards for general populations. Indeed, many of today's well known environmental carcinogens were identified first through studies conducted on workers and the workplace such as those conducted among uranium miners.[200]

One of the earliest of these studies was conducted in 1775 when London surgeon Percivall Pott reported a high level of scrotal cancer known as "soot-wart" among chimney sweeps in London. At that time, young men and boys were used to "sweep" because they were small, and when their clothing was removed, they were able to crawl naked through the narrow chimneys of London and remove the soot. As they cleaned, however, they came in direct contact with a number of chemicals that today are known carcinogens. This is believed to be the first evidence of the topical danger of certain chemicals. It appeared that the mere act of touching certain compounds was in itself sufficient to cause disease as the chemicals were soaked into the skin and absorbed by the tissues.[201]

A century later, similar cancers were reported by other scientists who were studying workers in the gas plants of Germany and the oil shale fields of Scotland. At about this same time, other studies confirmed that compounds of tar, soot and the oils known today as polycyclic aromatic hydrocarbons caused cancer in laboratory animals. When all of this information was combined, scientists realized that the compounds that caused cancer in animals in the second study were the same agents responsible for the cancers found among workers in the first study. This new information also helped explain the cause of "soot wart" that was so prevalent a century earlier among the English chimney sweeps of London.

The combination of this new evidence and the continued concern generated by Dr. Pott's initial 1775 publication prompted the chimney sweeps' guild of Denmark to take preventative action by issuing a personal hygiene guideline that urged guild members to take daily baths. Indeed, the British Medical Journal of 1892 published the report "Why Foreign Sweeps Do Not Suffer From Scrotal Cancer" which stated that the sweeps of northern Europe who followed the guideline appeared to benefit, while the English sweeps who ignored the guideline continued to experience high rates of scrotal cancer.[202]

It was these centuries' old studies that became the model for today's research investigating workplace environments and possible carcinogens. Modern day research, which follows the same steps, includes: 1) the observation of unusual cancers or a high incidence of common cancers among groups of workers; 2) searching for and profiling the responsible agents; 3) confirming these agents also cause cancer in laboratory animals and; 4) the introduction and implementation of preventative programs.[203]

Today, the following of this formula has identified several workplace hazards. One of the most significant findings, of course, is the evidence linking asbestos with lung and other respiratory cancers. Indeed, in the United States extremely high rates for lung cancer along the southeast Atlantic coast have been linked to asbestos exposure in shipyards that employed thousands of workers during World War II.[204]

Similarly, high rates of bladder cancer among men living in the northeast and the Great Lakes region have been attributed to industrial chemical and petrochemical exposures. Hazards that increase cancer risk also have been found among truck drivers exposed to motor exhausts and farmers exposed to herbicides. In addition, such research has identified many other harmful agents, including metals such as chromium, nickel, arsenic and cadmium. Harmful solvents such as benzene and methylene chloride, which is found in waxes, film, plastics as well as propellant hair sprays, deodorants and air fresheners, have been identified.[205]

So, too, have a variety of "probable human carcinogens" such as perchlorothylene and trichlorothylene which are chemicals often found in paint and spot removers, dry cleaning solutions, wood cleaners and adhesives. This is important research that's instrumental in the overall effort to uncover the causes of human cancer. For not only does it strive to create safe workplaces, it also increases a society's ability to identify those carcinogenic and possible carcinogenic environmental agents that threaten the general population as well.[206]

Diet

In the developed regions of the world where a variety of foods are typically abundant, diet is one of the easiest cancer risk factors to control. Most people are now aware that diets low in fat, high in fruits, vegetables, fiber and grains appear to reduce the risk for many cancers. What many may not be aware of is that science estimates improper diets may be responsible for a staggering thirty-five percent of all cancer deaths.

Fat

First, the most conclusive studies pertaining to diet and cancer risk appear to be those that examine the role of dietary fat. To begin, diets high in fat have been linked to several cancers including those of the breast, colon, prostate and possibly pancreas, ovary and endometrium.

Several studies have been conducted both among the populations of countries where low fat diets are standard and among the populations of countries who consume diets high in fat. When compared, the incidence and mortality rates for breast, colorectal and prostate cancer were consistently higher in the latter. Yet, it appears that some of these cancers are influenced by one's total fat intake while others are influenced by the specific type of fat consumed.[207]

First, fats are classified according to the structure of their building blocks, which are known as "fatty acids." All fatty acids are molecules composed primarily of carbon and hydrogen atoms. Fatty acids also are either saturated or unsaturated, and break down into three basic categories of saturated fat, monounsaturated fat and polyunsaturated fat. The number of "bonds" that join the carbon atoms in the hydrocarbon chain determines the category into which each fat belongs. For example, saturated fat is characterized by single bonds in that it has the maximum possible number of hydrogen atoms attached to every carbon atom. Thus, it is said to be "saturated" with hydrogen atoms.[208]

In contrast, monounsaturated fat is characterized by one double or triple bond per molecule because it's missing one pair of hydrogen atoms in the middle. Polyunsaturated fat is characterized by more than one double or triple bond per molecule because more than one pair of hydrogen atoms is missing. Saturated fat is usually solid at room temperature and is the most difficult fat for the body to break down. It's found mostly in animal fats, such as red meat, whole milk products, butter, cheese and some plant materials including cocoa butter and coconut oil. The second most difficult fat to digest is the monounsaturated fat found in poultry, many nuts and olive oil. The third and easiest to digest is polyunsaturated fat, found commonly in foods such as fish, corn, walnuts, soybeans and sunflower or safflower seeds.[209]

Of course, no discussion of fat would be complete without mentioning trans fat. Also known as "partially hydrogenated oil," this type of fat has received a lot of press in the last few years. It's a type of unsaturated fat that can be either monounsaturated or polyunsaturated. The result of a process called "hydrogenation," trans fat is made when manufacturers add hydrogen to vegetable oil to increase the product's shelf life.[210] While breast and colorectal cancer appear to be linked to one's total fat intake for most individuals, postmenopausal women appear to have a positive correlation between their risk for breast cancer and their intake of saturated fat in particular.[211]

Furthermore, these same women appear to have an increased risk for colon cancer when their total intake of saturated and monounsaturated fat is increased.[212] While one's daily caloric intake of fat, regardless of type, only requires thirty percent to provide the essential fatty acids or EFAs needed for physiological well being and energy, the average person typically attributes nearly thirty-seven percent of her or his caloric intake to fat. This excess, of course, results from the intake of several sources of fat common in many diets, including the added fats and oils used as spreads, dressings, sauces, cooking fats, salad oils, whole dairy products and meats.[213]

This is a tricky field, however, because fat intake has a positive correlation with caloric intake.[214] Again, this means that as the amount of fat in one's diet increases, the amount of calories consumed also increases. So, the question we need to ask is whether it's really the overall fat one consumes that contributes to an increased cancer risk, or is it the number of calories one consumes that's responsible?

It's well documented that individuals with a greater body weight put themselves at a greater risk for certain cancers. If we take a moment to analyze this, we need to know that in any diet, fat has the most concentrated source of energy of all the nutrients.[215] Along with this concentrated energy, however, comes nine calories per gram of fat. This is substantial when compared to the four calories per gram from either carbohydrates or protein. As a result, a decrease in fat intake is always accompanied by a decrease in caloric intake, and this results in a loss of body weight. So, even if one states that calories are the responsible factor for increased cancer risk, those calories are mostly contributed by fat. Therefore, a decrease in one, be it fat or calories, logically means a decrease in the other, and either way, a decrease in cancer risk is the end result.

Fiber

The protective benefits of a diet high in fiber have been loudly applauded. Fiber is defined as those food plants that are resistant to the enzymes produced by the human digestive tract. In fact, there are two different categories of fiber, those that are water soluble and those that are water insoluble.[216] The former refers to foods that are easily dissolved in water and the latter, of course, refers to those foods that cannot be dissolved in water. The important characteristic of all fiber is that it cannot be dissolved or absorbed easily by the body and, as a result, it's forced through the intestinal tract through the process of digestion. Because it's eliminated quickly from the body, it helps maintain regularity and helps keep the colon free of harmful material or bacterial buildups.

As a result, fiber clearly appears to reduce the risk of colon cancer by maintaining a healthy intestinal tract, yet fiber also may reduce the risk for other cancers as well, including those of the breast, mouth and stomach. It must be acknowledged, however, that high fiber foods also contain a variety of nutrients that may be the trigger for this risk reduction rather than the fiber. Similarly, high fiber foods also contain less fat, a fact that may be the key to the risk reduction. It may not be the fiber itself, therefore, which is the important protective element when discussing cancer risk reduction, but rather one of these other factors or a combination thereof.[217]

Fruits and Veggies

Similarly, the role of fruits and vegetables in the reduction of cancer risk has come under close scrutiny. It has been found that populations in countries that consume diets high in fruits and vegetables do tend to have a reduced risk of certain cancers.[218] These foods, in addition to being high in fiber, also contain nutrients such as vitamin C, vitamin A and carotenoids. Consumption of these foods appears to provide protection from cancer of the lung, colon and rectum, breast, oral cavity, esophagus, stomach, pancreas, uterine cervix and ovary. Conversely, the risk for these cancers, especially those of the respiratory and digestive tracts, doubles for individuals with a low fruit and vegetable intake.[219] Again, whether it's the fiber in these foods or the nutrients that are responsible for the risk decrease remains uncertain.

To begin, vitamin C is probably the most familiar and well-studied nutrient and is commonly found in citrus fruits and juices as well as green vegetables. It's believed that vitamin C offers significant protection from disease and cancer for the esophagus, oral cavity, stomach, pancreas, rectum and cervix. Indeed, studies also report that vitamin C offers protection from breast and lung cancer as well. In addition, carotenoids have been found to reduce the risk for some cancers, including lung cancer, where the protective effect has even been found to extend to cigarette smokers.[220]

Carotenoids are the orange, yellow and red unsaturated pigments found in foods such as carrots, sweet potatoes and cantaloupe and in dark green leafy vegetables such as broccoli, spinach, Swiss chard and collard greens. These carotenoids are important because they also include beta-carotene, alpha-carotene and lutein. Beta-carotene and alpha-carotene are "provitamins" that are converted into vitamin A within the body, as is lutein. It's believed that five servings of these foods each day is sufficient to trigger their protective effect against disease and certain cancers.[221]

Many of these nutrients are known also as antioxidants, which are agents that appear to help protect body cells from harmful oxidation and neutralize the effects of free radicals. Of all the antioxidants, the best known are probably vitamins C and E, and beta-carotene. The protective effect of these antioxidants, however, is a subject not fully understood and requires clarification. It isn't clear, for example, which antioxidants offer the most protection or how much of the antioxidant is needed to trigger the protective effect.[222]

It also isn't clear if antioxidants are helpful by themselves or if they must be combined with other antioxidants or nutrients to provide protection. All we know is that five or six of the above foods should be consumed on a daily basis, and these servings should reflect a variety of the recommended foods to gain maximum benefit. This is the current guideline for all individuals who actively desire to reduce their risk for developing virtually all cancers.

Finding these guidelines somewhat difficult to maintain, however, many individuals rely upon supplements to achieve these dietary goals. Unfortunately, the use of antioxidant supplements is a practice that may not be as beneficial as one might think. First, evidence supporting the theory that such supplements lower one's risk for chronic disease is preliminary and has not yet been "proven" in clinical trials. Second, researchers don't know if some antioxidants offer greater protection than others, or if their protective effect is the result of a combination of several antioxidants, or how much of each antioxidant is required on a daily basis to gain benefit. Third, the protective effect of antioxidants may not even be triggered unless they're combined with the other nutrients found in recommended foods.

Finally, research has not yet clarified what risks may be associated with the long-term use of dietary antioxidant supplements. For although vitamins C, E and beta-carotene are not generally toxic, studies with individuals regarding antioxidant supplemental use usually last less than six months. As a result, there is no clear evidence that long-term use and especially excessive long-term use in which large amounts of these supplements are consumed is risk-free over one's lifetime.[223]

It's important to remember that these products are called supplements–not substitutes. It may be advisable, therefore, to adhere to the current dietary guidelines for consuming the proper foods as much as possible. With the exception of an effective multivitamin, especially a calcium-packed one for women, such products should be used in moderation and only to supplement a healthy, balanced diet.

The high fiber foods of vegetables and fruits as well as grains also contain numerous other vitamins and minerals associated with their apparent protective effect. For example, vitamin E appears to reduce the risk of certain cancers, including those of the mouth and stomach. Selenium also appears to reduce the risk for some cancers. In fact, studies conducted in China among populations chronically deficient in a number of nutrients confirm that individuals who received daily supplements of beta-carotene, vitamin E and selenium over a period of five years had a significantly lower cancer-related death rate.[224]

It's unclear, however, which nutrient is the significant factor in this research as it could be any one or a combination of two or all. In addition, beta-carotene and vitamin E appear to reduce the risk of lung cancer among cigarette smokers. Similarly, calcium, which is found in dairy products and dark green leafy vegetables, may help protect males against colorectal cancer. Other evidence, however, fails to show that beta-carotene helps prevent lung cancer among cigarette smokers and that beta-carotene and vitamins C and E help prevent adenomatous polyps, which can be the beginning of colorectal cancer.[225]

There are numerous studies that have tried to compare the cancer rates and differing diets among countries worldwide. Unfortunately, there are so many variables involved in this comparison that strong evidence supporting any theory is difficult to establish. It's apparent, however, that countries whose populations share a high fat and low fiber diet tend to be modern and affluent countries such as those of northern Europe and North America. It also is apparent that these nations share a higher risk for several specific cancers and that certain features of a Western diet are contributing factors to a large but uncertain proportion of all cancers. Industrialized parts of the world differ in many ways from the less affluent and less developed regions. As a result, this greater cancer rate may not be as dependent upon diet as it is upon other factors that are common to affluent countries and rare in less developed countries.

In conclusion, we know that diet plays an important role in the development of certain cancers. We don't have a full understanding, however, of how or why some dietary factors appear to either increase or decrease one's risk for these certain cancers. This is a field that remains elusive and complex. The study of dietary fat, calories, meat intake, fiber, vitamins and body weight and their relationship to cancers of the colon, breast and others is far from complete and requires extensive additional analysis.

Headline:

Aspirin Prevents Breast Cancer

This headline, which appeared in a popular women's magazine a few years ago, clearly is not true. While it's true that aspirin and other NSAIDs or non-steroidal anti-inflammatory drugs appear to *help* prevent breast cancer, no one product or vitamin or nutrient can in and of itself prevent breast or any other cancer. The battle against all cancers, including that of the breast, is regrettably much more complicated than this headline might have us believe. New studies, however, have revealed that women who take aspirin regularly *after* experiencing breast cancer may be fifty percent less likely to suffer a recurrence of the disease *or* to die from it. Should this finding be substantiated in the years to come, it is nothing short of phenomenal.[226]

Alcohol

Yes, drinking alcoholic beverages can contribute to cancer in human beings, but this statement requires clarification on many levels. First, there are only a few cancers that appear to be directly linked to alcohol consumption including oral, pharyngeal, esophageal and laryngeal.[227] Oral cancers can occur anywhere on the inside of the mouth, although they usually occur on the bottom of the mouth or on the bottom and side of the tongue. Pharyngeal cancer affects the pharynx which is basically the inside wall of the throat. Esophageal cancer occurs in the tube that leads from the back of the mouth directly into the stomach known as the esophagus, and laryngeal cancer affects the larynx or "voice box" which is located at the top of the throat.

Alcohol also appears to be linked to the development of liver cancer.[228] It's believed that the alcohol alters liver functioning in a way that decreases the liver's ability to deactivate certain carcinogens. This theory, in fact, may well account for the fifty percent increased cancer related mortality rate found among alcoholics and heavy drinkers. Finally, there is additional although somewhat weaker evidence that links alcohol abuse to the development of breast and colorectal cancer.

Second, the risk for developing any of the above-mentioned cancers depends primarily upon the amount of alcohol consumed and to a lesser degree, the type of alcohol consumed. Clearly, the risk for these cancers increases as the level of alcohol consumption increases with heavy drinkers and alcoholics sharing the greatest risk. If our Cancer Blueprint is applied, especially to the four primary risk cancers of the mouth, esophagus, pharynx and larynx, we can see that much of the tissue of these organs comes into direct contact with the alcohol.

We also can see that many of these tissues are exposed to irritants in the alcohol that over time may weaken these tissues, making them more susceptible to disease, including cancer. Indeed, the link between these four cancers and alcoholic beverages suggests it's the common ingredients in all alcohols such as ethanol that are the responsible irritants.[229]

It also is believed that the risk for some of these cancers varies as the type of alcohol consumed varies. Esophageal cancer in particular appears to be linked to the intake of specific alcoholic beverages in different countries around the world. For example, the Calvados region of northern France has high rates of esophageal cancer that are linked to the consumption of local apple brandies. In Brazil there's evidence that links an increased risk of esophageal cancer to a beverage known as "cachaca." This popular drink, believed to have been discovered in the sixteenth century by a Brazilian slave, is a distilled spirit derived from fermented sugarcane juice. Similarly, the fact that the coastal areas of South Carolina in the United States have led the country in esophageal cancer mortality for decades appears to be directly related to the regular consumption of the area's homemade "moonshine" whiskeys. Finally, home-brewed rum in Puerto Rico has been linked with high rates of not only esophageal cancer, but with oral cancer as well.[230]

The common thread among these beverages is that each is a particularly potent and virulent form of alcohol that hasn't gone through the usual process of distillation or aging. As a result, they may contain more of the carcinogens that have proven harmful to body tissues. The distillation process appears to be quite important in ascertaining the potential cancer risk of a liquor. For, indeed, evidence suggests that the risk for oral and pharyngeal cancer is greater from the abusive consumption of other "hard" liquors such as gin, bourbon and even beer, than from the consumption of wine.

It's true that recent evidence appears to suggest that non-alcoholic beer may reduce the DNA damage that can lead to certain cancers in animals, yet the possible anti-cancer benefit in normal beer for humans remains unconfirmed. It also is true that hops used in the production of beer contain xanthohumol, a compound that appears to help inhibit a protein that has been linked to a variety of cancers including that of the prostate. The beneficial effect of this compound, however, remains inconclusive as one would have to consume a huge amount of beer to test the theory and the negative impact of such a study on an individual would probably outweigh the positive.[231]

It's important to understand that alcohol may act as a topical carcinogen as well as a systemic one. This means that the harmful effects of alcohol simply may occur when the alcohol comes into direct contact with tissue as well as when it's ingested into the digestive system.[232]

If we take cancer of the larynx, for example, we're talking about a cancer that can affect either the extrinsic larynx or the intrinsic larynx. The extrinsic larynx is the outer surface of the organ, and the intrinsic larynx is the deeper, inner tissue of the organ. It's the extrinsic larynx that makes contact with the alcohol during drinking and heavy drinkers share an unusually high risk for cancer of the extrinsic larynx while the risk for cancer of the intrinsic larynx among these individuals is far less. This indicates that mere topical exposure to alcohol may be sufficient contact to induce the development of certain cancers. In addition, reports also link the long-term use of mouthwashes that have a high alcoholic content with an increased risk of oral cancer.[233] This evidence also implicates the harmful topical effect of carcinogens as mouthwashes are seldom swallowed. And while these studies are fairly recent, the harmful effect of topical exposure to carcinogens, of course, was first suspected and documented centuries ago in England among the chimney sweeps.

While the amount and type of alcohol clearly play roles in the development of certain cancers, the risk is greatly increased when combined with other specific factors. For example, individuals who also smoke cigarettes increase their risk for oral, pharyngeal, esophageal and laryngeal cancer far above the risk associated with these cancers and alcohol consumption alone. When alcohol and cigarette smoking are combined, they form a potent combination that increases one's risk for each of these four cancers. Evidently, the effect of alcohol on these cancers is greatly enhanced by tobacco, as the risk for developing oral- related cancers is about thirty-five times greater among heavy consumers of both. And in the United States alone it's estimated that seventy-five percent of all oral and pharyngeal cancers are due to the combination of excessive drinking and smoking.[234]

It's important to remember that the key to preventing alcohol-induced cancers is to exercise moderation in the consumption of alcohol. And while alcohol abuse and tobacco use create a dangerous combination, a reduction in either of these activities will substantially reduce one's risk for each of the related cancers.

Tobacco

Cigarette Smoking

Tobacco use, especially in the form of cigarette smoking, is today the most preventable cause of excess mortality in the United States and many of the world's other industrialized countries. Over the last century it's been estimated that approximately one hundred million people died worldwide from tobacco related cancers. Indeed, today more individuals die prematurely from cigarette smoking than those who die prematurely from automobile accidents, drug abuse, AIDS and alcohol abuse combined. Medically and scientifically, it's the most recognized "cause" of cancer with causal relationships documented between cigarette smoking and eight major cancers, including those of the lung, larynx, oral cavity, esophagus, bladder, kidney, pancreas in both sexes and cervical in women.[235]

In addition, there also may be a relationship between cigarette smoking and stomach, liver, prostate and colorectal cancer. The common thread between all of these cancers and cigarette smoking is reduced to three factors, including 1) the number of cigarettes smoked daily, 2) the age one begins smoking with younger smokers bearing the greater risk and, 3) the number of years one smokes, with the risk increasing with every additional year.[236]

With such overwhelming evidence linking cigarette smoking to so many cancers it's important to explain why tobacco use is harmful. When tobacco burns, it produces a smoke that contains thousands of chemical agents. Of these thousands of agents, sixty today are known to be carcinogens, co-carcinogens or tumor promoters.[237]

First, a carcinogen is an agent that in itself "causes" the development of or increases the risk for cancer.[238] Second, a co-carcinogen is an agent that alone doesn't transform a normal cell into a cancerous one, yet when combined with another agent does become capable of "causing" cancer.[239] And third, a tumor promoter is an agent that may increase the growth of a cancer that already exists or increase the risk of developing cancer in tissue already susceptible to disease.[240] Clearly, when one smokes one is exposing her or himself to a barrage of harmful agents that, working alone or together, increases the risk for developing a variety of cancers.

Of all the cancers associated with cigarette smoking, lung cancer is the most common. In fact, lung cancer has the dubious distinction of being responsible for more than one out of every four cancer deaths each year in the United States alone and is the number one cause of cancer mortality around the world. Yet, the risk for lung cancer is not only great with those who smoke, it increases among those who simply live or work with those who smoke.[241]

Environmental tobacco smoke, or ETS, is now considered a significant "cause" of lung cancer in nonsmokers. In fact, nonsmokers who live or work with smokers share a risk for lung cancer that's thirty to fifty percent higher than nonsmokers who don't. For example, ETS, which also is known as secondary or passive smoking, is believed to be responsible for three to six thousand nonsmoker deaths from lung cancer each year in the United States alone. While these figures may seem small compared to the number of lung cancer deaths of actual smokers, the number is large when compared to lung cancer deaths caused by other indoor and outdoor pollutants.[242]

To illustrate, studies indicate that the risk of developing lung cancer for individuals exposed to asbestos fibers through their living or working environments is less than one in one million. By comparison, the lung cancer risk for people exposed to ETS is estimated to be more than one hundred times greater than twenty years' exposure to chrysotile asbestos common in buildings of the past few decades. Nevertheless, the efforts made to remove asbestos from contaminated buildings have been enormous compared to the efforts to remove and prevent ETS from contaminating working and living environments.[243]

Headline:

Lung Cancer Risk Greater For Black Cigarette Smokers[244]

There is evidence to suggest that in certain situations, there's a disparity for developing lung cancer between black and white cigarette smokers. It appears that black smokers with a parent or sibling who developed lung cancer at an early age have a greater chance of developing the disease than white smokers with the same family history.

In a study conducted over a thirteen year period from 1990 to 2003, cigarette smokers overall were found to have twice the risk of developing lung cancer after the age of sixty if they had close relatives who developed the disease before the age of fifty. Of this group, however, approximately twenty-five percent of the black participants developed lung cancer compared to seventeen percent of the white participants. The reason for this disparity is not clearly understood, and further research is obviously necessary. Yet, these preliminary findings do seem to indicate that genetics may play a role in the development of lung cancer, and that blacks may be more susceptible to the disease in general or more vulnerable to the harmful effects of smoking in particular.

Other Tobacco Use

Unfortunately, the dangers of tobacco are not limited to cigarette smoking alone. Individuals who use tobacco in a variety of ways face an increased risk for many diseases, including cancer. Pipe and cigar smokers, for instance, share an elevated risk for oral cancers as well as cancers of the larynx, pharynx and esophagus. Indeed, not only is their risk for these cancers equal to the risk shared by cigarette smokers, it often exceeds that of cigarette smokers. And while the risk of lung cancer among pipe and cigar smokers is marginally lower than that for cigarette smokers, the lung cancer risk equals that of cigarette smokers if the smoke is inhaled.[245]

Moreover, individuals who use smokeless tobacco in the form of snuff face an increased risk for oral cancers such as that of the cheek and gum as well as cancers of the larynx and esophagus. Although this use doesn't involve exposure to tobacco smoke, nitrosamines have been detected in snuff and in the saliva of snuff users.[246]

As we recall from our discussion on water pollution, nitrosamines are compounds formed by the reactions of nitrates with amines. To be more specific, nitrates can be produced either in the intestine by high nitrate foods such as vegetables or in the saliva by bacteria. Amines also are organic derivatives of ammonia that are naturally produced in the body and in and of themselves are harmless. When these two substances combine, however, they produce nitrosamines, which are potential carcinogenic compounds.[247]

In this case, we have nitrosamines in both the snuff itself and the saliva of snuff users, a fact that may account for the increase of certain cancers in these individuals. In conclusion, it appears that all forms of tobacco use from the inhalation of tobacco smoke to the use of smokeless tobacco are dangerous, and in many cases, deadly.

The cost to society from cancer deaths related to tobacco use alone is phenomenal. In the United States, for example, the nearly one third of all cancer deaths linked directly to cigarette smoking is only the beginning. To this figure we must add approximately 14,000 more deaths related to pipe and cigar smoking among men. As a result, approximately twenty-three percent of all cancer deaths among American females are attributed to cigarette smoking and the combination of cigarette, pipe and cigar smoking accounts for nearly forty-two percent of all cancer deaths among American males. As impressive as these figures are, they don't begin to reflect the true cost to society from tobacco use, which also includes disease and death resulting from heart disease, emphysema and bronchitis.[248]

When discussing the different layers of risk associated with cancers, tobacco use is the most obvious and easily linked. Yet, it's also a "lifestyle" factor that can be altered or eliminated. Either choice will greatly reduce one's risk for developing many diseases, including cancer. In fact, within one year of quitting smoking, the risk of developing heart disease is reduced by almost fifty percent.

The risk for lung cancer also is reduced although the risk reduction doesn't occur as quickly. Yet, within ten to fifteen years after "quitting the habit," the overall health of a former smoker doesn't differ significantly from the health of one who has never smoked. For the continued risk of developing tobacco-related cancers among former smokers depends upon the length of time one smoked, the length of time one has ceased to smoke and the state of one's health when one quits the habit.[249] Clearly, if all cancer deaths linked to tobacco use were eliminated from cancer mortality rates, all societies would experience a substantial decrease in the overall cancer rates and deaths.

Part 3:
Cancer: Up Close and Personal

Most Common Cancers[250]

U.S. Figures Based Upon Estimates from 2008

Men:		**Women:**	
	Prostate		Breast
	Lung		Lung
	Colorectal		Colorectal
	Urinary		Endometrial
	Non-Hodgkin's		Non-Hodgkin's
	Melanoma		Thyroid
	Kidney		Melanoma
	Oral Cavity		Ovarian
	Leukemia		Kidney
	Pancreatic		Leukemia

Most Common Cancers

Worldwide Figures Based Upon 2007 Data[251]

Men:		**Women:**	
	Lung		Breast
	Prostate		Cervical
	Stomach		Colorectal
	Colorectal		Lung
	Liver		Stomach
	Esophageal		Ovarian
	Urinary (Bladder)		Endometrial
	Oral Cavity		Liver
	Non-Hodgkin's		Esophageal
	Leukemia		Leukemia

Most Deadly Cancers

U.S. Figures Based Upon 2008 Estimates

Men:		Women:	
	Lung		Lung
	Prostate		Breast
	Colorectal		Colorectal
	Pancreatic		Pancreatic
	Liver		Ovarian
	Leukemia		Non-Hodgkin's
	Esophageal		Leukemia
	Urinary (Bladder)		Endometrial
	Non-Hodgkin's		Liver
	Kidney		Brain and Nervous System

Most Deadly Cancers

Worldwide Figures Based Upon 2007 Data

Men:		**Women:**	
	Lung		Breast
	Stomach		Lung
	Liver		Cervical
	Colorectal		Stomach
	Esophagus		Colorectal
	Prostate		Liver
	Leukemia		Esophageal
	Pancreatic		Ovarian
	Urinary (Bladder)		Pancreatic
	Non-Hodgkin's		Leukemia

If Basal and Squamous Cell cancers were included in all cancer statistics, cancer of the skin would be the most common cancer of all.[252]

Cancer statistics are collected in a number of ways and reflect a variety of information. They can vary significantly from one month to the next, or from one year to another. Further, even when statistics are collected in the same way and compiled for the same reason, during the same time frame, they can differ depending upon the source doing the collecting and compiling. As a result, determining the most common or deadliest cancers remains an inexact science. Yet, while the order of cancers in each category may vary from one source to another, the type of cancers remains surprisingly consistent.

For practical reasons, we cannot discuss every cancer implicated in the above lists. We will, however, make a good faith effort to discuss several of the major cancers that impact both females and males, of all ages, around the world. And while we've touched upon some of the following information in our previous discussion of risks, we will now discuss it from the perspective of the disease itself. Such cross-referencing will enhance our overall understanding of both and the ways in which they interact in our daily lives. As a result, the "big picture" will be easier for us to see.

Chapter 10:
Breast Cancer

Breast cancer is the most common cancer among the world's women with the majority of cases occurring in developed and industrial countries. The breast cancer rates, for example, in the United States are among the highest in the world, with the highest incidence rate at one time occurring in the San Francisco Bay area.[253] Unfortunately, breast cancer holds the distinction of being the second most deadly cancer for all women regardless of the country in which they reside.

Although breast cancer can occur rarely in men, this cancer is considered primarily to be a woman's disease. In the United States, for example, approximately fifteen hundred men annually are diagnosed with the disease while the rates of breast cancer among women are approximately one hundred times greater.[254] Accordingly, the following discussion will focus primarily upon breast cancer in women, although the procedures for the detection and treatment of male breast cancer parallel much of this discussion.

To begin, both female and male fetal development are fairly identical until the end of the first trimester when the sex of the fetus is believed to be determined. Both females and males are born with nipples because this particular tissue develops during the first trimester before the fetus continues to develop as either a female or a male. At the end of the first trimester, if the fetus develops as a female the additional female physical characteristics will form and, if the fetus develops as a male, the additional male physical characteristics will form.

After birth, the female breasts remain basically the same as those of the male until the age of puberty, sometime between the ages of nine and thirteen, when female breast development begins. This occurs when female hormones are released into the body in increasing amounts by the hypothalamus, pituitary, adrenal glands and ovaries. When developed, the female breast is composed of fatty tissue that contains as many as twenty groups of milk producing glands. In turn, each group of these glands contains a milk duct that runs to the nipple, which protrudes from the areola, the darkened circular area in the center of the breast.[255]

There are several different types of breast cancer. The most common is known as **ductal** breast cancer, a type that accounts for approximately eighty percent of all breast cancers. **Lobular** breast cancer affects the nipples of the breast and accounts for approximately ten percent of all breast cancers. **Inflammatory** breast cancer, or IBC, accounts for approximately one percent of all breast cancers, although it unfortunately remains the most deadly. And, approximately fifteen additional types of breast cancer account for the remaining nine percent of occurrences.[256]

As with many cancers, a woman's risk of developing breast cancer appears to be related to both genetic and environmental factors. The incidence rates for this cancer increase significantly with age as the majority of cases occur in women over the age of fifty. Surprisingly, the rate also increases for women of a higher socioeconomic status who are married and live in urban rather than rural areas. In addition, in the United States, the rate increases further for women who live in northern states as opposed to women in southern states.[257]

Since the early 1970s the incidence rate of breast cancer has increased dramatically. It's important to note that this increase is largely associated with the detection of low stage tumors and that it took place over a period of time when the use of mammography also increased by about seventy-five percent. These facts together strongly suggest that a large part of the increase in breast cancer incidence is due to the success of routine screening and early detection.[258]

It has long been recognized that the reproductive events in a woman's life are factors that greatly affect a woman's risk for developing breast cancer. The importance of these events is determined by the age of the woman at the time the events are experienced. The most consistent factor in a number of different populations around the world appears to be the woman's age at the time of her first full-term pregnancy. Women giving birth for the first time before the age of twenty have less risk than women who give birth for the first time after the age of thirty or women who have never borne a child. Indeed, women in these two latter groups share a risk that's two to three times greater than those women in the first group. There also is ample evidence to suggest that subsequent births are related to a further reduction in a woman's risk.[259]

Additional evidence suggests that women whose pregnancies are terminated either through miscarriage or abortion also may have a greater risk for developing breast cancer.[260] This research remains controversial, yet the findings appear logical if we remember that a full-term pregnancy interrupts a woman's overall exposure to estrogen for a longer period of time, thereby decreasing her risk for the disease. A terminated pregnancy, on the other hand, restores a woman's exposure to estrogen more quickly, and this increase in exposure, as compared to the decrease in exposure resulting from a full-term pregnancy, may slightly increase one's risk.

Although reproductive events are important in assessing risk, there is less evidence that periods of lactation provide a woman with more protection. In addition, there appears to be an increase of risk related to the number of years a woman experiences menstruation. The earlier the onset of menstruation, and the later the onset of menopause, the greater the risk. Women who have experienced endometrial or ovarian cancers also appear to have an increased risk for developing breast cancer as well. All of the above factors, however, appear to be related to a woman's hormonal balance such that her risk for developing breast cancer is changed in one way or another.[261]

Because of this relationship between endogenous hormones – those that occur naturally in the body – and breast cancer risk, there also has long been concern about the use and risk of exogenous hormones, those that are added to the body. As we know, hormone replacement therapy, or HRT, is a program where the sex hormones estrogen and progestin are administered to women experiencing uncomfortable symptoms of peri-menopause, menopause or post-menopause and whose bodies have naturally stopped producing these hormones partially or completely.

There is evidence to suggest that the risk for breast cancer among women who are long-term users of HRT and women who are on or have received high doses of estrogen may be higher. Similarly, while the relationship between the use of oral contraceptives and breast cancer is still in debate, evidence also suggests there may be a possible increase in breast cancer risk for women under the age of forty-five who have been long-term users of oral contraceptive and for women who began taking oral contraceptives at a young age.[262]

Finally, the relationship between breast cancer risk and oral contraceptives that combine the hormones estrogen and progestin, known as the combination pack or "combo," is even less clear. What is clear is that the roles of oral contraceptive use and hormone replacement therapy and breast cancer are subjects that require a great deal more study and research to properly guide each woman to make the best choice for herself.[263]

Interestingly, several studies also indicate that early female development may contribute to an individual's risk for breast cancer.[264] To understand these findings, let's analyze them by starting with the information we already have concerning estrogen. Clearly, both the natural production and the artificial addition of estrogen may increase a woman's risk for breast cancer. Early female development refers to the age at which a female begins to menstruate and develop adult female breasts. This phenomenon occurs when the female hormones such as estrogen begin to regulate the female growth into adulthood. If this occurs at an early age, it indicates that such females have more estrogen in their systems at an earlier age than perhaps do their peers. It follows that if such females experience more years of estrogen production, their risk for developing breast cancer also may increase.

Moreover, early human development is often associated with diets that are abundant and often high in fat. And such diets are more common in the industrialized nations of the world where, indeed, breast cancer among women is more prevalent.[265] Factoring all these elements together we can, once again, make sense of research the findings of which may initially appear confusing and odd. Indeed, it appears that the common thread linking many breast cancer risks is the amount of estrogen a woman is exposed to over her lifetime. For when the production of estrogen is limited or interrupted, be it by childbirth, late start of menses or early menopause, a woman's risk for this particular cancer decreases.

Genetics and family medical history, of course, is by now a familiar cancer risk that plays an important role in determining a woman's risk for breast cancer. If a woman's mother, sister or daughter has had breast cancer, her risk increases approximately two to three times. If two of these first-degree relatives have had breast cancer, a woman's risk becomes six times greater than the average woman's.[266]

Additionally, if the first-degree relative was diagnosed at an early age or experienced bilateral breast cancer, which involves both breasts, a woman's risk may be even greater. Once again, genetic inheritances where multiple members of the same family are affected by a common cancer are referred to as "clusters." In the case of breast cancer, such family clusters appear to be related to two genes–BRCA-1, which was first reported in 1994 and BRCA-2, both of which are found primarily in women of Ashkenazi Jewish heritage.[267]

While scientists recently have detected four additional genes that appear to be related to the development of breast cancer, it's estimated that approximately eighty-six percent of women with an inherited mutation in one or both of the BRCA-1 and BRCA-2 genes in particular will develop breast cancer by the age of seventy. Heredity, or family clusters, however, is only one factor that contributes to breast cancer and overall accounts for only five to ten percent of all breast cancers in women the world over.[268]

Headline:

Deadly Breast Cancer Linked to Race[269]

There is evidence that indicates younger, pre-menopausal African American women experience higher rates of an aggressive basel-like breast cancer than Caucasian women. The higher rates of this form of breast cancer among these women may help explain why black women in America share a greater risk of developing fatal breast cancer than white American women. This is especially interesting considering the fact that these black women actually share a lower overall risk of developing breast cancer than their white counterparts.

Indeed, in one particular study of five hundred breast cancer patients, thirty-nine percent of the pre-menopausal black women had the deadly form of basel-like cancer compared with fourteen percent of post-menopausal black women, and sixteen percent of white women of various ages. This information clearly contradicts the long held theories that African American women are more likely to die from breast cancer because they receive poor care or seek treatment late.

Moreover, an additional study of more than two thousand women indicated that black women overall developed more aggressive tumors than their Hispanic and Caucasian counterparts. In part this finding is attributed to a type of tumor known as an estrogen-negative or ER-negative tumor. Such tumors aren't dependent upon estrogen for their development and are extremely difficult to treat. Unfortunately, it appears that African American women have a greater tendency to develop ER-negative breast cancers and high-grade tumors than Hispanics or Caucasians.

Similarly, women who have a history of benign breast disease also may be at greater risk for developing breast cancer. One such disease known as atypical hyperplasia appears to indicate a higher risk in women, as may cystic mastitis, fibrosis and other benign conditions that cause unusual cysts or denseness in the breast tissue. Indeed, women who have particularly dense breast tissue may experience a risk three to four times greater than women who do not. An increased risk of breast cancer also exists for women who have already been diagnosed with endometrial or ovarian cancer and for those who have experienced a previous breast cancer.[270]

There is little, if any, controversy about the role of radiation exposure and a woman's risk for breast cancer. Without a doubt, exposures to high doses of radiation increase a woman's risk for breast cancer as she matures, even if the exposures occurred during infancy. Harmful radiation exposures such as those already discussed, however, should not be confused with the low dose radiation exposure of a mammogram. The exposure from this procedure is considered minimal, and the benefits of mammography greatly outweigh any possible risks, especially in women fifty years or older. In younger women, the use of mammography will depend primarily on each woman's medical and family history as well as her doctor's advice.[271]

The risk of breast cancer not only increases as a woman becomes older, but some studies suggest it also may increase as a woman's weight and body mass increase. This risk applies primarily to postmenopausal women who may experience weight gain or changes in weight distribution at this time in their lives. On the other hand, separate research indicates that lean premenopausal women are at a greater risk for developing breast cancer prior to menopause.[272] While again this information may appear confusing, a simple analysis may help clarify the issue.

First, most studies agree that a woman's risk for breast cancer increases as she becomes older. This is not surprising, as we already know that the risk for cancer almost always becomes greater as we age. It also is true that some women experience changes in their total weight and weight distribution as they get older and go through menopause. If a greater risk exists for these women, however, it could be due to many different factors. It might be due to long-term use of estrogens or hormone replacement therapy. It might be due to an increase in the estrogen level that occurs as a woman's weight increases. It might be due to other physical conditions that occur with age and that hinder good health inhibiting the body's immune system and resulting in a greater susceptibility to disease.

Moreover, with a great weight increase, a woman could experience a number of potential physical problems in addition to cancer risk. Possibly most important, breast cancer can be more difficult to diagnose in women with greater body weight because it's harder to see or feel tumors in breast tissue that's denser.

Similarly, it is easier to detect tumors and anomalies in women who have less body weight because they usually have less breast tissue. As a result, abnormal conditions may be seen or felt at an earlier stage. This also may explain the studies that indicate lean premenopausal women share an increased risk for breast cancer. It may not be that the risk is actually greater, or that they experience more breast tumors, but that more breast tumors are detected earlier and more often in lean women. It follows, therefore, that the incidence rate of breast cancer detected in premenopausal women who are leaner may indeed be higher, but not necessarily that their risk is greater.

It also is possible that heavier women may have an equivalent number of breast tumors as leaner women, but that those tumors simply go undetected until later in life. The fact that breast cancer is usually detected later in women with more body mass may, unfortunately, account in part for the high mortality rate from this cancer. For the most important factor in the successful treatment of this cancer, as with all cancers, is early detection.

Another area of concern and contradiction is the role that dietary fat plays in a woman's risk for developing breast cancer. It does appear that the incidence rates for this cancer are higher in Western industrialized nations while the rates are lower in Asia, Latin America and Africa, and several studies have attempted to explain this geographical difference. Some of these studies suggest that the increase in the West is due to the high fat diets typical of industrialized nations. Other studies, however, appear to show little if any relationship between fat intake and the occurrence of breast cancer.[273]

We need to remember, however, that this incidence difference may be related to many factors other than dietary fat, including the possibility that detection and reporting methods in less industrialized nations may not be as efficient or common as those of the world's industrialized nations. If this were true, it would logically follow that women in less developed countries may indeed have the same levels of breast cancer, but that the cancer is not being detected as frequently as it is in more developed countries.

This controversy extends to immigrants who migrate from countries where the breast cancer rate is lower to countries where the rate is higher. A few years ago, some studies found that women who migrated from countries where less dietary fat was consumed, Japan in particular, to countries such as the United States where the fat intake was greater, didn't increase their risk for breast cancer significantly even after adopting the higher fat diet of the adopted country. This finding, of course, suggested that diet and fat intake was not as important in determining breast cancer risk as, perhaps, one's genetic background. Conversely, other studies indicate that migrant women from countries where the rate of breast cancer is low, such as Japan, assume the higher incidence rate of the country to which they immigrate.[274] And, these results appear to state just the opposite, that international differences in the rates of breast cancer are not the result of genetic factors as much as, perhaps, diet and fat intake.

Yet, none of these results necessarily indicate that genetics, or diet and fat intake, is a controlling factor in the development of these breast cancers. It's possible that immigrant women from specific genetic and cultural backgrounds whose incidence rate increased after moving to a new country not only adopted a high fat diet, but perhaps increased alcohol use, or postponed having children, or began receiving large doses of estrogen, ceased physical activity or as mentioned above, simply had more access to procedures that detect breast cancer in the first place.

Moreover, additional research indicated that Japanese women who live in the United States appear to have a significantly lower recurrence rate of breast cancer than other women.[275] This, of course, once again suggests that genetic background may be an important factor in determining one's risk for this particular cancer. In any case, it's always important to remember that many factors may be involved in explaining the increase or decrease of breast cancer in women the world over, and that research, especially that which appears to be contradictory, should be questioned and analyzed carefully.

Fat intake is still significant, however, in that women whose diets contain high fat levels may have more body weight. More body weight not only increases the level of estrogen that a woman's body produces, estrogen exposure being a known risk factor for breast cancer, but it also may hinder the ability to detect breast cancer at an earlier and more treatable stage. For overall, the maintenance of a healthy body weight through a balanced diet and regular physical exercise will only benefit a woman and reduce her risk of developing many cancers, including that of the breast. Indeed, it's believed that physical exercise is an important factor in reducing the breast tissue's exposure to circulating estrogen.[276]

There are dietary factors other than fat, however, that may play a more significant role in the risk of breast cancer. There's fairly consistent evidence that excessive alcohol use may increase a woman's risk for developing this disease.[277] This increase is small, however, and may be due to the **leaching effect** alcohol may have on the body's store of nutrients.[278] To explain, excessive alcohol can deplete the body of necessary vitamins and minerals, which can decrease the body's immune systems and increase the body's susceptibility to infection and disease. Surprisingly, however, recent studies have suggested that the reasonable consumption of red wine actually reduces a woman's risk for breast cancer,[279] as due vitamins A, C and D.[280]

This information follows on the heels of research that indicates the reasonable consumption of red wine also reduces one's risk for heart disease. Indeed, many researchers now include red wine in the same category as other "cancer fighting" beverages such as lycopene-laden tomato juice, carrot juice and grape juice.[281] Research also indicates that the regular use of non-steroidal anti-inflammatory drugs, or NSAIDs, such as aspirin and ibuprofen may reduce one's risk for this cancer.[282] Finally, a healthy diet complete with foods rich in antioxidants appears to offer a protective effect from cancer of the breast as well as others.

It's important to remember that most of the factors known to be related to breast cancer today only increase a woman's risk by about two to three times.[283] Although this may sound significant, it's considered to be quite moderate. Multiple factors together, however, may increase a woman's risk significantly. It's important, therefore, for every woman to understand the effect of "layering" and to be aware of the multiple factors that may increase her particular risk. And while there may be many unknown factors that also contribute to one's breast cancer risk, dealing with the known and suspected factors is our logical starting point.

In addition, each woman must know the warning signs for breast cancer and be alert for their presence. These include lumps or thickening in the breast tissue, a discharge from the nipple or a refracted nipple, or any change in the contours of either breast. Also be aware of any changes in the skin surrounding the breast such as an unusual indentation in the skin, or a color or texture change in the skin of the breast. The diagnostic procedures recommended for early detection of breast cancer include regular self-examination at every age, yearly clinical examinations and mammography yearly or bi-yearly for older women according to their personal levels of risk. The treatments for breast cancer may include one or a combination of procedures, including surgery involving a radical or simple mastectomy or lumpectomy, external radiation and internal brachytherapy, cryotherapy, drug and hormone therapy and chemotherapy. Indeed, molecular testing can help predict the risk of breast cancer recurrence and who will benefit from chemotherapy.[284]

Harmful:	Helpful:
Estrogen Exposure	**Diet**
HRT	**Carotenoids**
High Dose	**Vitamins A, C & D**
Long-Term Use	**Antioxidants**
Early Menstruation	
Late Menopause	
Oral Contraceptives	
Long-Term Use	
Early Physical Development	
Heredity	
Benign Breast Disease	
Radiation Exposure	
Diet	
Animal Fat	
Excess Body Weight	
Inadequate Physical Exercise	
Alcohol Abuse	

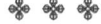

Headline:

White or Red–Does the Color Really Matter?[285]

Serge Reynaud first documented the health benefits of wine in his 1991 work *French Paradox*. This paper focused on the fact that the French, in spite of their typically rich cholesterol heavy diet, suffer significantly less coronary disease than other populations with similar high fat, high cholesterol diets. Reynaud concluded this result was due in large part to the daily consumption of wine in the French diet. Now, apparently Dr. Reynaud personally advocates red wine, yet his paper didn't specify any difference between red or white wine; it simply distinguished between wine and other alcoholic beverages. Also, this initial research was conducted in relation to cardiovascular disease, not cancer.

More studies conducted on the health benefits of wine have found that it contains several antioxidants that help reduce the damage caused by the body's free radicals and inhibits the process that leads to the growth and spread of cancer. Indeed, wine contains the strongest antioxidants in nature, including resveratrol, quercitin and epicatechin, all of which are approximately five times stronger than vitamin E. The primary and most beneficial antioxidant in question, however, is resveratrol, a compound found in the seeds and skins of grapes.

Red wine apparently has a higher concentration of resveratrol than white because the seeds and skin ferment in the juices of the grapes during the wine making process. In contrast, while white wine also contains resveratrol, the seeds and skin are removed early in the wine making process which reduces the total concentration of resveratrol in the final product. Based upon this information, some researchers believe that red wine, especially Pinot Noir and Merlot, offers the more protective qualities.

Other researchers have found that even though red wine contains more resveratrol than white, the resveratrol molecules in white wine are smaller and, therefore, are more easily absorbed by the body. Indeed, some research indicates that while free radicals were reduced in red wine drinkers by ten percent, free radicals were reduced in white wine drinkers by thirty-four percent. This, of course, leads to the alternate conclusion that the antioxidant value of white wine actually may be more effective than that of red. Another recent study suggests that white wine has no health benefit whatsoever. Yet, another actually associated white wine consumption specifically with an increase in lung cancer, although the increase was slight and only thirty-nine wine drinkers were studied.[286] Clearly, opinions differ on this subject.

Still, we must consider that the benefits of red wine are perhaps better known simply because red wine has been the subject of more research. In any event, it's true that both red and white wines contain resveratrol and other powerful antioxidants and both, when consumed in moderation, *may* minimize DNA mutations and help prevent leukemia as well as breast, colon, prostate and skin cancer.[287]

Chapter 11:
Colorectal Cancer

Worldwide, colorectal cancer is the third most common cancer among women and the fourth most common cancer among men. It also is the fifth most deadly cancer among women and the fourth most deadly among men. In the United States, colorectal cancer is the third most common and third most deadly cancer for both women and men.

Colorectal cancer affects the large intestine. This is the lower section of the overall intestine and is distinct from the upper, small intestine. Of this lower portion, the first five or six feet are referred to as the "colon," and the last five or six inches is referred to as the "rectum." The tissue of the colon and the rectum is anatomically and physically so similar that it's often difficult to determine in which part of the intestine a tumor has developed. For this reason, cancer of the large intestine, the colon or the rectum, is often referred to as "colorectal" cancer.[288]

The large intestine, a vital component of the human digestive system, is housed between the small intestine and the rectum. As food enters the small intestine, the necessary nutrients and vitamins are absorbed into the wall of the small intestine and are passed back into the bloodstream. The excess liquid in the small intestine then flows into the large intestine where most of it is reabsorbed through the intestinal wall. What remains is primarily waste material containing undigested and unabsorbed water, food and fiber. It's this material that moves through the large intestine into the sigmoid colon in the lower left abdomen, then into the rectum to be expelled by the body.

Colorectal cancer usually begins as a polyp, a benign growth that occurs in the lining of the intestine. There are many different varieties of polyps and most are basically harmless. The most common of these is called a **hyperplastic polyp**, a small growth that usually measures less than a quarter of an inch. Although it poses no cancer risk, this type of polyp should nevertheless be removed as it can grow and possibly interfere with digestion.

Another type that occurs in childhood is called a **juvenile polyp**. This benign growth isn't precancerous either, but it should nevertheless be removed to avoid other potential problems. And the last major group of polyps that remain noncancerous are **inflammatory polyps**. These are polyps that result from an injury to the intestinal lining or from inflammation caused by other medical conditions such as ulcerative colitis, a chronic disease that attacks the lining of the colon.[289]

On the other hand, the category of polyps of major concern is called the **adenomatous polyps**. Adenomatous simply means an abnormal growth that occurs in the tissue covering an internal or external organ. These polyps have the potential to become cancerous growths if they go undetected and untreated. This group of polyps is separated into three subgroups including **tubular**, **tubulovillous** and **villous adenomas**. The most common of these are tubular, polyps that also are the smallest of the three at approximately half an inch. Villous are less common and larger at one inch in diameter or greater. Tubulovillous are adenomas that contain characteristics of each of the other two. They all present a significant health risk and should be removed as soon as discovered.[290]

Similar to breast cancer, the highest rates of colorectal cancer in terms of incidence and mortality are found in the more industrialized countries of the world, including North America, northern and western Europe and New Zealand, while the lowest rates are found in Asia and Africa. While colorectal cancer in the United States accounted for fifteen percent of all diagnosed cancers fifteen years ago, the rates today are decreasing thanks in part to successful screening procedures.[291] Moreover, the majority of deaths from colorectal cancer, including those in the United States, appear to be concentrated in regions where great industrial activity takes place or has taken place.[292]

In the United States, these regions include the north Atlantic Coast, New York, Massachusetts, New Jersey and the urban areas of the Great Lakes.[293] At first glance, therefore, it appears that the higher rates of colorectal mortality may be related to occupational factors. Unfortunately, there is too little data on this relationship to reach a firm conclusion. Furthermore, it also is possible that certain industries have a harmful, lasting effect on the environment related to higher colorectal rates in individuals living in the region, whether or not those individuals actually work in a suspect industry.[294]

The role of the environment is often questioned when discussing the risk factors associated with specific cancers. For example, when a rapid rise in a particular cancer occurs in a certain region, environmental factors are the first to become suspect. In the case of colorectal cancer, for instance, environmental factors have been thought to play a role in migrating individuals who appear to adopt the cancer rate of the country to which they immigrate.

Studies have found, in fact, that individuals migrating from Greece and Yugoslavia to Australia reflected during their lifetime the higher colorectal cancer incidence rate of Australia rather than the lower rate of their native countries. Upon further examination, however, these findings may be due in part to factors other than the environment, such as a new diet, increased fat intake or decreased physical activity, all of which are risk factors for this particular cancer. To date, the relationship between colorectal cancer and the environment remains unclear.[295]

The relationship between colorectal cancer and other factors, however, appears to be clearer. First, unlike some cancers there appears to be a strong relationship between colorectal cancer and diet. Diet, in fact, may be one of the most important factors when determining one's risk for colorectal cancer. Information regarding diet also may be more reliable as it's a risk factor that's more easily controlled in a research environment. Clearly, diet is a factor that varies considerably from one part of the world to another and from one population group to another. It also is a factor that changes within individual countries and populations over time.[296]

The food that one consumes, and the numerous elements contained in the food, comes into direct contact with the intestinal tract and gastrointestinal epithelial tissue of every individual during the digestive process. From the early research of England's chimney sweeps to today's current studies it's clear that the direct contact of human tissue with certain substances can promote the development of cancer. Clearly, therefore, the food one consumes may be a significant layer in determining one's susceptibility to colorectal cancer as a topical factor as well as a systemic one.[297]

First, there's strong evidence that the consumption of fat promotes tumors in the tissues of the large intestine, a finding supported by numerous international studies. There are, of course, different kinds of fat. In women, studies have found that those with a higher daily intake of animal fat have twice the risk of developing colorectal cancer than women who consume less animal fat. In particular, there appears to be a strong relationship between colorectal cancer and the consumption of red meat, which, of course, has a high fat content. Further studies among female health care professionals found that women who consumed more red meat and less chicken and fish developed a risk for colorectal cancer two and a half times greater than women who consumed less red meat.[298]

When studying fat intake, however, men appear to be at more risk than women for developing colorectal cancer. Studies among male health care professionals indicated that those who regularly ate main dish meals of red meat, including beef, lamb and pork, had three times the risk of developing colorectal cancer than men who ate these foods less than once a month. Moreover, those male health care professionals in the highest category of fat intake also ran twice the risk of developing precancerous polyps, the adenomas, than those in the lowest category of fat intake.[299]

Here it's important to note that "red meat" is defined as meat relatively dark in color when raw. This darker color is apparent in foods such as beef and lamb and is typically found in animals that subsist primarily on a diet of grasses and other green vegetation. Color, however, also is influenced by other factors, including the sex and age of the animal, as well as the amount of exercise the animal receives. For these factors determine the amount of the protein **myoglobin** produced and found within the tissues of different animals. The more myoglobin that's present within the tissues, the darker the tissues are in color.[300]

In contrast, "white meat" is defined as meat light in color when raw. Typically, animals that subsist on diets that include a variety of foods greater than just green vegetation produce "white" meat as they lack the prerequisite amounts of myoglobin that create darker flesh. White meats, which include fish and poultry, generally are more tender than red meats, usually require a shorter cooking time and often contain less fat.

Technically, pork is included in this definition of white meat as pork is derived from animals that consume a variety of foods. Pork is obtained from animals that lack the myoglobin necessary for darker flesh and is relatively light in color when raw. Studies that attempt to identify the effects of dietary fat typically include pork with the red meats. For the fat content of pork, or for that matter any meat, is determined by the particular cut in question, and most pork contains more fat than the other white meats of fish and poultry.[301]

One wishing to adhere to a low fat diet, however, must remember that not all fish and poultry are low in fat either. The dark meat of a chicken thigh, for example, may contain more fat than a small beef filet. And other fowl dishes such as pheasant or duck also contain high levels of fat. In all cases, the skin of any fowl should be avoided if one is committed to lowering one's fat intake.[302]

It's important to understand, however, that all meats may present an increased cancer risk if they've been cooked at high temperatures through broiling, grilling or frying. High temperatures break down the amino acid creatinine in meats forming chemicals called **heterocyclic amines**, or **HCAs**. While these chemicals haven't been found conclusively to increase the cancer risk for humans, they have been linked to cancer development in animals.

Furthermore, there's concern that the smoke resulting from fat dripping onto hot coals during grilling exposes us to additional chemicals such as **polycyclic aromatic hydrocarbons**, or **PAHs**. These compounds form in the smoke and are deposited on and absorbed back into the meat as it cooks. So while the white meats of fish and fowl usually appear to reduce one's risk for certain cancers, they too may become harmful when cooked at high temperatures in the above ways.[303]

Accordingly, it's advisable to cook meats at lower temperatures, especially red meats, through roasting or stewing. If, however, one still chooses to grill, one should choose lean meats that will drip less and cause fewer flare ups, raise the grilling surface higher from the heat source, lower the gas or wait for the charcoal to burn low, avoid the charred or blackened portions, and consume well done meats cooked at high temperatures occasionally rather than regularly. While the best ingredients have yet to be determined, the process of marinating meat before grilling can decrease the formation of HCAs by approximately ninety-six percent.[304]

Foods that do contain higher levels of animal and other fats are harmful in part because fat is a dense material. It's more difficult for the body to digest fat than other foods. In addition, it appears that when one consumes more fat, one's system excretes more bile acids to aid in the digestion of that fat. Fat also promotes the growth of bacteria within the colon and, unfortunately, these bacteria have the ability to convert the bile acids to carcinogens. Therefore, the more fat one consumes, the more bacteria and bile are produced which, in turn, may promote the production of more carcinogens in one's system.[305]

While the connection between a high fat diet and colorectal cancer is well established, there is less evidence that individuals with a low fiber intake are at more risk. It's true that countries with the highest dietary fiber consumption per person tend to exhibit the lowest rates of colorectal cancer, and a majority of studies indicate that the fiber found in vegetables appears to have a protective effect.[306] It also is true that vegetables are a primary source of fiber in industrialized countries. This protective effect, however, hasn't always been found to be true of fruits. While most studies have simply been inconsistent when determining the protective effect of fruits, some studies have actually shown an inverse relationship between the two. This means that some studies actually suggest that the more fruit one consumes, the greater one's risk for developing colorectal cancer may be.[307]

Similarly, some studies have failed to show that fiber from grains reduces one's risk for developing colorectal cancer.[308] Research, however, does indicate a stronger protective effect from fruit, vegetable and grain fiber when studying colon polyps. In other words, the protective effect of fibers may be more important in reducing one's risk for developing colon polyps, which, of course, may lead to colorectal cancer. Fiber, therefore, may be more important in the early stages of cancer development, during its carcinogenesis when polyps may be developing. Dietary fat, however, remains a key risk factor in the promotion of both polyp development and the growth of cancerous tissue.[309]

It also is important to consider the possibility that the more apparent protective effect of vegetables may not be due to fiber, but to specific anticarcinogens found in the vegetable or, perhaps, a combination of both. For example, folic acid is found in many vegetables and may in itself reduce the risk of colorectal cancer. Calcium also may have a protective effect against colorectal cancer as individuals with a higher calcium intake tend to exhibit a lower incidence rate for colorectal cancer.[310]

To a lesser degree, it's believed that vitamin D also reduces one's risk for this cancer. Now, although a clear relationship between alcohol use and colorectal cancer risk is inconclusive, alcohol may contribute to the risk again simply because of its "leaching effect" on the body. As discussed in the previous section, excessive alcohol can deplete the body of protective vitamins and nutrients, leaving the body mo[311]re susceptible to colorectal cancer as well as many others.

In addition, research that indicates the regular use of nonsteroidal anti-inflammatory drugs or NSAIDs offers a protective effect against breast cancer also suggests these products may offer a protective effect against colorectal cancer as well. While NSAIDs such as aspirin have been known to offer protection from heart attacks and stroke for a number of years, their cancer fighting qualities are now beginning to be recognized.[312]

Although the use of aspirin and ibuprofen may not be appropriate for everyone, they appear to reduce one's risk for colorectal cancer by inhibiting the development of colonic neoplasia, which is the growth of abnormal and possibly malignant cells within the colon. Now, recent research conducted over a twenty-year period suggests that while the use of aspirin does offer a protective effect from colon cancer, that effect is only significant after a decade of use. This research also suggests that low dose aspirin use doesn't possess the same effect as high dose aspirin use.

The problem with high dose aspirin use, which is defined as two or more aspirin a day, is that it also can result in abnormal and dangerous bleeding. Yet, this particular research was conducted among women only and as such, the results may not be representative of the population at large. Further, this research doesn't negate the fact that aspirin does offer a certain amount of protection from colon cancer in certain situations.

Indeed, additional research has found that one baby aspirin each day of eighty milligrams can reduce the risk for precancerous polyps, or adenomas, by nearly twenty percent in individuals who have had prior adenomas. The same daily use of low dose aspirin in individuals with advanced adenomas or colorectal cancer appeared to reduce the risk of advanced adenoma recurrence by forty percent. In fact, this research found that the daily use of a higher dose aspirin, or 325 milligrams, had a less protective effect that reduced the recurrence of typical adenomas by only four percent and the recurrence of advanced adenomas and colorectal cancers by only nineteen percent.[313]

There also is evidence of a small direct relationship between the risk of colon cancer and body weight.[314] In fact, it's believed that individuals who weigh more may have an increased risk for developing the disease. If we re-examine the evidence concerning fat and its impact upon the human body, this connection to colorectal cancer begins to make sense. First, an individual who has a greater body weight may consume more dietary fat than current guidelines suggest. Second, as previously mentioned, fat promotes the excretion of intestinal bile acids and the growth of colonic bacteria that can convert the bile acids to carcinogens. A heavier individual, therefore, who may consume more dietary fat, may indeed put her or himself at a higher level of risk for developing colorectal cancer.

In contrast, physical exercise has been shown to greatly reduce the risk of colorectal cancer. The more physical exercise one gets in the workplace and at leisure, the less risk one has for developing colorectal cancer. Exercise keeps the muscles of the physical body toned and keeps the organs in good working order. It aids the digestive system in its job of absorbing the nutritious elements of one's diet and eliminating the harmful ones.[315]

If the intestinal tract isn't working properly, toxins and harmful elements may accumulate in the large intestine and increase its exposure to potential carcinogens. As a result, individuals who don't exercise regularly run a greater risk for developing colorectal cancer. Furthermore, this lack of exercise may contribute to a heavier body weight, and this combination of factors may increase an individual's risk for developing colorectal cancer.

Similar to breast cancer, heredity is an extremely important layer in determining one's risk for colorectal cancer. To the extent possible, every individual should know her or his family history as it pertains to this cancer. And once again, the most important family medical history is that regarding our first-degree relatives. If one's parent, sibling or child has a history of colorectal cancer, one's risk for also developing the disease becomes three times higher than the average individual.[316]

Indeed, families with such a history share a dominant pattern of inherited susceptibility, not only for colorectal cancer, but for developing intestinal polyps as well. As in the case of breast cancer, researchers have identified the mutated genes responsible for two conditions that may lead to colorectal cancer. The first condition is **familial adenomatous polyposis,** or **FAP**, a rare inherited condition, characterized by many, even thousands, of large intestinal polyps that frequently progress to cancer.[317] The second is called **nonpolyposis colon cancer,** or **HNPCC**, which is related not only to the development of colon tumors, but also to the development of tumors in other organs in family members often before the age of fifty.[318]

Similar to breast cancer, HNPCC is linked to two specific genes, which in this case are known as **MLH1** and **MSH2**. These two genes are actually **mismatch repair genes**, the function of which is to prevent DNA from making mistakes during replication. A family history of either condition is strongly indicative of a genetic predisposition to colorectal cancer that must be heeded. Lastly, women who develop colorectal cancer, which is believed to be the result of hereditary factors, also appear to have an increased risk for developing endometrial cancer at a later time in their lives.[319]

Colorectal cancer has many symptoms that may lead to early detection of the disease. These include any bleeding from the rectal area or any alteration of one's bowel habits. This refers to any unexplained diarrhea or constipation, or a feeling that the bowels aren't eliminating properly or completely. Abdominal cramping or bloating, an unexplained weight loss or anemia, also are classic symptoms of colorectal cancer.

If any of these symptoms should arise, there are many procedures available to help determine if the cause is cancerous or pre-cancerous. Among these are the seigmoidoscopy, colonoscopy, fecal occult blood test, CT scan, magnetic resonance imagery or MRI, and barium x-ray. Some of these procedures should be conducted on a regular basis for individuals over the age of fifty and on a regular basis for those under the age of fifty who have a prior personal or family history of colorectal cancer. It's important to note that the mortality rates for colorectal cancer have decreased recently for both males and females in many countries around the world. This decrease, however, is probably not a reflection of decreased incidence rates, but rather the result of early detection afforded to individuals by these procedures.

If colorectal cancer is detected in an individual, the treatment will usually involve one or more procedures including surgery, chemotherapy and radiation.

Harmful:	Helpful:
Diet	**Diet**
Animal Fat	Antioxidants
Well Done Meats	Folic Acid
Excess Body Weight	Calcium
Inadequate Exercise	Vitamin D
Heredity	NSAIDs

Chapter 12:
Esophageal Cancer–Silent

Among women and men around the world, cancer of the esophagus is the ninth and sixth most common cancer respectively. It also is an extremely dangerous and difficult disease as it's one of the "silent" cancers that all too often aren't detected until it's far advanced. As a result, this cancer is the seventh most deadly cancer among women and the fifth most deadly among men. While esophageal cancer isn't one of the most common cancers in the United States among women or men, it is, nevertheless, the seventh most deadly among American men.

The esophagus is a vital component of the human digestive system. It's a tube about ten inches long that extends from the back of the throat all the way down to the stomach. As food enters the esophagus, esophageal muscles begin a series of wave-like motions called **peristalsis** to move the food into the stomach.[320] The muscle that encircles the lower part of the esophagus near the stomach is critical in this process. This valve-like sphincter allows food to enter the stomach when it relaxes and opens. When it closes, food is prevented from flowing back, or regurgitating, into the esophagus.

Most esophageal tumors form in the middle and lower part of the esophagus and, unfortunately, most of these tumors are malignant. Further, because esophageal cancer is usually in an advanced stage of development by the time it's diagnosed, the rate of survival is low. And while it isn't a common cancer, it is particularly virulent, especially among males who are twice as likely to develop this cancer as women. In particular, males who drink or smoke heavily and are fifty to sixty years old have the greatest risk for developing this deadly cancer.[321]

As is the case with many cancers, esophageal cancer can affect either the outer skin cells of the esophagus or the deeper tissues. If only the outer cells of the esophagus are affected, the disease is called a squamous cell cancer, or cancer of the skin. If, however, the deeper tissues of the organ or gland are affected, the cancer is referred to as an adenocarcinoma– "adeno" simply meaning gland.

Among the western countries of the world, it appears that nearly eighty to ninety percent of all squamous cell cancers of the esophagus can be attributed to the use of tobacco and alcohol. While the use of tobacco and alcohol are less of a risk factor when determining one's risk for deep tissue adenocarcinomas of the esophagus, tobacco use remains a prominent layer of risk strongly associated with the development of all esophageal cancers.[322]

Interestingly, the association between esophageal cancer and tobacco use remains constant whether the use is in the form of smoking cigarettes, cigars or pipes.[323] Indeed, one doesn't have to inhale tobacco smoke before the tobacco becomes a health threat. When one smokes cigarettes, cigars and pipes, and to a different degree when one chews tobacco, the residue from the tobacco or from the tobacco smoke comes into contact with the tissues of the mouth. The inside of the mouth is composed of soft, moist tissues called mucous membranes. These membranes absorb certain elements of the tobacco and the smoke and transport this material down into the deeper tissues of the throat, larynx and esophagus.

As one continues to use tobacco and expose oneself to the carcinogens in the product, the harmful materials accumulate in the body tissues. If we apply our Cancer Blueprint, we can understand that this harmful accumulation over time will irritate and weaken the tissues of the esophagus. As a result, the cells of the tissue may become more susceptible to disease, infection and the harmful invasion of free radicals. If this occurs, the cell and its DNA may be damaged which, in turn, may result in the uncontrolled growth of additional damaged cells and cancerous tissue.

It appears that in regions of the world where tobacco use is commonplace, it's the tobacco that's most closely associated with the incidence rate of esophageal cancer. Yet, in those regions where the use of alcohol predominates over the use of tobacco, alcohol becomes the greatest risk factor. And, of course, when tobacco and excessive alcohol use are combined, the risk becomes significantly greater.[324]

In American studies, hard alcohol appears to carry the greatest risk for developing this cancer, although an excessive intake of beer has been found to contribute to the risk as well. It's clear that when the proof of the alcohol consumed increases, so too does the risk of developing esophageal cancer. As mentioned, it's the home-brewed alcoholic beverages, such as the apple brandies of France, the home-made rum of Puerto Rico, the cachaca of Brazil and the "moonshine" whiskey of the United States that carry an excessively high risk for this cancer.[325]

Indeed, in the United States, approximately ninety percent of African American patients affected with this cancer report drinking moonshine whiskeys on a regular basis. As a result, the rates for esophageal cancer among African American males are unfortunately among the highest in the world.[326]

Although esophageal cancer is more common in men than women, this doesn't necessarily mean that women are inherently less susceptible to this cancer. We know that the use of tobacco greatly increases one's risk for developing esophageal cancer. While tobacco is used by both men and women, its use for women is usually limited to cigarette smoking. On the other hand, cigar, pipe smoking and chewing tobacco are activities associated more typically with men. When all the statistics for tobacco use are combined, therefore, the overall result will probably indicate that the use of tobacco is greater among men than women. Logically, as a result, men overall would share a greater risk for developing this cancer than women.

Similarly, esophageal cancer risk increases with one's use of alcohol, especially the high-proof, home-brewed varieties. We know that men in regions of the world where the consumption of home-brewed alcohol is high have the greatest risk of developing esophageal cancer. This doesn't mean, however, that women are unaffected by these alcohols. Rather, it appears that the brewing and sampling of home-made alcohol around the world are "social" activities more dominated by the men of a community than women. This activity, of course, exposes men to a greater risk for developing esophageal cancer, although women who matched their male counterparts in the consumption of these alcohols would undoubtedly increase their risk as well.

Another factor that's important when discussing the effects of tobacco and alcohol use and the risk of developing esophageal cancer is simple nutrition. Studies indicate that cigarette smoking may contribute to a vitamin C deficiency. Similarly, the excessive use of alcohol has been linked to vitamin deficiencies of A, C, D and the B vitamins.[327] Due to this "leaching" effect, the use of either, and especially the use of both together, depletes the body's nutritional reserves and robs the tissues of necessary nutrients and vitamins. Obviously, therefore, diet plays a significant role in the development of this cancer. Clearly, the regular intake of foods high in the above elements will certainly help the body remain healthy and offer protection from the harmful effects of alcohol and tobacco use.

Additionally, studies that indicate socioeconomic factors play a role in the development of esophageal cancer may simply be the result of the inadequate diets and poor nutrition found in many parts of the world, for the rates of this cancer are far lower in the world's in-dustrialized regions. Indeed, esophageal cancer is the dominant cancer in some parts of the world with rates two hundred times greater than the rates of the United States and other industrialized nations. In regions of China and Iran, for example, where diets are limited and agriculture is impoverished, esophageal cancer rates are endemic.[328]

High rates also are reported in poorer areas of the world where carbohydrates that are deficient in micronutrients are the diet staple and fruits and vegetables are a rarity. Evidence from France, Italy, the United States and Iran offer further support indicating that when con-sumption of food groups like fruits and vegetables is reduced, the risk for esophageal cancer is increased. And the specific nutrients of carotene, ascorbic acid, riboflavin, niacin, thiamin zinc, magnesium, selenium and vitamin C appear to reduce one's risk for this cancer.[329]

Strangely, research also indicates that in less developed countries, the consumption of extremely hot beverages is considered a potential risk factor for esophageal cancer.[330] This is due to the apparent thermal injury that occurs to the tissue of the esophagus when such beverages are consumed. Although this may sound incredible, this too begins to make sense if we once again apply our Cancer Blueprint and examine the associated layers of risk.

First, this research was based only on the populations of some of the less developed regions of the world. In these less developed regions, it's also possible, if not probable, that the diet consumed by individuals living in the region may be deficient in a variety of nutri-ents, vitamins and minerals. As a result, the tissues of the body may be in a weakened condi-tion and susceptible to disease. If the tissues of the throat and esophagus in particular are in a weakened condition, they may be more vulnerable to the irritating effect of extremely hot beverages. And regular, continuous contact with the irritant may weaken the tissue cells to the point where they're incapable of fighting disease and infection. It's at this point that harmful agents may gain access to the individual cells, damage their DNA and begin the process of uncontrolled damaged cell growth.

If we were to add additional layers of risk, such as tobacco use and alcohol abuse, to inadequate diet, then the irritating and scalding effect of the hot beverages and their link to esophageal cancer becomes even easier to understand. Even without these additional layers of risk, however, it's important to remember that in the case of esophageal cancer any continuous problem that introduces irritants to the esophageal tissues, such as acid reflux disease or habitual vomiting due to eating disorders, may set the stage for an invading growth of cancer.

It appears that heredity once again may play a role in the development of esophageal cancer. It's believed that some individuals are more susceptible to the effects of tobacco and alcohol due to racial and hereditary factors. If one is more susceptible to the harmful effects of tobacco and alcohol, it follows that one also would be more susceptible to developing the diseases "caused" by tobacco and alcohol. If so, it may be this suspected genetic link that's responsible, at least in part, for the excess of squamous cell esophageal cancer in African American males compared to similarly affected Caucasian American males.[331]

Symptoms of esophageal cancer include unexplained weight loss, regurgitation of food and vomiting of blood. Difficulty swallowing may be the most obvious symptom, but because swallowing becomes more difficult slowly over a period of time many individuals delay seeking medical advice. For this reason, many cancers of the esophagus that might have been detected early go untreated and spread, making treatment more difficult and less successful. Like all cancers, early detection of esophageal cancer is of key importance to one's survival.

And while esophageal cancer often grows silently and proves deadly, it's one cancer the risk for which can be greatly reduced and possibly prevented through simple adjustments to one's lifestyle. First, by avoiding tobacco use the risk for this cancer drops dramatically. Second, by consuming less alcohol, especially hard alcohol and certainly the home-brewed varieties, the risk drops further. And third, by adding fruits and vegetables whenever possible to one's diet, the rates of incidence and mortality could become some of the lowest of all cancers. If one is diagnosed, however, treatment for this cancer may include surgery, radiation, laser endoscopy and, of course, chemotherapy.

Harmful:	Helpful:
Tobacco Use	Diet
Alcohol Abuse	Antioxidants
Poor Nutrition	
Heredity	

Chapter 13:
Kidney Cancer

The statistics for kidney cancer are similar to those for esophageal cancer in that this cancer is much more common in men than women. Indeed, kidney cancer doesn't even appear as one of the ten most common cancers in incidence or mortality for women. Worldwide figures rank this cancer as the fifteenth most common. Yet, in the United States where sixty percent of kidney cancers occur in men, it's the seventh most common cancer among men and the tenth most deadly.

The kidney is a small organ located in the torso usually right below the waist. Most humans are born with two kidneys whose primary function is to remove excess fluid and waste from the blood. Simply put, blood enters each kidney, then passes through its filtering system. The blood cells, the proteins, large particles and some of the water remain in the bloodstream. Other matter, including a large amount of water, is filtered into a part of the kidney called the tubule. The tubule then decides what portion of this matter will be expelled from the body as urine and what portion will be reabsorbed into the blood and used by the body. Waste products such as uric acid, excess water, salt and calcium will remain in the tubule until it's passed to the bladder to be eliminated as urine. The matter that can be used by the body will be absorbed into the tubules and returned to the bloodstream to nourish the body.[332]

Of malignant kidney tumors, approximately seventy percent develop into renal cell cancer with another fifteen percent developing into renal pelvic cancer. Renal cells are located in the main area of the kidney and accordingly, this is where renal cell cancer develops. Renal pelvic cancer, on the other hand, develops in the lower part of the kidney where urine collects before it enters the ureter. Finally, the ureter is the tube that passes urine into the bladder, and it's this area that's affected by the remaining fifteen percent of kidney tumors.[333]

It's easier to study renal cell kidney cancer than renal pelvic or ureter cancer simply because the former accounts for more than two-thirds of all kidney cancers and the latter two, at fifteen percent each, are considered relatively rare.[334] This makes the collection and analysis of data regarding renal pelvic and ureter cancers more difficult. All three cancers affecting the kidney, however, appear to share a number of risk factors.

Once again, tobacco use is at the top of our list and is considered to be the number one risk factor for developing these cancers. Cigarette smoking in particular is linked to each cancer; however, this link appears to be the strongest with renal pelvis and ureter cancers. Of renal cell cancers, only about thirty percent among men and approximately twenty-five percent among women are attributed to cigarette smoking. Yet, these numbers increase significantly for renal pelvis and ureter cancers with about seventy percent among men and forty percent among women being directly linked to smoking. Surprisingly, however, renal cell carcinoma appears to be linked strongly to the smoking of pipes or cigars, with these smokers sharing a much greater risk for developing this cancer in particular.[335]

Whatever form one's tobacco use takes, the major cancer researchers around the world agree that kidney cancer can best be prevented by eliminating the use of tobacco. If, for example, cigarette smoking alone were eliminated in the United States, approximately one third of all renal cell cancers and more than one half of renal pelvis and ureter cancers could be prevented.[336] This means that the incidence of kidney cancers in the United States would drop by nearly fifty percent simply by eliminating this one layer of risk. Moreover, this figure could increase significantly if tobacco use were eliminated or limited in those regions of the world where smoking is even more commonplace than it is in the United States.

Additionally, the use of analgesics, especially pain relievers that contain phenacetin, also has been linked to renal pelvic and ureter cancers. Similarly, but to a lesser degree, the renal cells in the middle section of the kidney are susceptible to the long-term use of such analgesics. Indeed, the excessive use of these analgesics also has been linked to a fairly rare type of kidney cancer called transitional cell cancer. This type of tumor can occur in the main body of the kidney itself or in the ureter. This rare cancer may account for nearly ten percent of all kidney cancers and is the one kidney cancer that occurs more in women than in men, usually striking women of middle age. In response to this evidence, the United States banned over the counter sales of analgesics containing phenacetin in the late 1970s.[337]

There are additional risks associated with these cancers, which include the use of prescription diuretics that recent studies have linked to the development of renal cell cancer. Renal cell cancer also is believed to be influenced by body weight, a finding supported by virtually all research regarding this cancer. While it appears that this association is more prevalent among women, heavier individuals of both sexes appear to be at a greater risk for developing renal cell cancer.

In contrast, neither renal pelvis nor ureter cancer appears to be affected by an increase in body weight. Renal cell cancer also appears to be linked to one's intake of red meat, with the risk for this cancer increasing as the amount of red meat consumed increases. Further, there is some evidence that asbestos-exposed workers and coke oven workers in steel plants have higher mortality rates for all the kidney cancers, although such occupational studies are difficult to assess because of the relative rarity of renal pelvic and ureter cancer. While the risk factors for these three cancers may differ somewhat, they're similar in that none appear to be affected by beverages such as caffeinated coffee, tea or even alcohol.[338]

Renal cell kidney cancer also appears to be hereditary in some cases. Evidence indicates that individuals affected by an inherited condition known as **von Hippel-Landau disease** are at a greater risk for developing renal cell cancer. Von Hippel-Landau is a medical condition that attacks the capillaries in parts of the brain and interferes with the necessary blood supply. Although the connection is unclear, a relationship does appear to exist between this disease and renal cell carcinoma.[339]

Furthermore, those patients on dialysis and who suffer from late stage renal disease also are at a greater risk for developing renal cell cancer. This finding, of course, is easy to understand if we again apply our Cancer Blueprint. Renal disease affects the renal cells in the middle of the kidney and inhibits the kidney's ability to remove waste products from the blood. It weakens the renal tissues and the renal cells, making them more susceptible to additional disease and infection. In such a weakened state, these cells become vulnerable to invading harmful agents that can damage DNA and lead to cancerous growths.

Although kidney cancer usually strikes men and women of middle age, it also can occur in children. When kidney cancer occurs in children, it's usually a type of cancer called **Wilms' tumor**. This cancer actually accounts for approximately ninety-five percent of all the kidney cancers affecting children under the age of fourteen. It's similar to adult renal cell cancer in that it also affects the child's renal kidney cells and is in essence a "sub-type," or childhood type of renal cell cancer. Most of the children affected by this type of cancer are diagnosed before the age of seven, usually during routine examinations when a mass is felt in the abdomen.[340]

Some of the symptoms associated with kidney cancers include blood in the urine or pain in the flank area, which is the lower side of the back. Any abdominal lump or mass that becomes obvious to touch or sight also should be immediately questioned. And, of course, any unexplained weight loss, unusual fatigue or fever may be indicative of kidney or a number of other cancers.

Treatments for kidney cancers vary from surgery, radiation, chemotherapy and immunotherapy depending upon the type of cancer and the extent to which it has or has not spread.

Harmful:

Tobacco Use

Alcohol Abuse

Analgesics

Phenacetin

Diuretics

Excess Body Weight

Diet

  Red Meat

Asbestos

Heredity

Helpful:

Diet

  Antioxidants

Headline:

French Fries Cause Cancer[341]

Not exactly. An initial study conducted in 2002 concluded that certain foods, including potato chips and French fries, contained a possible carcinogenic substance called acrylamide. Actually, the presence of this substance has less to do with the food itself and more with the way in which the food is prepared. It's believed that acrylamide is formed when asparagine, an amino acid found in certain starches and grains, reacts with sugars when exposed to high heat.

Known as the "Maillard Reaction," this formation can occur not only in foods that are fried but in those that are roasted or baked as well. While baked foods have long been considered healthier than fried foods because they're produced with little or no hydrogenated oils or saturated fats, the amount of acrylamide in some baked foods has been found to exceed the amount found in fried foods.

Indeed, acrylamide is found in significant amounts in a variety of foods, including cereal, bread and bagels, baby food, pre-cooked and processed foods, home cooked meals and even roasted coffee. Acrylamide also is sometimes used for treating water, and as a result, the Environmental Protection Agency in the United States regulates the amount of the substance to remain less than 0.12 micrograms for each eight ounce glass. Unfortunately, there are no similar regulations when it comes to food.

The question remains as to just how harmful acrylamide really is. Until 2004, research conducted with human beings only included the study of acrylamide in regard to cancers of the bladder, colon and kidney and no significant link between a moderate intake of the substance and an increase in these cancers was found. Critics, however, insist that the research should have included cancers of the lung, testicle, breast and uterus because these are the cancers linked to acrylamide intake in animals.

For the moment, the jury is still out as to whether or not acrylamide poses a true cancer risk for humans. Accordingly, this headline is confusing and apparently premature. More research is clearly indicated, and until more is known one can protect oneself simply by 1) consuming more raw vegetables, fruits and nuts; 2) steaming or boiling vegetables if they must be cooked; 3) avoiding deep fried foods and limiting the consumption of processed foods.

Chapter 14:
Leukemia

Worldwide, leukemias are the tenth most commonly occurring cancers. Worldwide, these cancers are the seventh most deadly among men, and the tenth most deadly among women. In the United States, leukemias are the ninth most common cancers and the sixth most deadly among men. Among American women, these cancers are the tenth most common cancers and the seventh most deadly.

Leukemia is the name given to the family of cancers that affect the body's blood-forming tissues, including the bone marrow and the lymph system. Leukemias begin as an abnormal white blood cell, which quickly progresses to more white cells. These abnormal cells eventually reach high concentrations in the bloodstream, bone marrow and lymph system and begin to interfere with the normal functioning of the body's vital organs. At this point, the amount of abnormal white cells is so high that the growth of healthy white blood cells and the production of red blood cells and platelets in the bone marrow are suppressed. An imbalance occurs as these abnormal cells become more and more abundant and the healthy cells become scarce.[342]

As a result, the body's ability to fight infections and harmful agents becomes compromised and the immune system becomes weakened. With an insufficient amount of red blood cells, the vital organs don't receive enough oxygen, and without a healthy amount of platelets the blood looses its ability to clot. Accordingly, individuals with leukemia become susceptible to infections, fatigue, abnormal bleeding and bruising which is, of course, bleeding below the surface of the skin. Unfortunately, without successful treatment, leukemias will prove fatal.

Again, cancers are usually named for the body part in which they begin, and leukemias are classified by the type of white blood cell they affect. All white blood cells are called leukocytes, yet there are three categories of leukocytes that include the granulocytes, the lymphocytes and the monocytes. While new forms of leukemia are constantly emerging and the affect each has on the white blood cells is varied and unpredictable, the most common leukemias affect the granulocytes and lymphocytes. The granulocytes are formed in the bone marrow, and the cancer that affects these cells is called myelocytic or myelogenous leukemia.[343] The lymphocytes are formed in the lymph system as well as the bone marrow, and the cancer that affects these cells is called lymphocytic leukemia.

Leukemias also are classified as "acute" or "chronic." Acute leukemias are those that progress quickly and are characterized by their effect upon the immature white blood cells called "blasts." Chronic leukemias are those that grow more slowly and are characterized by the effect they have upon the mature white blood cells as well as the immature blasts.

There are five major types of leukemias, although several subtypes exist as well. These five, although each is known by several different names, include 1) acute lymphocytic leukemia (ALL), 2) chronic lymphocytic leukemia (CLL), 3) acute myelocytic leukemia (AML), 4) chronic myelocytic leukemia (CML) and, 5) adult T-cell leukemia (ATL). For our purposes we'll refer to these five leukemias as ALL, CLL, AML, CML and ATL. While leukemia accounts for approximately one third of all childhood cancers, it remains largely an adult cancer with ten times more adults being diagnosed with it than children. Although the different leukemias usually strike a specific age group, the common thread is that each of the leukemias strikes and kills more males in each age group than females.[344]

Specific

Acute Lymphocytic Leukemia (ALL)

This cancer is sometimes called "childhood leukemia" because it usually strikes children under the age of fifteen. While the most common cancer among children remains tumors of the brain, one third of childhood cancers are leukemias and the most common of these is ALL. It's acute, therefore it's a leukemia characterized by its effect upon the immature white blood cells called "blasts." It also is lymphocytic, which means it's characterized by the effect it has upon the lymphocytes or white blood cells formed in both the lymph system and the bone marrow. This cancer can develop quickly in a matter of weeks or it can take several months to present itself. As with all leukemias, it reduces the body's ability to protect itself from harmful foreign materials and hinders the blood's ability to clot. As a result, the symptoms include bleeding, bruising, anemia and unexplained fever and infections. Clearly, immediate treatment is necessary, which today may include a combination of chemotherapy, radiation therapy and possibly a bone marrow transplant. It appears that those individuals who are younger and whose white blood cell count is lower at the time of diagnosis have the best chance of being cured. Indeed, treatment of this cancer in children between the ages of two and ten is one of the great success stories in the treatment of any cancer.[345]

Chronic Lymphocytic Leukemia (CLL)

This cancer is the most commonly occurring leukemia among older adults and is rarely seen in individuals under the age of thirty. Indeed, CLL is the most common form of leukemia in the Western world. It's a chronic leukemia, which means that it's a slow growing cancer characterized by its effect upon the mature white blood cells as well as the immature "blasts." It also is lymphocytic, which means the white blood cells formed in the lymph system and the bone marrow are affected. Although all leukemias strike males more often than females, the ratio of males with CLL to females is more pronounced than with other leukemias.

The symptoms of CLL develop slowly in most cases and include fatigue, bleeding, infections and weight loss. Swollen lymph nodes as well as pressure under the left ribs from enlargement of the spleen also may be present. Because of its slow growth, some individuals with CLL may live comfortably for many years, even without treatment. Once treatment begins, however, it may include chemotherapy and the use of corticosteroid drugs. In addition, if the spleen has become too enlarged or begins to interfere with the body's immune functions, its removal through a splenectomy may be advised.[346]

Acute Myelocytic Leukemia (AML)

The most common leukemia among young and middle-aged adults is AML. This again is an acute leukemia and thus grows rapidly. It's a myelocytic leukemia as well, which means it's characterized by the effect it has upon the granulocytes, or immature white blood cells or blasts, formed in the bone marrow. The onset of AML can be rapid and, unfortunately, without immediate treatment it can prove fatal within a matter of weeks. The symptoms include fatigue due to anemia, bruising or unexplained rashes, headaches or seizures and related vision problems. Unexplained weight loss and swollen lymph nodes are always suspect, and in the case of AML, the gums also may become swollen or overgrown. An AML diagnosis typically is based upon a differential count of the white blood cells as well as a complete cell blood count and a bone marrow analysis. The treatment may include chemotherapy, various anticancer drugs and antibiotics, and in some instances a bone marrow transplant.[347]

Chronic Myelocytic Leukemia (CML)

CML is a leukemia that tends to strike middle-aged adults more than any other age group. It's a chronic leukemia that develops and grows slowly. It also is a myelocytic leukemia that again is characterized by its effect upon the granulocytes or immature white blood cells formed in the bone marrow. Known as a "silent" leukemia, approximately one third of all individuals affected by CML experience no outward symptoms of the disease even at the time of diagnosis.

Although CML develops slowly, however, it's characterized by a crisis phase that usually occurs three to five years into the disease's development. This crisis results from a high concentration of blasts in the blood and bleeding under the skin due to a lack of platelets. At this point, CML is extremely resistant to treatment. When symptoms do present in CML, they include fever, infections, anemia, weight loss and swollen lymph nodes. One also may notice pressure or pain under the left ribs from an enlarged spleen, bleeding or the appearance of small red spots on the skin.

If CML, however, develops without presenting noticeable symptoms, its presence may only be suspected when a routine blood test produces abnormal results. Should this be the case, further tests typically will include a differential count of the white blood cells, a complete blood cell count and an analysis of an enzyme called leukocyte alkaline phosphatase. Diagnostic procedures also will include a test to determine if the individual possesses the **Philadelphia Chromosome**, an abnormal chromosome that develops when two different chromosomes break off and then reattach themselves in the other's position, a chromosomal translocation found in approximately ninety-six percent of individuals with CML.[348]

In some cases a bone marrow sample may be taken and, indeed, at one time, CML couldn't be cured without a bone marrow transplant. Today, however, a new drug known as **imatinib mesylate,** or **ST1571,** has been approved as a first line treatment for patients affected by CML. Marketed as Gleevec, this drug works by blocking an abnormal enzyme characteristic of the disease, and when combined with high dose chemotherapy, full body irradiation and additional drugs such as interferon, a bone marrow transplant may not be necessary.[349]

Adult T-Cell Leukemia (ATL)

Unlike other leukemias, ATL is a fairly new cancer only recognized a few decades ago. It also differs from other leukemias in that it appears to be caused by a virus. The virus in this particular case is the previously discussed virus known as human T-cell lymphotropic virus type 1, or HTLV-1. This leukemia is lymphocytic, which again means that it's characterized by its effect upon the white blood cells. ATL, however, differs from the other lymphotropic leukemias in that it only affects the white blood cells of the lymph system and not those of the bone marrow. Specifically, ATL affects the white blood cells derived from the thymus, an organ that's a part of the lymph system.

Again, ATL is named for the part of the body in which it begins, and in this case T-cell stands for those white blood cells formed in the thymus, known also as "helper" cells or "T-helper" cells. These T-cells are an essential part of the body's lymph system and are instrumental in fighting harmful and foreign agents and bacteria. Generally, ATL occurs in "clusters" of individuals and is called "adult" because the virus usually strikes adults and is spread through contact activities typically associated with adults, such as sexual intercourse and intravenous drug abuse.[350]

Individuals of all ages, however, can become infected with ATL through blood transfusions, and children can become infected perinatally or through breast feeding from an ATL-infected mother.[351] The course of treatment for ATL includes a variety of drugs and experimental procedures that may allow an individual to live with the disease for many years yet, because ATL is a fairly new cancer, research on the disease is limited and the long-term prognosis is unfortunately unclear.

General

The environment, both at home and in the workplace, is believed to be one layer of risk that must be considered when examining leukemia. In the case of AML for instance, the incidence increase in males fifty years and older may be due to occupational exposure in industrialized regions. It's believed that the chemical benzene in particular is related to the high rates of AML among certain industrial workers. These individuals were exposed to this chemical through their work in shoe, leather, rubber and chemical manufacturing.[352]

Indeed, early studies estimated the rate of AML among these workers was approximately two to ten times greater than average. The incidence rate for AML also was greater among individuals working in petroleum refineries and chemical plants, as well as those employed as pressmen, printers and painters. Farmers in some regions where the rate of AML is increasing also may be more at risk due to exposures to pesticides used in the care of livestock and crops.[353]

In addition, scientists have long suspected environmental causes of childhood leukemia. This suspicion, however, is difficult to substantiate because cancer in children is still considered fairly rare, with one or two children in 10,000 developing the disease. Nevertheless, there is some evidence that childhood leukemia is linked with parental exposure to chemical or metal manufacturing, hydrocarbons and other occupational factors. Such parental exposures are thought to occur during the child's early fetal development or even before conception.[354]

Moreover, it's believed that childhood exposure to environmental toxins such as pesticides, solvents and other household chemicals is linked to the development of childhood leukemia.[355] Similarly, the environment is always suspect when the cancer rate within a particular region, a particular population or a certain period of time increases noticeably. As previously discussed, these cancer clusters are often associated with environmental conditions such as hazardous waste sites or contaminated groundwater. For example, contaminated water sources from a chemical known as chromium 3 have been held responsible for several cancer clusters that developed in parts of the United States over the last decade.[356]

Specifically, radiation has long been suspect as a significant risk factor in the development of many cancers, including leukemia. Much of the earlier research investigating radiation focused on Japan, for example, where adults and children were exposed to high levels of radiation resulting from the atomic bombs of World War II. There, the leukemia rates increased noticeably in the five years following the exposure. Children, however, who were born to women pregnant at the time of this exposure didn't share this increased incidence rate.[357]

Overall, the evidence concerning the relationship of leukemia and accumulated radiation from nuclear sites and fallout from nuclear weapons remains in controversy. Some studies conducted among children whose exposure to radiation came from fathers employed in the nuclear industry at some time indicated the rates of leukemia increased. Other studies, however, failed to indicate an increase in leukemia in such children.[358]

Similarly, several studies conducted in the United States show there's a relationship between leukemia and nuclear weapon fallout, while other studies dispute this finding. Moreover, additional American studies that focused on 113 counties that bordered sixty-two nuclear plants found no increase in adult or childhood mortality from leukemia compared with control counties. Finally, European countries haven't found increases in childhood leukemia since the 1986 nuclear accident in Chernobyl in the former Soviet Union.[359]

As strange as it sounds, it appears that the harmful effect of ionizing radiation from simple diagnostic procedures such as x-rays is much better documented than the harmful effect of nuclear radiation. This doesn't mean that nuclear radiation is in any way less harmful. It simply may be that nuclear radiation lacks the long-term research that has been afforded other forms of radiation. Clearly, this may change In light of the nuclear emergency that occurred in Japan in 2011.

At this time, however, ionizing radiation remains one of the most extensively studied carcinogens in science and has been associated with every type of leukemia except CLL, which normally targets the adult population.[360] During the 1960s, for example, diagnostic x-ray exposure of women during pregnancy was associated with a fifty percent increase in childhood leukemias. Studies conducted in the decades since, however, indicate the relationship between leukemia and x-ray exposure to be less convincing and, of course, less of an issue now that ultrasound is the preferred diagnostic procedure for monitoring pregnancy.[361]

The link between radiation therapy, or radiotherapy, and different types of leukemia, however, appears to remain constant. Those individuals at risk include patients who have been treated with radiation for ankylosing spondylitis, a chronic inflammatory disease of the spine and joints, and Hodgkin's disease. This risk also applies to women who have been treated for cervical, uterine and breast cancer or for heavy menstrual bleeding due to benign medical conditions.[362]

In contrast, it appears that children who have been treated with radiation for other cancers don't have the same increased risk as their adult counterparts. Children, however, run a greater risk if they've been radiated for fungal infections of the scalp or for large thymuses in infancy. In contrast, radiation from radon exposure doesn't appear to increase the risk in children for developing leukemia and in particular ALL.[363]

Evidence also suggests a hereditary risk factor associated with leukemias as approximately five to ten percent of leukemia patients report other close relatives with leukemia or a similar blood malignancy. Furthermore, most of the acute leukemias such as ALL and AML appear to share a pattern of atypical chromosomal conditions. Indeed, children with Down's syndrome or other conditions involving chromosomal anomalies share an increased risk for developing ALL as well as other leukemias.[364]

Unfortunately, research hasn't yet discovered the genetic or environmental factors responsible for familial leukemias or for the individual chromosomal anomalies linked to leukemia. There are, however, a few cases involving chromosomal anomalies where the anomaly has been linked to exposure from ionizing radiation, benzene, pesticides and drugs in certain chemotherapy treatment.[365]

While cancer clusters have been linked to various environmental conditions over recent decades, "leukemia clusters" have been linked to specific viruses as well. Indeed, the human T-cell lymphotropic virus type 1 was the first human leukemia virus ever discovered.[366] To review, HTLV-1 is a retrovirus that contains its own DNA information. Unlike other viruses, therefore, once HTLV-1 or any other retrovirus enters a normal cell, its DNA becomes integrated into the normal DNA of the host cell. As a result, a retrovirus has the ability to actually change the cellular composition of a human being in a fundamental way.[367]

HTLV-I affects the lymphocytes, which again are the white blood cells that form in the bone marrow and the lymph system. We also know that HTLV-I targets the lymphocytes called T-cells, which are derived from the part of the lymph system called the thymus, an organ located in the neck near the thyroid gland. These T-cells are essential in destroying or neutralizing foreign and harmful cells and substances. When these T-cells are attacked and destroyed, the human body's immune system is severely damaged and becomes susceptible to many diseases, including adult T-cell leukemia.[368]

In this way HTLV-I is similar to the human immunodeficiency virus known as HIV. Both attack and weaken the human body by targeting the "helper" T-cells that are so necessary for the proper functioning of the body's defense system. Additionally, both are spread through intravenous drug abuse, sexual intercourse, blood transfusions, breast-feeding and perinatally from an infected mother to her child.[369]

It appears that HTLV-I is responsible for the leukemia clusters that commonly appear in regional populations of the world, including southern Japan, the Caribbean and parts of Africa. Furthermore, these leukemia clusters also appear in immigrants who have migrated from these regions to other countries of the world, including the United States.[370]

It's an unfortunate fact that certain treatments for various immune-related diseases and some cancers also have been linked to the development of leukemia. Just as excessive radiation exposure to x-ray procedures has been found to be detrimental to the future health of an individual, so too has the use of certain drugs. For example, AML is one leukemia that has been linked with the use of the class of chemotherapy drugs called alkylating agents. While this particular class of drug is useful in the treatment of many cancerous and noncancerous conditions, it also creates a chemical reaction in the body tissue that interferes with cell growth and division.[371]

These alkylating agents often are used in the treatment of an initial primary cancer, such as childhood ALL, yet contribute to the development of a secondary primary cancer such as AML as the individual ages. Similarly, children who have received high doses of topoisomerase inhibitors in primary cancer treatment appear to be at higher risk for a secondary acute myeloid leukemia or AML. Children who have been treated for Hodgkin's disease with some chemotherapy treatments and radiation also have an elevated risk of developing a secondary primary malignancy.[372] There also may be a possible link between some leukemias and the growth hormone chloramphenicol, certain fertility drugs, maternal exposures to some oral contraceptives and diethylstilbestrol or DES.[373] And, while some of these risks have been substantiated, others are only suspected and clearly require further research and study.

The relationship between non-ionizing electrical and magnetic fields and the risk of developing leukemia is another that remains unclear. While many studies fail to support a relationship, once again other studies may indicate a link. For example, research that appears to show that electricians, power line workers and electronics workers exposed to non-ionizing electrical and magnetic fields may share a slight increased risk for AML.

Specifically, this appears to be the case in Canadian and French utility workers who exhibited a small increase in the incidence of AML in certain studies. Additionally, some evidence suggests this small increase in risk may be shared as well by children who have been exposed to residential magnetic fields. It's important to realize, however, that if an increase exists in these cases it's small and, therefore, extremely difficult to substantiate.[374]

Finally, the roles of diet, exercise and cigarette smoking in relation to the development of leukemia are difficult to assess. Unlike some cancers, leukemia doesn't appear to be linked directly with specific dietary factors such as fat intake.[375] It's important, however, to remember that a balanced diet can only help an individual maintain health, protect against illness and help the body fight invading and threatening diseases. The same is true of alcohol. Although there's no evidence of a direct link between alcohol use and leukemia, the "leaching" effect of alcohol can deplete the body of necessary nutrients and vitamins leaving it in a weakened state more susceptible to disease and illness.

Nor is there clear evidence that an association between cigarette smoking and a higher risk for leukemia. This appears to be particularly evident with maternal cigarette smoking before pregnancy and its lacking association with childhood leukemias in offspring. Surprisingly, however, some studies have found an increased risk for childhood leukemia that is linked to the father's prenatal smoking habits.[376]

Once again as with many cancers, the causes of leukemia remain to a large degree unknown. It's a complex malignancy that strikes the fundamental building blocks of the human body. As such, it's a virulent adversary that medical research continues to study in the hope of finding more complete and accurate answers to the many questions it raises.

Of course, the symptoms for leukemia will vary somewhat depending upon the type. There are several, however, that appear to be common to most types including weight loss, fever, fatigue, night sweats and frequent infections.

Harmful:

Environment

    Benzene

    Parental Exposure to Toxins

    Pesticides & Chemicals

    Water Pollution

    Chromium 3

Ionizing Radiation

Heredity

Viruses

    HTLV-1

Alkylating Agents

Drugs

    Chloramphenicol

    Fertility drugs

    Maternal Use of Oral Contraceptives

    Diethylstilbestrol (DES)

Paternal Tobacco Use

Helpful:

Diet

    Antioxidants

Chapter 15:
Lung Cancer

Lung cancer is the most common cancer found throughout the world today. Among the world's women, it's the fourth most commonly diagnosed and the second deadliest. Among the world's men, it's the most commonly diagnosed cancer as well as the deadliest. In the United States, lung cancer is the second most common cancer among both women and men, falling behind breast cancer for women and prostate for men. Lung cancer remains the deadliest cancer among both sexes, claiming more women's lives than breast cancer and more men's lives than prostate cancer. Historically, lung cancer strikes men more often than women, although female deaths from lung cancer are increasing because the numbers of women who smoke tobacco are increasing.

The lungs are a pair of soft, spongy organs located in the human chest area. They're protected on all sides by the rib cage and perform the major function of the respiratory system, which is to provide oxygen to the blood while relieving it of carbon dioxide. The air finds its way to the lungs through the nose and mouth, then through the back of the throat or pharynx, through the voice box or larynx, and down the windpipe or trachea. The trachea branches into two air passages called bronchial tubes that continue to branch into smaller and smaller passages called bronchioles. The smallest of these bronchioles contain air sacs. It's the blood vessels that carry the blood to the air sacs where carbon dioxide is released and oxygen is absorbed.[377]

The human body possesses several defense mechanisms that prevent certain materials from entering the lungs and causing harm. Small hairs found in the nose help filter some of these materials while special cells in the trachea and bronchial tubes continue to catch other foreign material, such as dust and bacteria. When harmful materials invade the lungs, some or all of these defense mechanisms, as well as the organs, may be compromised and may lose their ability to function properly.

While there are at least twenty different types of lung cancer, there are four basic groups into which each can be placed. The first, squamous cell carcinoma, usually arises in the cells lining the large air passages of the lung called the bronchial tubes. This type of lung cancer accounts for about twenty-five percent of lung cancers and like most "squamous" cell cancers, it's one of the easier to identify early because it begins on the surface of the tissue and because it develops in the central part of the lung.[378]

The second type is called adenocarcinoma, a lung cancer that begins in the lining of the smaller air passages or bronchioles. Again, "adeno" means "gland," and this type of lung cancer forms in the gland or deeper tissue of the bronchioles unlike the squamous cell cancer that forms in the surface lining of the bronchial tubes.

Adenocarcinoma of the lung is the most common of the lung cancers. It accounts for about thirty-five percent of all lung cancers and is more difficult to identify at an early stage, not only because it develops in deeper tissues than squamous cell cancer, but also because it develops in the periphery of the lung rather than in the center. It also may spread faster to the lymph glands of the lung, then to the bloodstream, which can then carry the cancer cells to other organs in the body. There also is a subtype of adenocarcinoma of the lung called "bronchioloalveolar" cell carcinoma, which is fairly rare and accounts for only about five percent of all lung cancers. Bronchioloalveolar cell cancer affects the air sacs in the lung and seldom spreads to other parts of the body.[379]

The third type of lung cancer is large cell carcinoma, which also appears in the periphery of the lung and spreads to other parts of the body through the bloodstream. It accounts for about twenty percent of lung cancers, which leaves the fourth type of lung cancer called small cell carcinoma responsible for the remaining percentage.

This last type also is known as "oat" cell carcinoma, so named because it resembles oats under the microscope, and affects the bronchial tubes by compressing them. It's an aggressive cancer, yet because it occurs in the central part of the lung it can be identified at an earlier stage. It also is a cancer that occurs primarily in men who are heavy cigarette smokers.[380]

Indeed, lung cancer is one disease the etiology or "cause" of which has been linked directly to tobacco smoke with cigarette smoking in particular considered the major "cause" of all lung cancers. Smoking was first suspected as a carcinogen in the 1920s and 1930s and is today substantially documented in numerous studies around the world as a leading "cause" of cancer. It's believed to be responsible for about eighty-five percent of all lung cancer deaths in the United States alone.[381]

In fact, in these cases the risk of death from lung cancer is determined by the number of cigarettes smoked each day, the number of years one smokes and even one's inhalation patterns. If one's daily usage is reduced and if one smokes filtered, low tar cigarettes the risk is slightly lowered although it still remains higher than the risk shared by nonsmokers. Once one stops smoking, however, their risk of death from lung cancer drops fifty percent in ten years compared to those who continue to smoke.[382] Furthermore, if one stops smoking after lung cancer has been diagnosed, the risk for developing a second lung cancer is greatly reduced.

Yet, the cancer risk from cigarettes is not exclusive to those individuals who actually smoke, for environmental tobacco smoke or ETS has been shown to increase the risk of developing lung cancer among nonsmokers. It's believed that nonsmokers exposed to ETS or passive smoking experience a lung cancer risk equivalent to smoking one tenth to one cigarette per day. It does appear, however, that the risk of lung cancer for cigar and pipe smokers is lower than cigarette smokers, which may be due, perhaps, to less inhalation of harmful smoke.[383]

As discussed, radon is an inert gas produced from the radioactive decay of the uranium and radium which is found everywhere in the earth's crust. Because radon itself is radioactive, it may "cause" lung cancer. Several studies conducted with underground miners exposed to radon show an increased risk for lung cancer, which becomes greater with the length of each individual's radon exposure. Indeed, such studies suggest that radon may "cause" as many as 24,000 lung cancer deaths each year. Radon also may enter the home environment by seeping through cracks in the foundation of a house, through a sump pump hole or by dissolving in drinking water. Once again, the carcinogenic effect of radon exposure is greater when paired with tobacco smoke, just as the carcinogen effect of asbestos, or alcohol, is greater when paired with tobacco smoke.[384]

In the workplace, indeed, the greatest threat to an individual appears to be exposure to airborne asbestos, which may cause lung cancer, mesothelioma, a cancer of the chest lining, and another lung disease called asbestosis. Occupational conditions are an important consideration when discussing these diseases, and the risk for developing any of them increases greatly for those employed in certain industries, including miners and workers in the shipyard, textile, insulation and cement industries.[385]

Of these three diseases, however, lung cancer is the major disease resulting from asbestos exposure. For example, individuals who worked in United States shipyards during World War II, even for short periods of time, have an increased risk of developing lung cancer from their exposure to asbestos. In addition, other occupational materials that raise concerns and may be associated with an increased risk of lung cancer include chromium, nickel, mustard gas, chloromethyl ethers and inorganic arsenic.[386]

Also of important environmental concern is the role that air pollution plays in the development of lung cancer. Air pollution in general and certain materials in particular have long been suspected as factors in the development of lung cancer, yet establishing a direct link has been difficult to do. One element of air pollution, however, a material called benzo(a) pyrene, does appear to be related to an increased risk for lung cancer.

This substance was researched in the 1980s when excessive rates of lung cancer were noted in China. It was discovered that in both urban and rural areas there was an excessively high level of air pollution found in Chinese homes due to the use of heating and cooking coal, and a major component of that air pollution was the element benzo(a)pyrene. It's believed today that this substance, combined with excessive cigarette smoking, was responsible for China's high rates of lung cancer.[387]

We also know that byproducts produced from fossil fuels, such as the gasoline used to power our automobiles, contribute to air pollution. It hasn't been concluded, however, whether or not these byproducts increase the risk for lung cancer. Once again, the most notable of these byproducts are the polycyclic aromatic hydrocarbons or PAHs. Although PAHs have long been suspected carcinogens, studies haven't conclusively established a link between them and lung cancer. This is because air pollution is caused by many different materials, many of which may be carcinogenic. As a result, it's simply too difficult to isolate only one substance, such as PAHs, and determine its direct effect on the human body and the risk of lung cancer.[388]

Further, ionizing radiation remains a risk factor for lung cancer just as it does for so many other cancers. Over several decades, many studies have been conducted with individuals who have been exposed to high doses of ionizing radiation. Most of these studies conclude that as one's level of exposure to radiation increased, so too did their risk for developing many cancers, including those of the lung. During the intensive studies conducted after World War II among atomic bomb survivors in Japan, the incidence of lung cancer was found to have greatly increased. And, of course, the risk is greater among patients who have received high doses of radiation therapy for both malignant and nonmalignant medical conditions than for patients who have not.[389]

It also is apparent that certain lung ailments and diseases increase an individual's risk for developing lung cancer. Among these is tuberculosis, which can scar the lung tissues and leave them extremely vulnerable to future cancers, a fact that's not surprising if we apply our Cancer Blueprint. In addition, it appears that lung cancer runs in families.[390] At present, no specific gene has been identified with the development of lung cancer. Yet, certain noncancerous diseases of the lungs can indicate a particular weakness in the tissues. This particular weakness may be genetic, and if so, one with a family history of lung diseases may be more susceptible to cancer of the lung as well as other diseases such as tuberculosis.

While there are many layers of risk associated with lung cancer, however, there also now exists strong evidence to suggest that dietary factors may help offset those risks. It's believed that many vitamins, including vitamins A, C, E and selenium, offer a protective effect against lung cancer. Beta-carotene is also thought to reduce one's risk for developing lung cancer. This evidence is most consistent in studies that examine the link between lung cancer and the consumption of fresh fruits and vegetables, including the yellow and orange foods such as carrots and sweet potatoes and the dark green, leafy foods such as spinach and broccoli.[391]

Indeed, the risk in those individuals who consumed the greatest amounts of these foods was reduced by fifty percent compared with those who consumed the least amounts. It isn't completely clear, however, if it's the beta-carotene that is responsible for this risk reduction or if it's another element of the food or another carotenoid found in the food that's responsible.[392] Regardless of which element offers this protective effect, it's astounding that a higher intake of fruits and vegetables actually helps decrease the risk for a malignancy that more often than not is "caused" primarily by cigarette smoking.

The symptoms of lung cancer may include difficulty in breathing with a shortness of breath, chest pain or hoarseness when speaking. A persistent cough with discharge or the coughing up of blood also are possible signs of lung cancer. In addition, any unexplained fever, weight loss or loss of appetite should be questioned and immediately investigated.

If lung cancer has been diagnosed, there are three treatment options that vary according to the type of lung cancer. Individuals with squamous cell, large cell or adenocarcinoma of the lung may be candidates for surgery if the cancer hasn't spread to other parts of the body. This surgery would probably include removal of the affected lung. In cases where removal isn't possible, laser surgery may be performed. If the cancer is small cell carcinoma, which spreads quickly, or any of the other three types that has also already spread, treatment will probably include chemotherapy, radiation or a combination of the two.

Harmful:	Helpful:
Tobacco Use	Diet
Heredity	Antioxidants
Radon	Vitamins A, C & E
Asbestos	Selenium
Air Pollution	Beta-carotene
Benzo(a)pyrene	
Polycyclic Aromatic Hydrocarbons (PAHs)	
Ionizing Radiation	

Headline:

Beta-Carotene May Increase Risk of Lung Cancer[393]

Wait a minute! Beta-carotene is supposed to be good for us. Right? So, when we encounter claims like this that appear to fly in the face of common sense, we need to dig a little deeper to see what's really going on. First, numerous studies have been conducted to determine the beneficial effect of vitamin A and beta-carotene on human health. As these studies confirm, it's difficult to isolate the nutrients of a food known to offer protection from disease.

It's not completely clear if the beta-carotene in a carrot, for example, is the primary beneficial nutrient or not. It's not clear if beta-carotene offers protection by itself or if it must be combined with other nutrients to be beneficial. It's not clear if beta-carotene helps prevent lung cancer in cigarette smokers or not. It's even less clear that beta-carotene supplements provide protection from certain cancers and other diseases. Yet, the headline in question is disturbing as it states that beta-carotene actually may increase one's risk for lung cancer.

The first step in analyzing this particular statement is to understand the difference between a "primary prevention" study and a "secondary prevention" study. In the former, research is conducted among individuals who are generally representative of the population, relatively healthy and who don't exhibit any obvious pre-existing risk for the disease under investigation. In the latter, research is conducted upon individuals who are already at an increased risk for developing the disease under investigation. While primary prevention studies may be preferable in many cases, the decades of data they require often make them impractical. As such, secondary prevention studies are typically more common.

In this case, the studies in question were secondary prevention studies conducted upon individuals who smoked. These individuals, therefore, already had an increased risk for developing lung cancer. In addition, the studies involved beta-carotene in the form of supplements rather than natural beta-carotene commonly found in produce. We also know that any benefit gained from supplemental beta-carotene is less clear than any benefit gained from natural beta-carotene. So, let's review. First, we're not really sure if natural beta-carotene in and of itself is the source for the benefits found in fresh fruits and vegetables. We're less sure about any possible benefit derived from supplemental beta-carotene. Second, natural beta-carotene in itself isn't known to increase the risk for lung cancer within the general population. Similarly, beta-carotene in supplemental form is not known to increase the risk for lung cancer within the general population. Third, as the study suggests, beta-carotene in supplemental form *may* increase one's risk for the disease if the individual already smokes. Or, beta-carotene in supplemental form *may* be rendered ineffectual if the individual already has an increased risk for lung cancer due to smoking.

In any event, this particular headline is misleading. Clearly, further evidence is necessary to substantiate this particular claim. Yet in the meantime, to be safe one should simply stop smoking and eat more fresh fruits and vegetables.

Chapter 16:
Non-Hodgkin's Lymphoma

Non-Hodgkin's lymphoma is the ninth most commonly occurring cancer among men throughout the world and the tenth most deadly. In the United States, it's the fifth most common cancer among women and the sixth deadliest. Among American men, non-Hodgkin's is the fifth most common cancer and the ninth deadliest.

To begin, lymphomas are cancers of the lymph system. The lymph system includes the spleen and the lymph glands, located throughout the body and connected by small blood vessels called lymphatics. Although lymphomas include a diverse group of diseases, they're usually classified as either Hodgkin's disease or non-Hodgkin's disease or lymphoma.

Non-Hodgkin's lymphoma, or NHL, affects the white blood cells of the human immune system. As discussed in our section on leukemias, the white blood cells are called leukocytes, which are divided into three groups, including granulocytes, lymphocytes and monocytes. All white cells defend the body against foreign matter. Two of these groups, the granulocytes and monocytes, respond to many different types of infection by engulfing the harmful material. The third type called lymphocytes are the white cells that only react to specific infectious agents. The lymphocytes contain B-cells that produce antibodies and T-cells that attack foreign and virus-ridden cells.[394]

It's the abnormal growth of these lymphocytes that characterizes all lymphomas, and in this case, non-Hodgkin's lymphoma. The tumors that arise in these lymphocytes as a result of NHL are classified according to their size. The level of aggressiveness of the malignant cells, which includes low grade, intermediate grade and high grade, also categorizes them. It differs from Hodgkin's disease in that it's far more common and often occurs in older individuals.[395]

Again, individuals who experience immunosuppression are at a greater risk for developing NHL than others. As mentioned, this includes those who have AIDS or are HIV positive, and those who have had organ transplants. Indeed, NHL is sixty to one hundred times more common in AIDS patients than in the general population, a fact related to the significant increase in NHL in many countries including the United States. AIDS, however, doesn't explain the increase of NHL before the AIDS epidemic surfaced, or the increase that continues in the absence of HIV infection.[396]

There are other immunodeficiency conditions related to this increase, including those that are both genetically and medically induced. Specifically, those who have undergone kidney transplants develop NHL forty to one hundred times more frequently than the general population.[397] Ironically it appears, therefore, that the advances in medical technology that have made life-saving organ transplants more common and accessible also may be a contributing factor to the increase in NHL.

In addition, viruses have been linked to the development of non-Hodgkin's lymphoma. In particular, HTLV-1, the retrovirus associated with certain types of adult T-cell leukemias, has been linked to the risk for and development of NHL. This virus, however, typically found in parts of the Caribbean and Africa, southern Japan and the southeastern United States, isn't believed to be a factor in the widespread increase of non-Hodgkin's. In contrast, the Epstein-Barr virus, or EBV, is believed to be a strong factor in the development of Burkitt's lymphoma, a childhood cancer common in central Africa. It also appears that when individuals who have acquired or genetic immunosuppression become infected with EBV, they develop a greater risk for non-Hodgkin's lymphoma as well. Whether or not a relationship exists between the Epstein-Barr virus and non-Hodgkin's lymphoma for the general population remains a matter still under investigation.[398]

Non-Hodgkin's lymphoma is greatly influenced by several factors found in the workplace environment. Many studies, for example, have found a strong association between the use of pesticides, herbicides and insecticides and a high incidence rate of NHL. Among the most potent of these products is 2,4-D, an herbicide the use of which is associated with a great increase in the rate of non-Hodgkin's lymphoma.[399]

For example, research conducted in farming communities in the United States, Sweden and Canada indicates the risk of developing NHL among farmers who used 2,4-D increased as much as eight times. Yet, the danger isn't confined to humans. Evidence also indicates that canine malignant lymphoma is greater in dogs whose owners use 2,4-D or commercial pesticide lawn treatments. Similarly, individuals who handle grain increase their risk for developing non-Hodgkin's lymphoma by approximately five times simply through their exposure to pesticides, organic solvents and grain dusts in the course of their work.[400]

Unfortunately, an increased risk for NHL isn't confined to the agricultural workplace. Other occupational workers who share a greater risk include rubber workers, vinyl chloride workers, chemists, petroleum refiners, dry cleaners and aircraft maintenance workers. While the specific industrial compounds responsible for this increase among such occupations haven't been identified, it's important to note that all share a workplace exposure to organic solvents.[401]

Many of us may recall reports of the last few years that claimed hair dyes "caused cancer" and that their use should be discontinued. As strange as it sounds, this is still a subject of controversy that needs to be clarified on several points. In studies conducted in the late 1980s and early 1990s, evidence linking hair dyes with lymphatic cancers such as non-Hodgkin's lymphoma was first reported. It appeared that individuals who used dark colored dyes over long periods of time or those exposed to hair coloring products through their occupations shared an increased risk for NHL that was two to four times greater than the general population.[402]

These studies, however, weren't conducted to examine hair-coloring products. They were conducted for other reasons, and this possible link was found entirely by accident. This means that the results of these studies lacked the professional detail and follow-up essential to determining a link, if any, exists. It's a fact that hair-coloring products sometimes contain compounds that can be carcinogenic and harmful to animals, yet the role these products play in the development of NHL and other lymphatic malignancies in humans hasn't been substantiated.[403]

One study conducted in the United States by the Federal Drug Administration found one substance known to be a human carcinogen called 4-ABP in some of the hair dye being tested. This substance, however, isn't an ingredient of hair dyes. Rather, this ingredient appears to be a by-product of the chemical process associated with the production of some dyes. If so, the issue is not whether such products contain carcinogens, but if the production or oxidizing process associated with the products can contaminate them in such a way as to produce carcinogens.

In 2004 a new study was published that once again questioned the safety of dark hair coloring products and linked their use to the development of bladder cancer, as well as non-Hodgkin's lymphoma. Yet, this study observed only women, and only women who used these products prior to 1980. This is important because in 1979 the formula for hair dyes was substantially changed by the industry in an effort to remove all suspicious substances from the products.[404] So, even if some relationship between cancer and hair dyes was suspected at the time, that suspicion would no longer be substantiated. Furthermore, many other factors could have contributed to this particular finding. For, indeed, additional studies conducted by institutions, including the American Cancer Society and Harvard University, have found no increased risk for cancer from the use of these products.

The carcinogens that some believe may be linked to hair dyes belong to a class of chemicals known as the aromatic amines. We know that the human body is usually able to detoxify these chemicals.[405] Yet, some humans lack the genetic ability to do so, and these individuals may, indeed, account for the findings of some studies that have linked hair dyes in the past to certain malignancies. Similar to much cancer research, this subject remains a tangled web of controversy. It's important, however, to continue the investigation of this possible risk as nearly sixty percent of women, ten percent of men and a growing number of teenagers and young adults continue to use hair-coloring products on a regular basis.

The symptoms of non-Hodgkin's lymphoma can occur over a period of time or they can appear quite suddenly. A slow onset of NHL may be characterized persistent fatigue, loss of appetite, fever and night sweats or chills. There also may be swelling of the lymph nodes and the abdomen. On the other hand, emergency symptoms of NHL may include a sudden, spiking fever, numbness in the arms and legs, incontinence and an unexplained mental confusion or drowsiness. In addition, a swollen abdomen may be the result of severe constipation, which also may indicate the presence of NHL.

If non-Hodgkin's lymphoma is suspected, it can be diagnosed through blood and urine tests, abdominal scans and a biopsy of the bone marrow. NHL may be treated by surgery to reduce the size of an existing tumor, chemotherapy and radiation therapy.

Harmful: **Helpful:**

Immunosuppression   **Diet**

Viruses   **Antioxidants**

   HTLV-1

   Epstein-Barr (EBV)

Environment

   Pesticides, Herbicides, Insecticides

   2,4-D

   Organic Solvents

   Grain Dusts

Chapter 17:
Ovarian Cancer–Silent

Ovarian cancer is the sixth most common cancer affecting women the world over with the highest rates during the last few decades occurring in the Scandinavian countries. It also is the eighth deadliest cancer among the world's women. In the United States, it remains the eighth most common cancer among women and the fifth most common cause of cancer death. Moreover, ovarian cancer is one of the "silent" cancers, which is usually in an advanced stage of development by the time it's discovered.

The ovaries are a pair of almond-shaped glands located in the abdomen, slightly above and to the side of the uterus, about five inches below the waist. The ovaries store the egg cells and also produce the female sex hormones estrogen and progesterone. Cancer of the ovaries usually occurs in the epithelial cells that surround the ovaries. Epithelial cells are those that cover the internal and external organs of the body. They're arranged in layers and are bound together by connective tissues. When cancer attacks these cells, both ovaries appear to be involved in about one third of the reported cases.[406]

Although there are always exceptions, ovarian cancer generally affects women over fifty and have experienced menopause. Ovarian cancer shares many of the same layers of risk with other cancers that affect women, including breast cancer. Indeed, reproductive and menstrual factors appear to be the greatest influences affecting a woman's chances for developing ovarian cancer. The risk is greatest for women who experience difficulty getting pregnant and for those who have never conceived.[407]

In contrast, women who have experienced three or four full-term pregnancies share about half the risk for ovarian cancer than women who have had none. This risk, in fact, appears to decrease about fifteen percent with each full-term pregnancy and decreases to a lesser degree with each incomplete pregnancy. Additionally, the risk for women who breastfeed their children decreases as the length of time women breastfeed increases.[408]

In the case of ovarian cancer, women who use oral contraceptives also reduce their risk by approximately five to ten percent for each year of use. The reproductive events in a woman's life that don't appear to increase her risk for ovarian cancer include her age at the birth of her first child, and her age at the start of menstruation or menopause. Nor does it appear that the risk for ovarian cancer increases for women who have undergone estrogen or hormone replacement therapy.[409]

Other layers of risk for ovarian cancer include a woman's medical history and the medical history of her family. As mentioned, the risks for ovarian cancer are similar to the risks for breast cancer, and for a woman who has already experienced breast cancer her risk for developing ovarian cancer as well may be increased by as much as seventy percent. This relationship between breast and ovarian cancer may be traced to the BRCA-1 and BRCA-2 genes. For an inherited anomaly in one or both not only increases a woman's risk for breast cancer, it also increases a woman's risk for ovarian cancer according to various sources by as much as twenty to fifty percent.[410] The syndrome HNPCC discussed in our section on colorectal cancer also poses an increased risk for ovarian cancer.[411]

This, of course, is of great significance when compared to the general female population, which has a one to two percent chance of developing ovarian cancer. Additionally, women whose mothers or sisters have had ovarian cancer share a risk that's three to five times greater than average for developing the disease themselves.[412]

As always, there's much speculation about diet and the risk it poses in relation to ovarian cancer. Evidence appears to suggest that a high fat diet may slightly increase a woman's risk for developing the disease.[413] There's another theory that women who lack the ability to metabolize glucose properly may have a greater risk as well, although this hasn't been supported by significant studies. Other dietary factors, including one's consumption of alcohol, coffee or even tobacco use, don't appear to have any relationship to a woman's risk for developing ovarian cancer.[414]

Additional factors associated with ovarian cancer risk include certain medical procedures, such as a tubal ligation or hysterectomy.[415] Indeed, both procedures appear to decrease a woman's risk for developing ovarian cancer, as well as providing her with a permanent method of birth control. A tubal ligation is a procedure in which a woman's fallopian tubes are blocked to prevent the eggs from passing from the ovaries to the uterus. A hysterectomy involves removing a woman's uterus, cervix and, in some cases, the ovaries. It doesn't appear to matter, however, whether the ovaries are removed or not with this procedure. In either case a woman's risk for ovarian cancer is decreased although the reasons for this decrease aren't fully understood.[416]

Finally, certain personal hygiene rituals may impact the risk for this disease. For example, there has been concern that the use of talcum powder in the perineal area may contribute to some cases of ovarian cancer.[417] If our Cancer Blueprint is applied, this particular concern may be easier to understand. It's possible that products we use on our bodies may cause irritations and even infections. If the product is used over a period of time, certain tissues may be exposed to irritants on a regular basis, which in turn may make those tissues more susceptible to future infections or disease.

It also is possible that products used externally on these tissues may find their way into the body cavities causing further irritation or infection and leaving the tissues vulnerable to attack by harmful elements. Yet, it's important to remember that if there is a causal relationship between products such as talcum powder and ovarian cancer, it's slight, and the number of cases that might be attributed to such factors is small.[418]

As one of the "silent" cancers, ovarian cancer produces few noticeable symptoms in the early stages and, unfortunately, the disease is often in an advanced stage of development by the time of diagnosis. As this cancer grows, however, it's possible for it to produce mild symptoms, including abdominal swelling and bloating or intermittent pelvic pain, symptoms that require serious attention and immediate follow-up with a pelvic exam. Indeed, most diagnoses of ovarian cancer are usually the unexpected result of routine pelvic exams. If an ovarian tumor is suspected during this exam, either a CT scan or an ultrasound test can confirm the suspicion. Yet, it's important to know that only one out of four ovarian tumors is cancerous.

If cancer is confirmed, treatment will involve surgery. Such surgery may be minimal with the removal of only the affected ovary and its fallopian tube. The advantage of this surgery is that it allows women of childbearing age to become pregnant in the future should they choose to do so. Unfortunately, because most ovarian cancers affect both ovaries, the required surgery usually involves the removal of the ovaries, the fallopian tubes and the uterus. Further, if the cancer has spread, the nearby lymph glands and tissue may be removed as well as sample fluid and tissue from the abdomen.[419] A combination of chemotherapy drugs and, in rare cases radiation therapy, also may be a part of a woman's complete treatment program for this cancer. And while such treatment may sound overwhelming and frightening, it's exactly this type of aggressive new surgery and follow-up therapy that's increasing the survival rate of women the world over diagnosed with ovarian cancer.

Harmful:

Difficulty Conceiving

Never Having Been Pregnant

Heredity

   BRCA I & BRCA II

   HNPCC

Diet

   Excess Fat

Possible Hygiene Habits

Helpful:

Full Term Pregnancies

Breastfeeding

Use of Oral Contraceptives

Tubal Ligation

Hysterectomy

Chapter 18:
Pancreatic Cancer–Silent

Pancreatic cancer is the thirteenth most commonly diagnosed cancer worldwide. It is the ninth most deadly among the world's women and the seventh most deadly among the world's men. In the United States, it's the tenth most common cancer among men and the fourth deadliest. While it is not among the most common cancers affecting American women, it is the fourth most deadly. This cancer affects men more than women and is uncommon before the age of forty. It usually strikes individuals around the age of seventy, and unfortunately, it also is one of the "silent" cancers that often remain undiagnosed until in an advanced stage of development.

The pancreas lies horizontally behind the lower part of the stomach. The pancreas, which is actually two glands, manufactures important secretions vital to the proper functioning of other body parts. First, as an exocrine gland, the pancreas produces and secretes digestive enzymes and alkaline agents. Together, these materials enable the pancreas and small intestine to break down nutrients that are then absorbed into the bloodstream. Second, as an endocrine gland, the pancreas produces and secretes the hormones insulin and glucagon that also are absorbed into the bloodstream and aid in the digestion of carbohydrates and fats.[420]

As a "silent" cancer pancreatic cancer, like ovarian cancer, usually remains asymptomatic until it's well advanced. Although this cancer will eventually present itself through weight loss and abdominal pain, the pancreas remains virtually an inaccessible part of the human body that makes diagnosis and treatment fairly difficult. The stage at which this cancer is diagnosed is in part determined by the part of the pancreas that's affected.

As mentioned, the exocrine gland of the pancreas produces the enzymes that aid in digestion. This gland, and the bulk of the pancreas, is composed of acinar cells, and when cancer strikes these cells, chances are the disease won't produce noticeable symptoms until late in its development. If, however, the cancer develops in an area of the pancreas situated near the common bile duct, a blockage may occur that may lead to a condition called jaundice. Jaundice is a noticeable yellowing of the skin and should this occur it might be the one symptom that alerts the individual to the dangerous condition and allows the cancer to be diagnosed at an early and hopefully treatable stage.[421]

Jaundice also may occur if the cancer occurs in the islet cells of the pancreas. These cells produce hormones that regulate several different bodily functions including blood sugar levels and the production of stomach acid. In addition to jaundice, therefore, this type of cancer also may produce diabetes-type symptoms such as high blood sugar. These symptoms, when combined with the typical weight loss or anorexia that occurs with many cancers, make islet cell pancreatic cancer easier to diagnose and accordingly, more survivable.[422]

Unfortunately, little is known about the causes of pancreatic cancer. It appears, however, that dietary and environmental factors may play a major role. First, there appears to be a link between pancreatic cancer and high fat diets. A diet high in fatty foods, such as meats and butter creates a higher risk for developing this cancer than a diet rich in foods such as fruits and vegetables.[423] This is easier to understand when we consider the fact that the endocrine gland of the pancreas is responsible for the digestion of fats and carbohydrates. As one's fat intake increases, the pancreas is forced to work harder to digest this increase. If this high intake of fat continues over a period of many years, the pancreas may reach a point where it becomes overworked and exhausted.

Similar to the physical body itself, once the pancreas or any living tissue becomes exhausted, it becomes weakened and more susceptible to invading infection and disease. Of course, another risk factor associated with a high fat diet may include an increase in body weight. And, if a lack of physical exercise is added to the equation, we have three factors that exacerbate one another and further complicate the harmful effects of a high fat diet.

Furthermore, research indicates that urban populations experience higher rates of pancreatic cancer than rural populations. This isn't surprising if we remember that the dietary habits of urban and industrialized regions typically include foods higher in fat such as meats and dairy products. We also know that a high fat diet is a significant risk factor for pancreatic cancer. If we compare the incidence rates of this cancer around the world, the highest rates occur among African Americans and the Maoris of New Zealand while the lowest rates occur in India and Thailand.[424]

Of course, this fact may be related to hereditary and environmental factors as well as diet, yet evidence also suggests that certain population groups such as the Seventh Day Adventists who consume more foods like beans, lentils and peas exhibit low rates of pancreatic cancer. Indeed, such foods are not only lower in fat, but they contain "protease inhibitors" which appear to provide protection from possible carcinogens. In addition to dietary fat, there's always concern about the effects of alcohol, coffee and tea and their relationship to various cancers. Yet, a link between these beverages and the risk for pancreatic cancer hasn't been confirmed and remains inconsistent at best.[425]

Certain environmental factors, however, have been more consistently linked to the risk for and the development of pancreatic cancer. In particular, the workplace environment appears to play an important role. For example, workers exposed to petroleum share a higher incidence rate for pancreatic cancer. Also, individuals who work as leather tanners, chemists, auto mechanics or manufacturers of photographic film and are exposed to certain chemicals have a higher risk for developing pancreatic cancer.[426]

There also are pre-existing medical conditions that may contribute to the growth of pancreatic cancer. One such condition is cirrhosis of the liver, a condition brought about by infection, disease or poison in which the tissue of the liver is irreversibly and progressively destroyed. When cirrhosis enters the cancer equation, other body parts such as the pancreas are forced to work harder to compensate for the liver's inability to function properly. This additional workload may again exhaust the pancreas, leaving it vulnerable and susceptible to disease, including cancer.[427]

Ironically, however, studies have shown that other medical conditions, including those that affect the pancreas directly such as pancreatitis, haven't been shown conclusively to contribute to the risk for pancreatic cancer. Similarly, some studies have been unable to establish a conclusive link between diabetes mellitus, a complex disorder of carbohydrate, fat and protein metabolism that directly affects the pancreas and pancreatic cancer.[428] Yet, other sources indicate that within three years of a diabetes diagnosis middle aged and older individuals may experience a risk for pancreatic cancer that is eight times greater than nondiabetic individuals.[429] Recent studies also have confirmed that a history of *chronic* pancreatitis does appear to carry an increased risk for developing pancreatic cancer.[430]

As with many cancers, however, the most important layer of risk for pancreatic cancer once again appears to be cigarette smoking. This use of tobacco is the only dominant risk factor whose link has been consistently established time and time again in cancer studies throughout the world. Indeed, individuals who smoke cigarettes share twice the risk for developing pancreatic cancer than individuals who don't smoke. Moreover, the risk is also greater for individuals who habitually smoke cigars rather than cigarettes, another indication that tobacco smoke doesn't need to be inhaled to pose a serious health threat.[431]

In addition to jaundice, weight loss and abdominal pain, the symptoms of pancreatic cancer also may include back pain, a lack of appetite, nausea and vomiting. Among these the most significant are, of course, jaundice and an unexplained weight loss that may average about twenty-five pounds. An ultrasound or CT scan may help determine if pancreatic cancer exists, as will a biopsy and microscopic examination of a sample of the pancreatic tissue. Ultimately, if a malignant tumor is found, it may be surgically removed if it hasn't spread or invaded nearby tissues. If surgery isn't advisable, chemotherapy and radiation may be. An **endoscopic retrograde cholangiopancreatography,** or **ERCP,** also may be used to clear any obstruction of the pancreas when surgery isn't an option. Finally, any pain resulting from this type of cancer can be controlled by a strong regimen of analgesics or by a celiac ganglionic block, which deadens the nerves leading to the pancreas.

Harmful:

Diet

    Excess Fat

    Excess Body Weight

    Inadequate Exercise

Environment

    Urban Societies

    Petroleum Exposure

    Chemicals

Tobacco Use

Medical Conditions

    Cirrhosis of the Liver

    Certain diabetes

    Chronic pancreatitis

Helpful:

Diet

    Antioxidants

Pro-tease Inhibitors

Chapter 19:
Prostate Cancer

Second only to lung cancer, prostate cancer is the most commonly diagnosed cancer among the world's men. It also is the sixth leading cause of cancer deaths among the world's men. In the United States, prostate cancer, which typically strikes men at the average age of seventy-two, is the most commonly diagnosed cancer and the second deadliest after lung cancer.[432]

The prostate gland is located in the pelvis at the base of the penis. It lies just under the bladder and surrounds the urethra, the tube that passes urine from the bladder out of the body. The prostate produces seminal fluids that play an important part in reproduction by protecting sperm after ejaculation and ensuring survival of the sperm within the female vagina. As men grow older, the prostate often becomes enlarged, a condition called hyperplasia, causing a variety of symptoms that range from simply annoying to severe.

Because of the location of the prostate gland, one of the first noticeable symptoms of an enlarged prostate is the inability to urinate properly. As the prostate grows, it puts pressure on the urethra, inhibiting the flow of urine into the urethra from the bladder. Such symptoms, however, may be caused by a benign enlargement of the prostate as well as a cancerous enlargement. In fact, the prostate enlargement that commonly occurs as men get older doesn't lead to cancer. It's important, therefore, to determine the difference as soon as possible to avoid allowing a cancerous condition time to spread.[433]

The cause of prostate cancer is unknown, although there are several suspected factors that appear to increase one's risk for the disease. First, heredity once again appears to play a major role. If one is impacted by the BRCA I and II genes (the same genes implicated in breast and ovarian cancer for women) one is at a greater risk for developing prostate cancer.[434] If an individual's parents, siblings, children or "first-degree relatives" develop this cancer, the individual and other male family members may share an increased risk for the disease.[435]

In this case, men who have fathers or brothers who have been diagnosed with prostate cancer, especially if these relatives where diagnosed at an early age, have the greatest risk of developing prostate cancer themselves. In addition, men with other relatives such as grandfathers or uncles who have had the disease also may share an increased risk for this cancer. In fact, it's estimated that five to ten percent of all prostate cancers may be directly linked to a family predisposition for the disease.[436]

Heredity, however, is only one of the suspected factors contributing to this cancer. It isn't clear if certain families appear to be predisposed to this disease only because of genetic makeup or if the predisposition is the result of shared environmental influences, or both. For example, prostate cancer is generally uncommon among Japanese males who live in Japan. Yet, for Japanese males who live in other parts of the world, such as the Hawaiian Islands, the rates for this cancer are higher.[437] This is one study, therefore, that supports the theory that immigrant populations are susceptible to the risk pattern of their adopted country, at least for this particular cancer. And even further, this suggests that one's environment may underscore or change one's risk for this disease regardless of the hereditary factors.

While there is weak evidence suggesting that certain chemical exposures in the workplace environments of rubber manufacturing, iron and steel foundries increase the risk of prostate cancer for male employees,[438] there's stronger evidence that links an increased risk for the disease to dietary factors. In fact, the highest rates of prostate cancer occur in countries where the populations generally consume greater amounts of dietary fat. This fat, once again often in the form of red meat, is believed to contribute to prostate cancer risk.[439]

In contrast, it's believed that certain fruits and vegetables offer protection from prostate cancer.[440] Surprisingly, high blood levels of retinol also appear to be linked with a decreased risk for this cancer although, strangely, high intakes of vitamin A may be linked with a greater risk.[441] Important research also is being conducted among low risk Asian males who consume a large amount of soy products.[442] Indeed, it's possible that the Japanese Hawaiians mentioned above increased their risk for prostate cancer not by changing their overall environment, but simply by changing their diet once in their new environment.

There also is the possibility that some cases of prostate cancer may be influenced by or result from a sexually transmitted agent. The reason for this speculation is that some cases of the disease appear to arise in individuals who have a history of greater sexual activity *and* frequency of venereal disease. To date, however, ongoing research has been unable to identify a responsible microorganism.[443]

In addition, it also appears that a history of benign medical conditions affecting the prostate, such as hyperplasia and prostatitis, may increase the risk of prostate cancer. Hyperplasia, of course, refers to enlargement of the prostate gland and prostatitis is an infection of the prostate gland that results in painful and frequent urination as well as painful ejaculation.[444] Again, an increased risk resulting from these conditions makes sense if we apply our Cancer Blueprint in that a body part exposed to many or continual irritations may become weakened and susceptible to a variety of diseases, including cancer.

Finally, it's believed that male hormones may play a significant role in the development of prostate cancer. Certain hormones, including the male androgenic hormone testosterone, are necessary for the prostate to develop and function properly.[445] If the hormonal balance is disturbed, a number of abnormal conditions affecting the prostate may occur. Similarly, the manipulation of these hormones is important in the treatment of prostate cancer once it has been diagnosed.

The common thread, therefore, between all of the factors suspected of increasing the risk for prostate cancer appears to be that each one may influence the male hormonal levels in some distinct manner. As a result, men who share a greater risk for the disease also may share a different hormonal pattern from men whose risk is low. Clearly, this is a complex field of study that requires an enormous amount of research to substantiate the preliminary, yet promising, evidence.

The incidence rates for prostate cancer have risen dramatically in the last few decades. This rise, however, doesn't necessarily mean that more men today are developing prostate cancer. While men are living longer, a fact that may account for some increase in the disease among older men, it's more likely that the rates of incidence have increased simply because the use of early diagnostic procedures has increased.[446]

Prostate cancer remains an enigma, however, in that the mortality rates for this disease also continue to rise regardless of the increase in early incidental discovery and detection of the disease. This fact may indicate, therefore, that even with the new diagnostic technologies, a real change in the overall risk for developing this cancer is occurring, but hasn't yet been recognized.

Overall, prostate cancer is more common in black men the world over than in white men. It also is more common in North America and northwestern Europe than in Asia, Africa and South America. As a result, the highest rates for prostate cancer are found among African American males and the lowest rates among Asian males.[447] If we combine the known layers of risk we've discussed, therefore, it appears to indicate that African American males who have a first-degree relative, who developed prostate cancer, especially at an early age, share the highest risk for developing prostate cancer. Conversely, our evidence suggests that Asian men who have no first-degree relatives with the disease and no family history of the disease share the lowest risk for prostate cancer.

Prostate cancer is extremely common the world over. As men age, abnormal conditions of the prostate will be experienced by most at one time or another. Indeed, some researchers theorize that if a man lives long enough, the development of prostate cancer is inevitable. Yet, prostate cancer also is one malignancy that can be completely cured if diagnosed at an early stage of development. It's especially important, therefore, for men over the age of forty or for men with a family history of prostate cancer to undergo a digital rectal examination in the course of their yearly physical checkup. This simple exam can detect prostate cancer at its earliest stage, before symptoms appear. Additional early detection procedures that can diagnose prostate cancer before any symptoms become noticeable include computer tomography, transrectal ultrasound biopsies, x-rays, urine analyses and the serum test for prostate specific antigen or PSA. It's the use of these techniques that's responsible for the early detection of prostate cancer and its extremely high survival rate.

Once symptoms do appear, a complete cure is less certain. When symptoms appear, they may be fairly noticeable and easily can be confirmed by the above medical procedures. Because prostate cancer results in pressure and pushing of the prostate on the bladder and the urethra, these symptoms may include a weak or interrupted urine flow, the inability to urinate or frequent urination, especially at night. One also may experience blood in the urine, pain with urination or continual pain in the lower back, pelvis or upper thigh.[448] Again, these symptoms may be indicative of cancer or one of several benign conditions. It is, therefore, necessary to take advantage of the available medical procedures to determine the nature and cause of such symptoms and improve the chances for survival should cancer be detected.

If the diagnosis is indeed cancer, there are a number of treatments that may be recommended depending upon a number of factors. If the cancer is "in situ" and hasn't spread to other parts of the body, surgery to remove the prostate or radiation therapy may be advised. Radiation therapy may be delivered in the traditional form or it may be delivered by implanting tiny radioactive seeds into the affected tissue. If the cancer has spread, treatment may involve hormonal manipulation through the removal of the testicles or by monthly injections of specific medications. Both of these procedures prevent the production of male hormones, which appear to promote the growth of the cancer. While every treatment will have side effects, each will succeed in either removing the cancer or retarding its growth.[449] Either way, each treatment improves one's chances for surviving this cancer, a result that greatly outweighs the negative side effects one might experience.

Harmful: **Helpful:**

Heredity   **Diet**

Diet   **Antioxidants**

   Excess Fat

   Excess Vitamin A

Hyperplasia

Prostatitis

Hormonal Imbalance

Headline:

Frequency of Sexual Activity Increases Risk of Prostate Cancer

Again, this particular claim requires clarification. First, lots of sex, or ejaculations through masturbation, doesn't appear by itself to increase a man's risk for developing this disease. Studies that indicate a possible link between greater sexual frequency and prostate cancer may be explained in other ways we've already discussed. Men who have had more sex, for example, may have been exposed to more sexually transmitted diseases. And sexually transmitted diseases, of course, may compromise the health of the prostate over time and make the tissue more susceptible to problematic conditions including cancer.

In addition, prostate cancer has been linked to a possible imbalance of hormones, including testosterone. Testosterone also is linked to one's sex drive. If an individual has a higher than average level of testosterone in his body, he also may possess a greater than average sex drive and as a result, engage in more sex. Therefore, while the amount of sex may not be the contributing factor, the increased amount of testosterone in one's system, or an increased exposure to STDs, *may* be the contributing factor. Further, the study supporting this finding was conducted primarily with Caucasian males, a sample group that may not be representative of males and prostate cancer risk in general.

In contrast, a study conducted in 2004 in the United States concluded that a lot of sex, or ejaculations, might actually *reduce* a man's risk for developing cancer of the prostate. Such a finding may be based in part upon the theory that frequent ejaculations, with a partner or without, may help reduce the formation of calcifications or "flush out" cancer causing chemicals believed to be associated with the disease's development. Strangely, however, this study was conducted with men few of whom reported having exceptionally high levels of sexual activity. Clearly, the need for more research on the subject is indicated and until then this headline remains questionable.[450]

Chapter 20:
Skin Cancer

There are three types of skin cancer. From the least to the most dangerous they're known as basel cell carcinoma, squamous cell carcinoma and melanoma, the first two of which also are referred to as the nonmelanoma skin cancers. As mentioned, statistics at this time only calculate the incidence rate of melanoma, yet if all three types were combined, skin cancer would be the most commonly diagnosed cancer in the world among both women and men. Because worldwide figures on the incidence rate of skin cancer are difficult to determine, we'll use statistics from the United States to illustrate the cancer's prevalence.

For example, it's estimated that approximately one million Americans will be diagnosed with some form of skin cancer this year. One in five will develop some form of skin cancer over her or his lifetime. More than half of all cancers diagnosed in the United States are skin cancers. And, more skin cancer is diagnosed each year in the United States than breast, colon, lung and prostate cancer combined. Indeed, melanoma by itself is the seventh most common cancer among American women and the sixth most common among American men.[451]

The skin is the largest organ of the human body, a dynamic organ that's constantly replenishing itself. An adult human body has about two square yards of skin that accounts for approximately fifteen percent of its total body weight. Each square inch of skin contains millions of cells, numerous oil and sweat glands, hair follicles, and special nerve endings that sense pain, heat and cold. Its average thickness is about one tenth of an inch and is composed of three layers, including the epidermis, the dermis and the subcutaneous tissue.

The epidermis is the top layer of the skin that's visible to the human eye. The epidermis manufactures new skin cells that take about one month to move upward to the outer surface. As these new cells move to the surface, they become smaller and flatter and become a lifeless protein called keratin. This keratin remains on the surface for a short period of time until it flakes off during the course of normal washing and daily friction.

About ninety-five percent of the epidermis is devoted to those cells that manufacture new skin cells. The remaining five percent are cells that produce a black pigment called melanin. These cells, known as melanocytes, number the same in people of all skin colors. It's the rate of melanin production and their degree of concentration, both hereditary characteristics, which determine the color of one's skin and offer protection from exposure to ultraviolet light.[452]

The dermis is the layer of skin found beneath the epidermis. This layer makes up about ninety percent of the total skin area, giving strength and elasticity to the skin. It consists of collagen, a bed of strong white fibers, and elastin, which is made of yellow, elastic fibers. It's this layer of skin that contains the lymph channels and hair follicles as well as muscle cells, nerve fiber and blood vessels. This is the layer of skin that grows thinner as one grows older, resulting in skin that becomes more transparent and less elastic.

Beneath the dermis is the third layer of skin, the subcutaneous tissue. This tissue consists mostly of fat through which the blood vessels and the nerve fibers run. This is where fat is manufactured and where the sweat and oil glands are located. This tissue also thins and disappears with age.[453]

The Nonmelanomas

Basel Cell Carcinoma

Each type of skin cancer affects the epidermis and basel cell carcinoma arises from the bottom of the epidermal layer. Basel cell is the most common form of skin cancer and accounts for approximately seventy-five percent of all skin cancers. When cancer attacks the basel cells, a bump, or flat spot, may appear on the skin. This cancer may spread or ulcerate in time, but it almost always remains a local growth rarely spreading to other parts of the body.

Basel cell cancer is usually found on unprotected areas of the skin that have been repeatedly exposed to ultraviolet radiation. This is the type of exposure that normally comes from habitual outdoor activity such as boating or swimming, and is often referred to as **recreational exposure**. Heredity is another layer of risk for this nonmelanoma with fair-skinned, blue or green-eyed and fair or red-haired individuals sharing the greatest risk. Basel cell carcinoma can be diagnosed by conducting a biopsy, which involves the removal and microscopic examination of a small part of the tissue.

If the tissue is found to be cancerous, the prescribed treatment will vary according to the size and location of the growth. This treatment may include cryosurgery, which freezes the affected tissue, scraping and cauterization, which burns the affected tissue, x-ray radiation or laser therapy. Such growths also may be surgically excised or removed by a process of microscopically controlled shaved excisions called **Moh's surgery**.[454]

Squamous Cell Carcinoma

Squamous cells are found in the middle layer of the epidermis just below the outer surface. Cancer of these cells is more aggressive than basel cell cancer and can spread to other parts of the body, including the lymph nodes and the internal organs. Again, this cancer is caused by the repeated recreational exposure to ultraviolet light and is influenced by the inherited traits of fair skin, blue eyes and blond or red hair. It also may arise at the site of a prior scar, burn or chronic inflammation or be triggered by precancerous skin conditions such as actinic keratosis, which is the result of sun damage.

In the early stages, squamous cell carcinoma may appear also as a flat spot on the skin or as a red bump with a hard or scaly surface. Once again, a biopsy of the growth will determine if a squamous cell cancer exists. Once again, the treatment will depend upon the size and location of the growth and whether or not the cancer has spread to other parts of the body. If the cancer has metastasized, chemotherapy may be required, and if a large portion of tissue has to be removed a skin graft may be necessary to replace the excised tissue.[455]

Melanoma

Melanoma is the most deadly of the skin cancers, yet fortunately it's also the least common. This cancer arises in the epidermis and attacks the cells that produce melanin. While the melanin cells only make up five percent of the epidermis, melanoma is an extremely aggressive cancer that requires prompt attention. If the melanoma spreads into the cells surrounding the initial site, it remains treatable. Without treatment, however, a far more serious condition will develop with the melanoma spreading to other areas of the skin or growing downward and invading the lymph nodes and internal organs.

There are four kinds of melanoma. The most common of these is called **superficial spreading melanoma**. This melanoma affects every age group and accounts for approximately seventy percent of all reported melanomas. It usually begins as a small lesion, which is a local abnormality in the tissue of the skin that's visible to the eye. This lesion may appear on an individual's arms, legs, or trunk and may have an irregular border with white, red, black or bluish colorations.[456]

The second melanoma is called **nodular melanoma** because it begins as a shiny, hard, rounded bump. This melanoma accounts for about fifteen percent of all melanomas and can occur anywhere on the skin, usually affecting individuals between the ages of twenty and sixty.

The third, **acral lentiginous melanoma**, is more common in older individuals accounting for about ten percent of reported melanomas. "Acral" refers to the extremities and in particular to the end or top of an extremity. In fact, while this melanoma can occur in the mucous membranes, it's most commonly found on the tips of the fingers and toes, the palms of the hands and the soles of the feet as a dark brownish or black lesion.

The last of the melanomas is called **lentigo maligna**, a cancer that usually affects individuals over the age of sixty. It accounts for approximately five to ten percent of the melanomas and is the result of overexposure to the sun. This damage to the skin actually may occur many years before turning cancerous and begins as a brownish spot or freckle that develops irregular darker spots over time.[457]

As is the case with other cancers, the reported incidence rate of melanoma is greater for those who have had prior melanomas. Additionally, it appears that the risk for developing melanoma also increases for those individuals who have experienced brain and breast cancer. Indeed, evidence supports the theory that melanoma in women shares some of the hormonal and reproductive risk factors associated with breast cancer.[458]

Dietary habits such as alcohol, tobacco and caffeine use haven't been confirmed as contributing factors to melanoma nor has excessive fluorescent lighting, which has long been suspect. Similarly, the use of oral contraceptives, hair dyes and pesticides as well as other occupational and environmental hazards do not appear to be linked to an individual's risk for developing melanoma.[459]

If, however, the presence of melanoma is suspected, it can be confirmed by a skin biopsy and, if there's reason to believe the melanoma has spread, further testing, including CT scans or x-rays may be conducted. Once diagnosed, melanoma treatment usually will require the surgical removal of the affected tissue. In some cases the nearby lymph gland also may be removed and because of the aggressive nature of melanoma, a large portion of the surrounding healthy tissue may require excision as well. This surgery may be followed by a skin graft to repair the site, and if the melanoma has spread further, the treatment may involve anticancer drugs and immunotherapy, chemotherapy or radiation.[460]

Personal Note

Knowing my Risk Profile also indicates an increased risk for skin cancer based upon my light coloring, fair skin and past sun exposure, I always schedule a complete body check with my dermatologist each year. Sure enough, during the several years between my diagnoses of colon cancer and breast cancer, I was diagnosed at different times with basel cell carcinomas as well. While this type of skin cancer is, of course, the least dangerous, it must be detected and treated before it develops into something more serious. As mentioned, it's true that skin cancers often are visible to the naked eye. Yet, this is not always the case.

For example, my first skin cancer, a basel cell located on my back, wasn't clearly visible even to my doctor. However, this area of my back itched, and had been itching for several weeks. Ultimately, upon closer inspection and a biopsy, the tissue in question was found to be an early stage basel cell cancer. It's important, therefore, to pay attention to any change in one's skin whether or not the area appears to look different, and have it checked by a professional as soon as possible.

General

The rate of incidence for all three skin cancers, basel cell, squamous cell and melanoma, has increased dramatically in several countries around the world, including the United States, and poses a major health concern to many populations. The greatest layer of risk for these cancers is the overexposure to sunlight and the effects of solar radiation.

Indeed, it appears to be UV-B exposure that determines the development of any of the three skin cancers. As mentioned, the nonmelanomas, basel and squamous cell cancer, appear to be related to the repeated overexposure to UV-B rays known as "recreational" exposure.[461] In contrast, melanoma appears to be related to intense, separate occurrences of UV-B exposure, such as blistering sunburns that occur in childhood and adolescence.[462]

When assessing this first layer of risk, it also is important to consider the risk associated with heredity and one's skin type and color. For instance, the highest rates of melanoma are found among light-skinned populations where the sunlight is intense, such as Arizona in the United States or Queensland in Australia. In light-skinned populations, most melanomas appear on the trunks of males, the lower extremities of females and the head and neck of both sexes. In dark skinned populations, melanomas appear most often on the light areas of the body, such as the soles of the feet and the palms of the hands.[463]

Again, this is because light skin contains less melanin, which makes it more susceptible to damage from ultraviolet exposure. As a result, those individuals who have lighter skin, which is usually paired with lighter hair and eyes as well, have less protection from UV-B and are, therefore, at greater risk for developing skin cancers. Individuals, who don't tan, tan minimally and sunburn easily also have a greater risk for developing skin cancers as do those who have freckled skin or whose skin is dotted with excessive moles.

Certain mole patterns are genetic and some "atypical" moles, those that look different from the norm, may increase the melanoma risk and become cancerous. A mole pattern is determined by the number of moles and the type of mole that appears on one's skin. Moles themselves are simply clusters of the melanin-producing cells called melanocytes. They're actually benign lesions, which means they're noncancerous, yet, they may change abnormally. If this should happen, and if the mole is not removed, it could become a melanoma.[464]

Fortunately, most moles that are called "nevi" are normal. "Dysplastic" nevi, however, are moles that are larger and flatter than normal nevi. These dysplastic nevi may have irregular or indistinct borders and may contain pink, red or brown areas. For family members who have dysplastic nevi, the risk for developing melanoma is greater than for members who don't have dysplastic nevi. That risk increases if dysplastic nevi or melanoma appear to run in the family and one or the other affects several members.[465]

For those individuals where both dysplastic nevi and a history of melanoma run in the family, the risk is greatest. Similarly, individuals who are born with or develop within one year of birth "giant congenital" nevi, or birthmarks, also are at a greater risk for developing melanoma. And of course, if an individual has had one melanoma, the risk is always greater for developing another.[466]

In addition to ultraviolet exposure and heredity, the site of a scar, burn or chronic irritation or inflammation may set the stage for cancer.[467] Again, this is a logical result in light of our Cancer Blueprint. In any area of the body, if the tissue has been damaged, it may become weaker and more susceptible to many problematic health conditions, including cancer. Now, if that same tissue is repeatedly damaged it becomes gradually weaker with each injury and more susceptible to invading harmful agents.

This is exactly what happens when skin is overexposed to the sun time and time again over many years, or when it suffers one or several severe sunburns when an individual is young. Although the human body possesses an enzyme that helps repair the cellular DNA damage caused by ultraviolet exposure, constant overexposure inhibits the ability of that enzyme to help and the result, of course, is an increased risk for both nonmelanomas and melanoma. Yet, like many cancers, melanoma can begin in perfectly normal tissue as well where the actual "trigger" lies in one or a combination of other physical conditions.

For example, individuals who experience immunosuppression are at greater risk for developing many cancers, including nonmelanomas and melanoma. Again, immunosuppression is an abnormal condition of the immune system, which inhibits the body's ability to respond to helpful antibodies and fight off harmful elements.[468] This condition may be a side effect caused by the use of certain drugs such as corticosteroids and the alkylating agent cyclophosphamide. It also can be intentionally caused as in the preparation of transplant patients to prevent rejection of donor organs and tissues, or unintentionally caused by irradiation or chemotherapy in the treatment of cancer.

Renal transplant patients, for instance, and those with Hodgkin's disease share an increased risk for skin cancers. Similarly, about fifty percent of individuals who have undergone a kidney transplant or are on anti-rejection drugs related to other organ transplants develop some type of skin cancer within ten years. Patients with xeroderma pigmentosum, a rare hereditary skin disease, also are at greater risk for nonmelanomas and melanoma because they lack the enzyme needed to repair UV-B damage.[469]

Harmful:

Ultraviolet Radiation

Heredity

Atypical Moles

Immunosuppression

   Renal Transplants

   Hodgkin's Disease

Xeroderma Pigmentosum

Chronic Skin Irritations

Helpful:

Diet

   Antioxidants

Chapter 21:
Urinary (Bladder) Cancer

Worldwide, cancer of the bladder is the seventh most common cancer among men and the ninth deadliest. In the United States, urinary (bladder) cancer is the fourth most common among men and the ninth deadliest.

The bladder is located in the pelvis just above the prostate gland in males and between the pubic bone and the uterus in females. It's the sac where urine is stored after the urine has passed through the kidneys and before it enters the urethra for elimination from the body. And although both males and females have a bladder and a urethra, the placement of these organs in each sex presents a different set of problems. It's this different placement in males, for example, that in part explains why males are four times more likely to develop bladder cancer than females.

There are several layers of risk associated with bladder cancer, yet it shares a dubious distinction with lung, esophageal and pancreatic cancer in that cigarette smoking appears to be the greatest risk. In the United States, for example, it's estimated that cigarette smoking is responsible for approximately half of bladder cancer deaths among males and about one third of deaths among females. Indeed, cigarette smokers develop bladder cancer about two to three times more often than non-smokers. Because one's risk for bladder cancer increases as the number of cigarettes smoked each day increases, heavy smokers increase their risk over non-smokers by two to five times.[470]

On the other hand, once an individual stops smoking their risk for this cancer decreases by as much as sixty percent.[471] Yet, cigarettes aren't the only culprits when evaluating the smoking risk for bladder cancer. It appears that the use of pipes and cigars also creates an increased risk, although to a lesser degree.[472] Once again, the belief that tobacco smoke remains harmless if not inhaled is a misconception made clear by the evidence for this cancer as well.

The environment also plays a significant role when evaluating the risks for bladder cancer. Certain chemicals in the workplace have been found to have a positive association with the disease. Aromatic amines, for example, have been linked to a number of bladder cancer cases among workers whose exposure was the result of their occupation. Two of these compounds are benzidine and 2-naphthylamine, both of which are potent bladder carcinogens. Individuals, therefore, who work in dye, rubber and leather industries where exposure to such compounds may occur, share an increased risk for the disease. Other occupations that may increase one's risk for this cancer due to chemical exposures include painters, printers, metal workers, textile workers and truck drivers.[473]

As with many cancers, the role of heredity must be examined as an important layer of risk for the development of bladder cancer. Again, if one has a first-degree relative including a parent, sibling or child who has experienced bladder cancer, the risk for also developing the disease may be higher for that individual. Further, a family history in which relatives other than first-degree relatives have experienced the disease also may indicate a genetic predisposition for the disease.[474]

Again, the signs to watch for in determining a family predisposition, even if first-degree relatives are not affected, include multiple cancers in one generation, cancer in more than one generation and cancer that strikes early in life. For even though the risk involved in these cases may not be as great as when a first-degree relative has been affected, an increased risk may exist nonetheless.

Certain aspects of diet also have been found to contribute to the risk for bladder cancer. One of the first dietary factors to be identified as a risk was a compound found in artificial sweeteners known as cyclamates. Indeed, in the United States the Federal Drug Administration removed cyclamates from the market in 1969 because of their substantial link to bladder cancer. Other artificial sweeteners used today often come under suspicion; however, none to date has been shown to be a definite health risk.[475]

Similarly, another substance that has commonly been suspected as a risk in the development of this cancer is coffee, or more precise, the consumption of caffeine. Current studies, however, indicate that if there's a link between bladder cancer and coffee drinking or the consumption of other caffeine products, the link remains weak.[476]

Medical conditions and prior medical treatments also may contribute to the risk for bladder cancer. Individuals who have a history of urinary tract infections and stasis, a condition where the flow of urine is frequently slowed or halted, may share an increased risk. Similarly, bladder infections that involve the parasite **Schistosoma haematobium** may increase one's risk. This parasite is particularly virulent and affects the bladder, urethra and pelvic organs causing painful and often blood-filled urination.[477] Our Cancer Blueprint again comes into play, in that tissue that's repeatedly assaulted by harmful or irritating elements or conditions becomes more susceptible to future infection and disease.

Unfortunately, bladder cancer also is linked to past treatment for other cancers. In this case, the anticancer drugs chloraphazine and cyclophosphamide are important elements in treating certain cancers yet may increase one's risk for developing secondary primary cancers, including that of the bladder. Finally, drugs used in pain management for cancer and other serious medical conditions may increase a patient's risk for bladder cancer if the drugs contained elements such as phenacetin.[478]

The symptoms for this cancer include difficult urination due to pain and frequency or inability to urinate. Blood in the urine and generalized pain in the pelvic area also may be experienced, although blood in the urine with no pain or discomfort is often the earliest recognizable symptom. Bladder cancer has many symptoms in common with typical bladder infections, or cystitis, so it's always advisable to receive a professional diagnosis as soon as possible.

Whether or not cancer exists will be determined through a number of procedures such as an **intravenous pyelography**, a detailed x-ray of the kidney and urinary tract, or a **cystoscopic examination** of the bladder. If a tumor is detected, a CT scan or magnetic resonance imaging may determine the stage of the cancer, while chest x-rays and blood tests will help determine if the cancer has spread.

The treatment for bladder cancer will depend upon the stage of the cancer and whether or not it has spread. In early stages the tumor may be removed through a cystoscope, while more invasive surgery may be required if the cancer has invaded surrounding tissue. In some cases, the bladder itself may have to be removed, which means that a surgical procedure called an **ileal conduit** must be performed to pass urine from the body through an opening in the abdominal wall. And, of course, any surgery may be followed by either chemotherapy or radiation therapy, or a combination of both.

Harmful:

Tobacco Use

Environment

  Aromatic Amines

  Benzidine

  2-Naphthylamine

Heredity

Diet

  Cyclamates

Medical Conditions

  Urinary Tract Infections

  Stasis

Parasites

  Schistosoma Haematobium

Alkylating Agents

  Chloraphazine

  Cyclophosphamide

Drugs

  Phenacetin

Helpful:

Diet

  Antioxidants

Chapter 22:
Uterine Cancer

When we speak of uterine cancer we're really speaking of two major types of cancer. The first is cervical cancer and the second is uterine corpus cancer, or endometrial cancer. Among the world's women, cervical cancer is the second most diagnosed cancer following that of the breast. It also is the third leading cause of cancer deaths among the world's women. While it's not one of the most deadly cancers in the industrialized countries of the world, it's extremely deadly in developing countries where eighty percent of all cervical cancer deaths occur. Endometrial cancer is the seventh most commonly diagnosed cancer among the world's women. In the United States, it's the fourth most common cancer among women and the eighth leading cause of cancer deaths.

The uterus is shaped like an upside-down pear and is located in the center of the female abdomen. This organ is approximately two and a half inches long in non-pregnant females, and is an extremely powerful muscle with thick walls. The main part of the uterus is called the corpus while the narrower end of the uterus is called the cervix. The cervix is the opening from the uterus that extends into the vagina. The cervical opening is usually small and also has thick walls. Accordingly, endometrial cancer affects the main part of the uterus while cervical cancer strikes the uterine tissue that forms the cervix.

Uterine Cervical Cancer

The cervix is the lower, narrow part of the uterus that forms the opening into the vagina, which in turn leads to the outside of the female body. This cancer attacks the tissue found in the cervical opening of the uterus to the vagina. And again, it's named for the part of the body in which it begins. While cervical cancer isn't one of the ten most common cancers in the United States and many other developed countries, when figures are combined from all countries, it becomes the most commonly diagnosed cancer affecting women around the world.

Cervical cancer is actually a squamous cell carcinoma. As we know, squamous cell cancers begin in the outer layer of skin, in this case, around the cervix. At this early stage, cervical cancer is called "in situ" which again means that the cancer hasn't metastasized or invaded nearby tissues. If the cancer, however, has spread and invaded the inner layer of cells, the cancer is referred to as "invasive." In situ cervical cancer occurs more frequently in women between the ages of twenty-five and thirty-five, while invasive cervical cancer is usually diagnosed in women over the age of fifty.[479] Fortunately both types of cervical cancer, if caught early, are among the most successfully treated of all cancers.

Sexual behavior and history are major considerations when evaluating a woman's risk for cervical cancer. First, women who have sexual intercourse at an early age appear to have an increased risk.[480] This may be because the cervical tissue, either before or during puberty, is developing or undergoing many changes that may make the tissue more vulnerable or susceptible to irritation and long-term damage. In addition to early intercourse, sexually transmitted diseases and certain types of human papilloma viruses appear to be major risk factors for both in situ and invasive cervical cancer.[481]

As a result, women who have many sexual partners are at greater risk for this cancer because the risk of acquiring a sexually transmitted disease or virus that affects the cervical area increases as the number of a woman's sexual partners increases. Furthermore, women whose partners have had many sexual partners are at a greater risk for developing cervical cancer. This phenomenon, referred to as the **male factor** is evidenced in husbands of cervical cancer patients who report they've had considerably more sexual partners than husbands of women who remain unaffected.[482]

There's much concern about the role of the human papillomavirus, or HPV, that causes genital warts in both men and women. There's considerable research that indicates HPV is related to the risk for cervical cancer as women who have HPV or whose partners have HPV have a higher than average risk of developing the disease. Yet, HPV isn't found in all women who have cervical cancer and women who have HPV don't always develop cervical cancer. As stated before, therefore, it's believed that HPV must be combined with other factors that may affect the cervical tissue such as the herpes virus, hormones or diet before HPV becomes a significant risk factor itself.[483]

A woman's choice of birth control also appears to affect her risk for cervical cancer. "Barrier methods" such as the diaphragm, sponge or condom lower the risk of cervical cancer because they lower the risk of contracting the infections and sexually transmitted diseases that are linked to cervical cancer. The role played by oral contraceptives in the risk for cervical cancer is less clear. While it appears that women who use oral contraceptives have a higher incidence rate for the disease, it may not be the contraceptive itself that directly affects the rate.[484]

For example, women who use this form of birth control also may have experienced sexual intercourse at an early age or may have had multiple sexual partners. Oral contraceptives also fail to protect women from sexually transmitted diseases. All three of these factors are directly linked to an increased risk for this cancer. Having stated this, however, research nevertheless appears to indicate that some excess risk still remains for women who use oral contraceptives even after adjusting for a variety of sexual and socioeconomic factors.[485]

New evidence also suggests that dietary factors may play a role in determining one's risk. In particular, an increase in vitamin A may offer protection against cervical cancer as may vitamin C and beta-carotene.[486] In contrast, a lack of folacin, one of the B complex vitamins, also may increase one's risk. This is especially interesting as the use of oral contraceptives has been found to deplete the amount of folacin in women who use that form of birth control.[487]

It's logical, therefore, that the increased risk for developing cervical cancer among women who use oral contraceptives may not be due to the pills themselves but, at least in part, to the negative effect the pills have on a woman's stores of folacin. In other words, the use of oral contraceptives may have a leaching effect, which may drain the body of necessary nutrients or vitamins such as folacin.

This leaching effect has already been mentioned when analyzing the role of cigarette smoking and alcohol abuse in the development of other cancers. Of the two, cigarette smoking is again implicated as an important layer of risk in the development of cervical cancer. In this case, neither the cigarette nor the tobacco smoke actually comes into contact with the cervical tissue. Components of the harmful carcinogens, however, have been found in the cervical mucous of women diagnosed with this cancer.[488]

Indeed, women who smoke for many years, or who smoke large quantities of cigarettes per day may double their risk for this disease.[489] It's possible, therefore, that the leaching effect of cigarette smoking also depletes a woman's stores of important nutrients and vitamins leaving her more susceptible to infectious agents, disease and cervical cancer.

Prior medical treatments and conditions also have been found to increase a woman's risk for cervical cancer. From the 1940s to the early 1970s a drug called diethylstilbestrol, or DES, was used by many pregnant women to prevent miscarriage. Unfortunately, there were many unforeseen side effects from the use of this drug, including an increased risk for a rare type of cervical and vaginal cancer in the daughters of women who were treated with DES. In addition, women who have compromised immune systems as a result of contracting HIV appear to share an increased risk for developing cervical cancer as do women who are organ transplant patients.[490]

The symptoms for cervical cancer may include abnormal vaginal bleeding that occurs between one's periods, after menopause or after intercourse. A vaginal discharge also may occur, and in the case of advanced cervical cancer, one may experience pelvic pain, backaches and general declining health. To determine if a malignancy exists, a simple Papanicolaou's test, or Pap smear, may be conducted as well as a colposcopy and biopsy. If the laboratory analysis of these tests finds evidence of cancer a **conization** or a **dilatation and curettage,** or "**D and C,**" may be performed to determine the stage of the cancer and whether it has spread from the cervix to the surrounding tissue.

As with many cancers, the treatment for cervical cancer will depend upon the size, location and stage of the tumor. If the tumor is in situ and hasn't spread, treatment may include cryotherapy, electrocoagulation, laser ablation or local surgery. If the cancer is invasive, however, a radical hysterectomy may be required. In this procedure the uterus and cervix, upper vagina, fallopian tubes and surrounding lymph nodes may be removed. The ovaries also may be removed unless the woman is younger, in which case one or both ovaries may be left intact. Regardless of which surgery is performed, it will most likely be followed by a course of traditional radiation therapy or a radioactive implant to destroy any remaining cancer cells in the area. Finally, if the cancer has spread to the lymph nodes in other parts of the body, chemotherapy also may be required.

Harmful:	Helpful:
Early Sexual Intercourse	**Diet**
Sexually Transmitted Diseases	**Antioxidants**
Multiple Sexual Partners	**Vitamins A & C**
Partners with Multiple Sexual Partners	**Folacin**
Viruses	
Human Papilloma (HPV)	
Oral Contraceptive Use	
Tobacco Use	
Drugs	
Diethylstilbestrol (DES)	
Immunosuppression	

Headline:

Quitting Smoking Could Reduce Cervical Cancer[491]

This appears to be true. A link between the carcinogens of tobacco smoke and cervical tissue has already been substantiated. Indeed, results of additional studies reported in 2003 found that the elimination of tobacco use among women could reduce the world's cervical cancer rate by as much as twenty-five percent.

Uterine Corpus Cancer–Endometrial

The main body of the uterus, or corpus, consists of two layers of tissue, the outer wall of muscle and the inner lining. The outer wall is called the myometrium and the inner lining is the endometrium. Most uterine cancers begin in the endometrium, thus their name. Endometrial cancer is one of the most common female cancers and one of the most curable. This cancer is rare in females under the age of forty-five, but rises quickly in post-menopausal females between the ages of fifty and seventy.[492]

Endometrial cancer is similar to breast cancer in that a woman's reproductive history is one of the most important risk factors. Specifically, a high and cumulative exposure to estrogen and hormonal imbalances appear to be the major risk factors for most types of uterine cancers be they endometrial or cervical. Indeed, the dramatic rise in endometrial cancer that occurred during the 1960s and the 1970s is believed to be the result of estrogen replacement therapy or ERT. As discussed, this unopposed estrogen use was a popular and common treatment at the time. Conversely, the dramatic fall in this disease by the late 1970s is believed to reflect the reduced usage of ERT that occurred at the end of the decade.[493]

Today, the use of Tamoxifen to treat breast cancer also may increase the amount of estrogen to which a woman is exposed and appears to increase her risk for developing endometrial cancer. As a result, exemestane and other drugs known as aromatase inhibitors are gaining favor as alternatives to the use of Tamoxifen.[494] Finally, a woman's estrogen exposure also may be increased due to early onset of menstruation, late onset of menopause or never having children.

In each of these situations the production of estrogen is either increased or uninterrupted for long periods of time. In addition, women who have been treated for infertility problems and failure to ovulate also share an increased exposure to estrogen over their lifetime. Ironically, one reproductive factor that doesn't appear to increase the risk for endometrial cancer even though it prolongs estrogen production is experiencing a first birth later in a woman's life. This is in contrast to breast cancer where late first births are a contributing factor to an increased risk. Yet, similar to ovarian cancer, women who have already experienced breast cancer appear to have an increased risk for developing endometrial cancer as well.[495]

In any case, women who use estrogens in different forms, and certainly those exposed to unopposed estrogen use, have an increased risk of developing endometrial cancer estimated to be five to ten times greater than women who do not. To help balance the harmful effects of estrogens on endometrial tissue, it has become common practice for estrogens to be given in combination with a progestogen, which is any natural or synthetic form of the female hormone progesterone.[496] While this practice appears to lessen a woman's risk for endometrial cancer, it may not remove it completely.

A woman's choice of oral contraceptive also appears to have a significant impact upon her risk for developing endometrial cancer. For example, oral contraceptives that include a program of strong estrogen used alone, then followed by a small exposure to weak progestin – again, in the form of natural or synthetic progesterone – have been linked to an increased risk for the disease and as a result, are no longer on the market.[497]

On the other hand, oral contraceptives that contain both estrogen and progestin have been found to decrease a woman's risk for the disease. In fact, women who use the "combination pill" may reduce their risk by approximately fifty percent compared to women who don't use the regimen. Further, the longer a woman uses the pills, the greater the protection appears to be. Indeed, for women who have never had children and are therefore at greater risk for developing endometrial cancer, use of the combination pill appears to have a significant and enduring protective effect.[498]

Endometrial cancer also appears to strike women who share a higher socioeconomic status around the world. Indeed, the highest rates of this cancer are found in North America and northern Europe, while the lowest rates occur in Asia and Africa. It also is true that North America and northern Europe are regions typically more industrialized and urban than parts of Asia and Africa.[499] The populations of such regions usually share an abundant diet. We also know that estrogen exposure over a woman's lifetime increases her chances for developing endometrial cancer that's similar to the risk for breast cancer.

If we combine all this evidence, therefore, we can deduce that women who live in these industrialized parts of the world may have an abundance of nourishment early and throughout their lives that may hasten physical development and the production of estrogen, a known risk factor for endometrial cancer. Evidence also suggests that high fat diets contribute to a woman's risk for the disease.[500] And, populations of industrialized regions normally consume more fat in their diets.

If our evidence is reliable, therefore, it becomes easier to understand why this cancer is more prevalent in some parts of the world than in others. It also is important to remember, however, that women who live in more industrialized regions of the world simply may have greater access to medical care and procedures that enable the cancer to be diagnosed more frequently than women who live in rural or undeveloped regions and as a result, lack the same medical access.

Similarly, women from higher socioeconomic regions whose diets may be higher in fat may share a greater risk for endometrial cancer because women who possess greater body weight produce more estrogen. So once again, it may not be that environmental or dietary factors directly affect a woman's risk for the disease, but rather that these factors directly affect the amount of estrogen a woman's body produces which, in turn, directly affects her risk for the disease.

Evidence also indicates that the incidence rate of endometrial cancer is more common in women who experience other medical conditions, including high blood pressure, diabetes and gall bladder disease. Yet, the common thread between these three conditions is that each occurs more frequently in heavier women. We also know that heavier female bodies produce more estrogen than lighter female bodies. As a result, it's more probable that the high rates of endometrial cancer aren't linked so much to women who experience these medical conditions as it's linked to the heavier body weight of a woman.[501]

In contrast, Stein-Leventhal syndrome is a medical condition that's directly linked to an increased risk for endometrial cancer. This is a syndrome that produces multiple ovarian cysts.[502] It's possible, however, that while anomalies take place within the ovaries, other parts of a woman's reproductive system are affected and weakened as a result. If so, and in accordance with our Cancer Blueprint, the uterus also may become susceptible to disease, infection and, of course, endometrial cancer.

The most common symptoms of endometrial cancer in pre-menopausal women include heavy bleeding during menstruation or bleeding between periods. After menopause, unexplained vaginal bleeding may be symptomatic of an early stage tumor, yet estrogen taken alone also can cause bleeding in post-menopausal women that's totally unrelated to cancer. And although some women with the disease also may experience a vaginal discharge, endometrial cancer may fail to produce any symptoms in its early stages.

If such symptoms are experienced, an endometrial biopsy or a "D and C" may be conducted to determine the cause. Fortunately, endometrial cancer is a slow growing malignancy likely to be localized when detected. If diagnosis confirms a malignancy, treatment commonly includes a hysterectomy, in which the uterus is surgically removed. In addition, a woman's fallopian tubes and ovaries may be removed to prevent the cancer from spreading to these tissues. Depending upon the stage of the cancer and whether or not it has spread, treatment may include radiation therapy, a radioactive implant or a course of anticancer medications.

Harmful:	Helpful:
Estrogen Exposure	**Diet**
Tamoxifen	**Antioxidants**
Early Menstruation	**Combo Birth Control Pill**
Late menopause	
Estrogen Replacement Therapy (ERT)	
Specific Oral Contraceptive Use	
Higher Socioeconomic Status	
Diet	
Excess Fat	
Excess Body Weight	
Medical Conditions	

What we call failure is not the falling down
but the staying down.

Mary Pickford

Headline:

Finger Length Linked to Prostate Cancer

Maybe. In December 2010 a Wall Street Journal article highlighted a report by the British Journal of Cancer in which more than 1500 prostate cancer patients and 3000 healthy men were studied over a fifteen year period. In each of these groups, researchers compared the length of each participant's second or index finger with the length of their fourth or ring finger on the right hand. It was found that fifty-seven percent of the men in the cancer group had index fingers that were shorter than their ring fingers. In the healthy or control group it was found that fifty-two percent of the men had index fingers shorter than their ring fingers. In other words, a longer ring finger may indicate a greater risk for this cancer. Based upon these findings, the researchers went on to postulate that men with longer index fingers were thirty-three percent less likely to develop prostate cancer. It also stated that men under the age of sixty had an eighty-seven percent lower risk for developing the disease. These findings echo those of an earlier study in which 366 Korean men shared a similar association between finger length and prostate cancer risk.

The logic is that finger length is believed to be the result of hormonal influences. And of course, we know that prostate cancer is linked at least in part, to hormones. It's possible that if the length of a man's ring finger is determined by the amount of testosterone, then a longer ring finger may be the result of a greater amount of or an excess of testosterone. If so, it's possible that this excess may influence a man's body in other ways as well, including increasing his risk for developing prostate cancer.

It's important, however, to examine this research more closely. First, the length of each participant's fingers was measured and reported by the participant himself. This means that several thousand men came to their own conclusion as to how long their fingers were. There was no control in this aspect of the study. Perhaps the measurements were consistent, perhaps not. Second, it's commonly acknowledged that men under the age of sixty typically have a lower risk of developing prostate cancer. And third, we must ask questions about the sample groups. What were the ages of the participants? What was the breakdown of nationalities? How many Blacks, Asians and Caucasians were represented? How did their family backgrounds, diets and environments compare?

As always, it's necessary to come to our own conclusions. Having a longer ring finger doesn't mean one will develop prostate cancer. Having a shorter ring finger doesn't mean one will not develop prostate cancer. This may be one piece of information to consider if the findings of this study continue to be supported by future studies. Until then, however, one must continue to stay informed, gather information and exercise common sense.

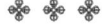

Part 4:
The Layering Effect–Revisited

Chapter 23:
Risk Analysis

Based on the previous sections, we now have a solid understanding of the most common cancers in the world and the various layers of risk associated with each. We also now have the tools that enable us to once again examine The Layering Effect and create a few more Risk Profiles. This time, however, we'll combine all the information we've discussed regarding the thirteen areas of known and suspected risk and the cancers they most commonly implicate. As a result, we'll go into much greater detail and create profiles that are much more complex than our initial profiles.

A. Profile #1

Our first individual is a thirty-year-old Caucasian female with light hair and green eyes. She lives in a city on the Australian seacoast where she worked as a lifeguard for many summers during her high school and college years. As a result, she experienced numerous sunburns, a few of which were quite serious.

She's an only child who has her mother's light coloring. She doesn't have her mother's excessive freckling, but she does have numerous moles on her torso and arms, some of which have irregular borders and vary in color. Her mother, who experienced two miscarriages and had trouble conceiving, was thirty-nine at the time of her daughter's birth.

Our individual used the combination birth control pill for three years beginning at the age of eighteen. She stopped this use when she contracted a sexually transmitted disease known as the human papilloma virus or HPV and changed to a barrier method of birth control. Our individual is now ready to have her first child, but after failing to conceive for two years she's now undergoing fertility treatments.

Our individual has never smoked cigarettes, but her father was a heavy smoker for several years and didn't quit the habit until her birth. She's in general good health and continues her active outdoor lifestyle in her current position as an on site investigator for the Australian Department of Agriculture, Fisheries and Forestry.

Initial Risk Profile

As in our earlier scenarios, we'll again begin our analysis at the top of our risk list examining those layers over which we have the least control, moving on to those over which we have the most control.

1) Heredity: From our information it's not evident that our individual has an increased risk for those cancers known to have a genetic link such as those of the breast or colon. There are, however, a few hereditary factors that may be linked indirectly to an increased risk for specific cancers. These include her genetic light coloring, atypical mole patterns and her possible inherited difficulty conceiving. The first may indicate an increased risk for all skin cancers, including basel cell cancer, squamous cell cancer and melanoma. The second may indicate an additional increased risk for developing melanoma, and the third may present an increased risk for ovarian cancer. Although these factors will surface again in our analysis, they remain important issues in our discussion of heredity and as such this layer of risk becomes the first in our profile.

2) Solar Radiation: Clearly, this factor is significant in our individual's profile. First, we know that ultraviolet solar radiation, or UV-B, alters the tumor suppressor genes in the skin, which makes the tissues more vulnerable to possible cancers. Our individual is a Caucasian with light hair and eyes, which in itself makes her more susceptible to the harmful rays of UV-B. In addition, she has a history of intense UV-B exposure as a result of her past work as a lifeguard and her current outdoor employment with the Australian government. She lives in an area where the rates of melanoma skin cancer are among the highest in the world, and the separate intense sunburns that she's experienced also increase her risk for developing melanoma. In addition, her history of regular or "recreational" UV-B overexposure and intermittent sunburns also puts her at a greater risk for developing basel and squamous cell skin cancers. Based upon this information, therefore, solar radiation becomes the second layer in our risk profile.

3) Air Pollution: Our individual lives in a city in an industrialized part of the world. In any city, pollutants are likely to be a regular feature of the environment. Air pollution in particular, however, is difficult to determine, for it's difficult to isolate the airborne elements that may be harmful. If we cannot identify these elements, we cannot effectively protect ourselves from them. In addition, the city in which she lives is on a seacoast where air quality typically is considered to be fairly good, and her employment with the Australian government keeps her outdoors in recreational areas. As a layer of risk, air pollution won't usually come into play unless one is employed in an occupation where the existence of air pollutant risks has been researched and substantiated. As a result, this layer will be omitted from our profile.

4) Water Pollution: Water pollution is similar to air pollution in that it's difficult to determine if harm exists without scientific evaluation. Unlike someone who may live in a rural area and obtain their water from wells and springs, our individual lives in an industrialized city where the water supplies typically are safe and inspected regularly. In all probability, this layer of risk is not of great import to this individual and will, therefore, not be added to our profile.

5) Pesticides/Chemicals: Again, it's possible that some of these factors may exist in our environment and in our homes in the form of household cleaners and solvents. They also may exist in our food supply as the result of industrialized spraying. While it's important to be aware of these possibilities, this layer of risk typically won't become an issue unless the individual is employed in certain industries or when she or he lives in a rural agricultural area of the world. As a result, this layer of risk will be omitted from our profile as well.

6) Viruses: In this case, our individual was exposed to the human papilloma virus or HPV. We know that exposure to this particular virus may put her at an increased risk for developing cervical cancer at some point in her life. Although it appears that HPV may be a co-factor that needs to be paired with one or a number of additional factors to lead to cervical cancer, it remains a notable risk. Our individual also may run an increased risk for developing skin cancers, oral cancers and cancer of the larynx because of her exposure to this virus. Accordingly, this risk will become the third layer in our profile.

7) Medical Treatments/Conditions: Our individual has numerous atypical moles on her body that are varied in color and have irregular borders. Such atypical moles need to be monitored as they may indicate an increased risk for developing melanoma. If this condition is diagnosed as "dysplastic nevi," our individual's risk for developing melanoma becomes an even greater risk. Either way, this risk will be included and becomes the fourth layer in our profile.

8) Ionizing Radiation: There is no indication that our individual has undergone any procedure that utilizes ionizing radiation. The typical x-rays involved in dental and medical examinations such as mammograms are virtually harmless and will normally be present in the background of every individual who lives in an industrialized part of the world. This risk, therefore, will be excluded from our profile.

9) Hormones: For every woman, this is a risk that must be examined very carefully. In this case, our individual used an oral contraceptive for three years. She used the combination method, however, which uses progestin to counteract any harmful effects the estrogen may create. There is a slight possibility that use of the combination pill increases a woman's risk for breast cancer. This slight risk, however, is usually related to use that began at an early age and continued for a long period of time. In this case, our individual was eighteen when her use of the pill began and her use was quite short-term. As a result, there is little reason to believe her use of the pill has increased her risk for developing breast cancer.

In addition, there's slight evidence that use of the combination pill increases a woman's risk for cervical and liver cancer. If so, this increase is minimal and based upon our individual's limited use this alone is probably not an issue. We cannot completely disregard the issue of cervical cancer, however, because she already has an increased risk for developing this cancer based upon her exposure to HPV.

On the other hand, use of the combination pill appears to offer protection from endometrial and ovarian cancer. Overall, her exposure to endogenous estrogen from use of the pill wasn't long-term and there is no other indication she was exposed to high doses of estrogen. Accordingly, the various risks and protections associated with use of the pill are probably not significant either way.

The fact that she hasn't been able to conceive and is undergoing fertility treatments, however, may be significant. First, the inability to conceive easily can be related to physical conditions stemming from either the male or the female. In our case, our individual is undergoing fertility treatments, which indicates that the underlying reasons for her inability to conceive are related to her. The treatments also indicate that the problem isn't the result of an infection, tumor, blockage or structural anomaly that may be corrected by medical procedures or surgery. Rather, the treatments indicate that the difficulty in this case may result from our individual's failure to release an egg, a condition known as **anovulation**.

Such difficulty is a complicated matter that ultimately appears to be linked to a woman's hormonal factors. Women who experience this difficulty, or women who have never conceived, share the greatest risk for developing ovarian cancer. This difficulty, as we already noted, also may be hereditary as indicated by her mother's reproductive history. Nevertheless, the possibility of cancer risk based upon hormonal factors typically will be a part of every woman's profile and in this case becomes our fifth layer of risk.

10) Occupation: Our individual works outdoors and is exposed to the elements, in particular, solar radiation. She also works in a part of the world where the UV-B rays of the sun are among the most intense. She's already at risk for developing all types of skin cancer based upon her genetic coloring and her atypical mole patterns. As a result, this risk will be added as the sixth layer in our overall profile.

11) Diet: At this time, this layer doesn't appear to present a risk for our individual. All our information suggests that she's healthy, active and physically fit. Assuming, therefore, that her dietary habits and body weight are properly maintained this layer will be excluded from our profile.

12) Alcohol: Again, this layer doesn't appear to present a risk to our individual's health. Based on the information we have we'll exclude this risk from our profile as well.

13) Tobacco Use: Our individual doesn't use tobacco in any form. Her father, however, was a heavy cigarette smoker at the time she was conceived and until the time of her birth. There is evidence that such paternal tobacco use at the time of conception may increase one's risk for developing childhood leukemias. Our individual, however, is thirty years old and as such has passed the stage at which this risk might be an issue. We will, therefore, mention this risk associated with tobacco use, but will omit this layer from our overall profile. In conclusion, our initial risk profile combines six layers of risk including **1) Heredity; 2) Solar Radiation; 3) Viruses; 4) Medical Treatments/Conditions; 5) Hormones** and **6) Occupation**.

One by one, we've now examined each of the thirteen layers of known cancer risks and have determined that six of these layers appear to be significant in some way to our individual. Now, it's our job to re-examine those six risks to see which ones our individual may be able to eliminate, reduce or control. We begin with **heredity**, which as we now know may indicate an increased risk for skin cancers and, based upon her inability to conceive which also may be genetically related, ovarian cancer. This layer of risk is one that cannot be removed, but may be mitigated through other means. As a result, it will remain in our risk profile.

Similarly, **solar radiation** is an environmental layer of risk that cannot be eliminated. In addition, the harmful exposure to UV-B rays our individual has experienced in her past cannot be removed. This past harm, however, may be mitigated by adhering to a healthy diet and continuing with her active lifestyle. She also can greatly reduce her current and future exposure to this harm by exercising common sense and implementing "sun safe" practices in her life. By wearing protective clothing and using a strong sun screen every day our individual can minimize her risk for developing future skin cancers even though past history, genetic predispositions and occupational factors increase her susceptibility. This layer will, therefore, remain in our profile, but it now will be controlled.

Again, the risk presented to our individual from **viruses** is based upon exposure that has already occurred. Her increased risk for developing cervical, skin, oral and laryngeal cancer as a result of this exposure will remain in our profile. Similarly, her **medical condition** of atypical moles is something that cannot be eliminated. Unlike her fair skin that can be protected from UV-B harm, her mole pattern indicates anomalies that already exist in her skin cells. Although aggravation to this condition may be prevented by "sun safe" practices, the underlying atypical structure of the skin tissue cannot be changed. Her increased risk for developing melanoma based upon this condition, therefore, will remain in our profile.

Our fifth layer of risk involves **hormones**. In this case, our individual hasn't experienced long-term or high dose estrogen, the hormone most commonly associated with a number of female cancers. Her use of birth control pills was limited. This indicates any harm or protection from their use would be limited as well and, therefore, probably not an issue. Similarly, infertility treatments themselves haven't been associated with an increase risk for developing certain cancers. The hormonal factors related to difficult conception, however, remain a fact for our individual and her increased risk for ovarian cancer. As a result, this layer of risk will remain in our profile as well.

Finally, we come to **occupation**, which is the sixth and final layer of risk in our profile. It appears that our individual has always enjoyed an active outdoor lifestyle, which continues to be reflected in her current occupation. As discussed, her outdoor work for the ADAFF increases her exposure to UV-B and her risk for skin cancers. While it's always possible our individual could find a new position that requires her to work indoors, it's probably not likely or even practical. Nor is it necessary, as "sun safe" practices will go a long way in affording her proper protection while she's in the field. As a result, we won't eliminate this layer of risk from our profile, but the potential harm it may create can be greatly reduced.

In summary, this individual's initial profile included six layers of risk that indicated possible tendencies for developing the following cancers:

Heredity>	**All Skin Cancers (Indirectly)**
	Ovarian Cancer (Indirectly)
Solar Radiation>	**All Skin Cancers**
Viruses>	**Cervical Cancer**
	All Skin Cancers

Oral Cancers
Laryngeal Cancer

Medical Treatments/Conditions>   **Melanoma**

Hormones>   **Ovarian Cancer**

Occupation>   **All Skin Cancers**

Adjusted Risk Profile

Now we'll combine each layer in our initial profile and add all the cancers that have been indicated as possible risks for our individual. In so doing, we'll see that the cancers implicated either directly or indirectly in our individual's profile include basel cell cancer four times; cervical cancer once; laryngeal cancer once; melanoma five times; oral cancers once; ovarian cancer twice and squamous cell cancer four times. Seven different cancers are implicated a total of eighteen times throughout this profile, and those that are indicated by heredity or appear more than once will probably present the greatest risk. The most significant risk for our individual, therefore, clearly appears to be for skin cancers, which appear thirteen times in her profile. Ovarian cancer appears to be her second most significant risk, yet after making the recommended changes, her adjusted profile will reflect the following:

Heredity	>>>>>>>>>>>>>>	**Heredity**
Solar Radiation		**{Controlled}**
Viruses		**Viruses**
Medical Condition		**Medical Condition**
Hormones		**Hormones**
Occupation		**{Controlled}**

Of the six layers of risk in our initial profile, four remain as factors. There are risks associated with heredity, viruses, medical conditions and hormones that cannot be eliminated. Our individual cannot change her genetic coloring, her past exposure to HPV, her atypical mole pattern or the fact that she has difficulty becoming pregnant. Yet, the cancers for which she may have the greatest risk appear to be basel cell cancer, squamous cell cancer and melanoma. By controlling the layers of solar radiation and occupation, she also indirectly mitigates the hereditary and medical conditions that contribute to the risk for these cancers. As a result, only cervical and ovarian cancers remain constant as potential risks. Even these potential risks can be mitigated by maintaining a healthy diet and regular physical activity.

In summary, our individual may not be able to eliminate all her possible risks for developing cancers, but she can greatly reduce some and mitigate others by exercising common sense, making informed decisions and incorporating simple lifestyle changes. Once

again, this profiling exercise cannot determine with certainty what risks and related cancers our individual may face during her lifetime. It can, however, identify some of the risks
and cancers for which she may be susceptible. Armed with this knowledge, she can defend
her health by adopting a participatory and pro-active role in cancer prevention, through
acknowledgment and action.

Headline:

Tanning Beds Cause Cancer[503]

This is another topic that has long been in debate. First, the light bulbs used in tanning beds
do emit an artificial source of ultraviolet light. When tanning devices were first introduced
in the 1970s, however, this ultraviolet light was composed mostly of UV-A rays. As we know,
UV-A radiation is implicated in the aging and wrinkling of the skin, but less implicated in the
burning and tanning of the skin that increases the risk of skin cancer.

Accordingly, many individuals considered indoor tanning "safe" for several years. Beds
that emitted UV-A light, however, weren't effective in providing the darker and faster tanning that the proponents of indoor tanning desired. As a result, indoor tanning devices
today use a combination of UV-A and UV-B light that replicates the light produced by the
sun. Artificial light that replicates natural sunlight also will replicate the damage that natural
sunlight creates.

Furthermore, recent research appears to indicate that long time exposure to the ultraviolet light of tanning beds does increase one's risk for developing skin cancer. Indeed, it
has been estimated by some studies that women who use tanning beds more than once a
month may increase their risk for developing melanoma by as much as fifty-five percent.

For fair-skinned individuals who desire the "healthy glow" of a tan, therefore, a safer
alternative may include the use of over the counter artificial tanning products, or spa treatments that literally "spray" one with an even and surprisingly realistic bronze tint. In addition, a synthetic hormone that instructs the melanocytes to make pigment without sunlight
is being developed. Known as Melanotan-1, this drug can tan the skin of the fairest individuals without exposing them to harm from ultraviolet radiation. It requires further testing,
however, as this drug at present can only be administered by injection and may result, in
addition to a tan, flushing, nausea and bloating.

B. Profile #2

Our second individual is a fifty-three-year-old African American male who lives in a
northeastern city in the United States. He's an on-site manager for a textile company that
manufactures insulation, a company with which he's been employed for thirty years. He

enjoys a diet typical of industrialized regions that includes a fairly large amount of red meats and dairy products. He's not overweight, however, and attributes this fact to his participation in a number of leisure time sports. He's always been a moderate to heavy drinker of bourbon and started smoking cigarettes and cigars habitually ten years ago. His grandfather had been diagnosed with adenomatous colon polyps on several occasions late in his life. They were removed, however, and his grandfather lived to the age of eighty-nine. His father, who recently turned eighty, was just diagnosed with prostate cancer.

As a child, our individual had a thyroid disorder for which he received radiation treatments and asthma that was treated with a program of corticosteroids. Throughout his adulthood, however, he has remained in good health with no specific ailments or physical problems.

Initial Risk Profile

Beginning at the top of our list, we again will examine those layers of risk over which we have the least control and progress to those over which we have the most. This, of course, means we'll start with heredity, our first and potentially most significant layer of risk.

1) Heredity: There are two factors in our individual's biography that trigger this particular layer of risk. The first is his grandfather's history of colon polyps, and the second is his father's recent diagnosis of prostate cancer. As we know, adenomatous polyps have the potential to become cancerous, and even though the condition was successfully treated, it may indicate a familial predisposition for developing these polyps. If a predisposition exists for developing these polyps, one also may exist for developing colorectal cancer, a cancer known to have significant hereditary risk factors. Moreover, colorectal cancer is more common in men than in women, a fact that also increases our individual's risk for this disease.

Similarly, hereditary factors appear to play a significant role in the development of prostate cancer, a disease with which our individual's father was diagnosed at the age of eighty. We know that an individual's risk for a specific cancer may increase if a first-degree relative has been diagnosed with the cancer. We also know that if the diagnosis occurred early in the relative's life, the cancer is even more likely to be hereditary.

In this case, only one of these factors applies to our individual. Yet, prostate cancer is known to be a genetically influenced cancer whose highest rates of incidence are found among African American males. As a result, our individual is clearly at an increased risk for developing both colorectal and prostate cancer and heredity, therefore, becomes the first layer of risk in our profile.

2) Solar Radiation: First, our individual lives in a part of the world not known for the intensity of its solar rays. Second, our individual doesn't work outdoors where he's exposed to the elements on a regular basis. Third, our individual is an African American whose darker coloring may not be as susceptible to the harm from UV-B rays as perhaps another individual with lighter skin, eyes and hair. Yet, harm from the atmosphere's free radicals can occur indoors as well as outdoors, and regardless of skin coloring, every individual, to a different degree, remains at risk for developing every type of skin cancer including basel cell, squa-mous cell and melanoma.

Moreover, our individual engages in a number of sport activities. If these activities take place outdoors, the need to practice good "sun sense" will be accentuated. This layer of risk will apply to virtually every individual regardless of skin coloring and in this case it becomes the second layer in our profile.

3) Air Pollution: As we mentioned in our above profile, air pollution typically won't become an issue for an individual unless she or he is employed in an occupation where harmful air pollutants have been studied and identified. In this case, our individual works in the textile industry in which insulation is manufactured. We know that this industry may expose him to airborne asbestos, which in turn may put him at a greater risk for developing cancer of the lung. His working environment also may expose him to harmful industrial emissions, exhausts and byproducts known to be associated with lung cancer in particular. Although it's difficult to assess the existence of air pollutants in one's living environment, the fact that our individual lives in a region of great industrial activity may well aggravate the risks he already may face in his workplace. Additionally, our individual smokes cigarettes and cigars, a factor that when combined with urban air pollutants further increase his risk for develop-ing lung cancer. Accordingly, these facts propel us to include this layer of risk in our profile.

4) Water Pollution: Similar to the risk of air pollution, water pollution is difficult to substan-tiate without specific scientific evidence. As mentioned, this layer of risk typically won't be activated unless the individual lives in an area where the wells and groundwater are vulner-able to nearby industrial runoff and contamination. Although our individual lives and works in an area of industrial activity, it's an urban area where the water is supplied and regularly inspected by city sources. Without further information, therefore, we'll omit this risk from our profile.

5) Pesticides/Chemicals: This is another risk that will usually not be included in one's pro-file unless there's specific information regarding the use of or exposure to such products in one's daily life. Typically, this may be the case if one lives or works in rural areas or in the agricultural regions of the world. It also may be implicated if one has experienced wartime chemical exposure or workplace chemical exposure.

First, our individual lives and works in an urban environment and is not associated with the agricultural industry in any way. Second, we have no information linking him to military operations or wartime activities during his life. And, with the exception of airborne asbestos, there is no indication he's exposed to other workplace pollutants linked to industry such as chemical solvents. As a result, we'll omit this risk from our profile as well.

6) Viruses: There is no evidence that our individual has ever been exposed to any of the viruses that have been linked to the development of certain cancers. This layer, therefore, also will be omitted from our profile.

7) Medical Treatments/Conditions: In contrast to the last three layers of risk, this one is implicated in our individual's profile. Medical treatments and conditions will include any procedure, drug therapy or pre-existing physical condition that has been linked to the development of any cancer. This layer doesn't include ionizing radiation or hormone exposure, both of which will remain separate risks to be examined independently.

In this case, our individual suffered from childhood asthma, an inflammation of the bronchial wall that restricts the flow of air and impairs one's ability to breathe normally. For this condition he was treated with corticosteroids, which are anti-inflammatory agents. Inflammation, however, is one of the body's defense mechanisms that typically occur in response to infection or injury. Corticosteroids suppress this natural tendency of the body to protect itself and inhibit the immune system from working properly.

From our earlier discussions, we know that immunosuppressants often produce unintended as well as intended effects. The use of corticosteroids in particular has been linked to an increased risk for developing non-Hodgkin's lymphoma, or NHL. This risk appears to be directly related to the amount and duration of one's exposure to these steroids. Even if our individual's treatment was brief, however, an increased risk for this cancer may exist and as such this layer becomes the fourth in our individual's profile.

8) Ionizing Radiation: This risk also is implicated in our profile and stems from our individual's childhood treatment of a thyroid disorder with radiation therapy. Unfortunately, such treatments appear to increase one's risk for developing both cancer of the thyroid and adult on-set leukemia many years after the exposure. This is another possibility that must be recognized, and a risk that becomes the fifth layer in our profile.

9) Hormones: To clarify, corticosteroids are drugs that are modified forms of the hormones cortisone and hydrocortisone, both of which are produced by the adrenal glands. When modified, these hormones create drugs whose strong anti-inflammatory effect is extremely useful in the treatment of many medical conditions. As such, corticosteroids are related to hormones and could be included in the discussion of this particular layer of risk. For our purposes, however, we'll consider them drugs to be included as a layer of risk in our section on medical treatments. As we have already done so, and because our individual hasn't used any other type of hormonal supplement or androgen, this layer will be omitted from our profile.

10) Occupation: Clearly, this risk applies to our individual and is cross-referenced and overlapped in our discussion of air pollution. He works in the textile industry manufacturing insulation, an occupation where airborne asbestos exposure has been linked to an increased risk for lung cancer. He has held this position for thirty years and regardless of recent workplace improvements that may have taken place, his probable exposure to asbestos has been fairly long-term. As a result, his increased risk for developing lung cancer may be significant.

In addition, there is evidence that the mortality rates for colorectal cancer are greater in areas of industrial activity. Although this link isn't completely understood, our individual works, and lives, in such an area. Further, an increased risk for colorectal cancer has already been implicated by his hereditary factors. As a result, occupational factors may not only increase his risk for lung cancer, but for colorectal cancer as well. This layer, therefore, will be added to our profile.

11) Diet: This factor also becomes an addition to our profile in that our individual consumes a diet high in animal fat from red meats and dairy products. Such a diet has been linked to a variety of cancers, including those of the colon, kidney, pancreas and prostate. As we know, our individual already may have an increased risk for developing colorectal and prostate cancer. His high fat diet will only aggravate any genetic predisposition he may have for these cancers and increase his risk for developing one, or both, as well as others. This layer of risk, therefore, becomes the seventh in our individual's profile.

12) Alcohol: Alcohol use and its links to cancer is a topic that requires specific clarification. First, there are only a few cancers that may be linked directly to alcohol use, and they include oral, pharyngeal, esophageal, laryngeal and liver cancer. Furthermore, this link is dependent upon the strength and the amount of alcohol consumed. First, our individual in this case is a moderate to heavy drinker, and he favors a "hard" alcohol, which is stronger than many other alcoholic beverages. These two factors may combine to increase his susceptibility to the four cancers mentioned above.

Second, based upon the amount of alcohol he consumes, he may be subject to the "leaching effect" of alcohol, whereby any positive attributes of the vitamins and nutrients contained in the foods he consumes is diminished. We already have established that our individual's diet presents a risk for developing certain cancers. This leaching effect caused by excessive alcohol use, therefore, can only make matters worse.

And finally, our individual also smokes cigarettes and cigars. When the negative effects of alcohol use are combined with the negative effects of tobacco use, the harmful elements of each is increased significantly. Because our individual may drink in excess, and has smoked for ten years, not only may his risk for alcohol-related cancers increase, his risk for tobacco-related cancers may increase as well. Based upon this information, alcohol will be added to our list of risks, becoming the eighth layer in our profile.

13) Tobacco Use: As we know, tobacco use, especially in the form of cigarette smoking, is associated with numerous cancers affecting males, including those of the bladder, colon, esophagus, kidney, larynx, liver, lung, oral cavity, pancreas and stomach. Our individual has smoked cigarettes and cigars regularly for a period of ten years.

In addition, the fact that alcohol and tobacco act as mutual "accelerants" for one another greatly increases the harmful effects of each. If the statistics hold true for him, therefore, he's at an increased risk for developing each of the cancers related to alcohol use as well as tobacco use. As a result, we're propelled to add this risk as the final layer in our profile, which now includes: **1) Heredity; 2) Solar Radiation; 3) Air Pollution; 4) Medical Treatments/ Conditions; 5) Ionizing Radiation; 6) Occupation; 7) Diet; 8) Alcohol** and **9) Tobacco Use.**

Again, our job now is to re-examine each layer of risk in our profile and once again determine which of these layers can be eliminated, reduced or controlled. We begin with **heredity**, which in this case indicates our individual may have genetic predispositions for both colorectal and prostate cancer. This layer cannot be eliminated, although he may be able to reduce his risk for these cancers by altering or eliminating other layers in his risk profile.

Similarly, **solar radiation** cannot be eliminated from our atmosphere or the risk profile for any individual. We know that skin coloring may dictate the degree to which an individual is susceptible to UV-B harm yet, some risk will always remain. This layer, however, can be controlled by exercising good "sun sense" which will greatly reduce the risk anyone may face for developing skin cancers.

The next layer implicated in our profile is **air pollution**. As mentioned, this risk won't usually be implicated unless certain factors exist in an individual's occupation. In this case, our individual has been employed for thirty years in an industry known for potential asbestos exposure. His past exposure to this pollutant cannot be changed, nor is he likely to alter the possible harm he may face from working and living in a region of high industrial activity.

His current workplace environment, however, can be controlled to prevent future harm, especially in light of new information and guidelines regarding asbestos exposure. Additionally, any harm from air pollutants in his urban location may be reduced if he eliminates the co-factor of tobacco smoke. Such steps can decrease his overall risk for lung cancer even though the risk cannot be entirely eliminated.

Medical treatments and conditions is another layer of risk that cannot be eliminated. Our individual's use of corticosteroids also occurred in the past and his increased risk for NHL as a result will remain. This possible harm, however, can be mitigated by altering other layers of risk in his profile. **Ionizing radiation** treatment also is something that occurred in our individual's past. Any increased risk he runs for developing either thyroid cancer or leukemia will remain as a result. Similar to his use of corticosteroids, however, past harm incurred by the radiation also may be mitigated by altering other risks for which he's profiled.

Any increased risk resulting from his **occupation** is another layer that our individual may not be able to eliminate or change. The risk of developing lung cancer as a result of his employment has already been mentioned in our discussion of air pollution. This risk overlaps, yet while he may be able to control his on-the-job exposure to airborne asbestos, he may not be able to actually change his job. Assuming this is the case, this layer of risk will remain in his profile.

Diet is a significant layer of risk in our individual's profile, yet it also is one that can be controlled. Consuming less red meat and dairy products could decrease his consumption of dietary fat. He can increase his intake of fruits and vegetables each day, the vitamins, nutrients and antioxidants of which will provide further protection. Doing so will decrease his risk for colorectal, kidney, pancreatic and prostate cancer, all of which are directly related to a high fat diet. Proper diet also will help mitigate any harm that may have occurred in the past by providing the body with the nutrients it needs to fight infection and protect itself.

With his physician's approval, he also may choose to increase his intake of calcium, which appears to decrease one's risk for colorectal cancer. For any reduction in the risk of colorectal, or prostate cancer in particular, is especially important as both have already been implicated in his profile as potential hereditary risks. The fact that he's not overweight and that he appears to exercise regularly also combine to lower his risk for many cancers. Proper diet, however, is essential as it can reduce his risk for virtually every type of cancer and can help mitigate those risks that cannot be eliminated, such as air pollution, past medical treatments, radiation therapy and occupation.

Alcohol is another layer of risk that's significant in this profile yet, like diet, it's one that can be controlled or eliminated. Alcohol use in itself is rarely a cancer risk unless the use is excessive and involves the consumption of hard alcohols with a high concentration of ethanol. Our individual easily could reduce his risk for the five alcohol-related cancers by drinking less or by substituting less potent alcoholic beverages in place of his preferred bourbon. Doing so also would reduce the leaching effect excessive alcohol use appears to have on the human body. Yet, the positive effect of making such changes will be greatly hampered unless our individual takes the necessary steps to eliminate his ninth layer of risk as well.

Our profile begins and ends with the most significant risks with which any individual may be confronted, heredity and **tobacco use**. Unlike heredity, however, tobacco use presents a risk that lies completely within the control of an individual. In this case, our individual's use of cigarettes and cigars will in all probability increase his risk for ten tobacco-related cancers.

Of these, colorectal cancer may be the most significant in that this cancer already has been implicated in his profile and overlaps in three layers of risk, including heredity, diet and tobacco use. His tobacco use also acts as a co-factor with urban air pollutants the combination of which may further increase his risk for lung cancer. It would, therefore, be advisable for our individual to stop smoking and also to avoid environmental tobacco smoke whenever possible.

Our initial profile included nine layers of risk. When we combine these layers, the cancers implicated by each often overlap and give us the following overview:

Heredity>   **Colorectal Cancer**
                                               Prostate Cancer

Solar Radiation>   **All Skin Cancers**
Air Pollution>   **Lung Cancer**

Medical Treatments/Conditions>   **Non-Hodgkin's Lymphoma**

Ionizing Radiation>   **Thyroid Cancer**
                                               Adult On-Set Leukemia

Occupation>   **Lung Cancer**

Diet>   **Colorectal Cancer**
                                               Kidney Cancer
                                               Pancreatic Cancer
                                               Prostate Cancer

Alcohol>   **Esophageal Cancer**
                                               Laryngeal Cancer

Liver Cancer
Oral Cancers
Pharyngeal Cancer

Tobacco Use>

Colorectal Cancer
Esophageal Cancer
Kidney Cancer
Laryngeal Cancer
Liver Cancer
Lung Cancer
Oral Cancers
Pancreatic Cancer
Stomach Cancer
Urinary (Bladder) Cancer

Adjusted Risk Profile

We can now analyze the types of cancers for which our individual appears to have an increased risk for developing. Those, of course, that overlap in our profile most likely will present our individual with the greatest risk. In summary, our initial profile indicated potential risks for colorectal cancer three times; esophageal cancer twice; kidney cancer twice; laryngeal cancer twice; leukemia once; liver cancer twice; lung cancer thrice; non-Hodgkin's lymphoma once; oral cancers twice; pancreatic cancer twice; pharyngeal cancer once; prostate cancer twice; skin cancers, including basel cell, squamous cell and melanoma once; stomach cancer once; thyroid cancer once and urinary (bladder) once.

The combined layers of risk present us with sixteen different cancers implicated in one way or another a total of twenty-six times. Once again, the risk may be the greatest for those cancers associated with heredity, those that appear more than once and those suggested by the combination of both alcohol and tobacco use.

Of the sixteen types of cancer, therefore, our individual's potential risk appears to be the greatest for colorectal, esophageal, liver, lung and prostate cancer. Colorectal cancer is indicated three times by heredity, diet and tobacco use; esophageal cancer twice by alcohol and tobacco use; liver cancer twice by alcohol and tobacco use; lung cancer three times by air pollution, occupation and tobacco use; and prostate cancer twice by heredity and diet. And while initial profiles may appear overwhelming, they can be altered in many ways to reduce the impact of the risks they present. In this case, after making the above-recommended changes we can create an adjusted profile that includes:

Heredity   >>>>>>>>>>>>>>   **Heredity**
Solar Radiation   **{Controlled}**
Air Pollution   **{Controlled}**

Medical Treatment	**Medical Treatment**
Ionizing Radiation	**Ionizing Radiation**
Occupation	**Occupation**
Diet	**{Controlled}**
Alcohol	**{Controlled}**
Tobacco Use	**{Eliminated}**

Of the nine layers of risk that appeared in our initial profile, only four – heredity, medical treatment, ionizing radiation and occupation – remain unchanged. This individual cannot eliminate his possibility of a genetic predisposition for both colorectal and prostate cancer. Similarly, he cannot change the fact that he has undergone treatment with corticosteroids or that he received radiation therapy. Assuming he's not able or willing to change his occupation, this layer of risk also remains in our profile.

There are five additional layers, however, that can be altered in ways that will reduce his risk for developing a number of different cancers. Of these five, solar radiation, while it cannot be eliminated, can be controlled so that the harm it may present virtually can be eliminated. Similarly, past exposure to air pollutants, especially in the workplace, cannot be eliminated, but steps can be taken to prevent harm from current and future exposure. Although his occupation remains in the profile, the risks it may present also are reduced greatly by controlling his exposure to workplace airborne pollutants as indicated in the third layer of his profile.

Diet, alcohol and tobacco use are all lifestyle risks the potential harm of which can be significantly reduced by asserting personal control over each. Proper diet is not only essential to reduce current risks, it will help mitigate the harm created by those layers of risk that cannot be changed, and those in which harm may have already occurred, such as medical treatments and ionizing radiation. In addition, by avoiding alcohol abuse and eliminating tobacco use completely, our individual will enormously reduce his risk for all twelve cancers implicated by the last three layers in his profile.

Once again, the Layering Effect is only an exercise in which we hope to shed light on the potential risks and cancers for which an individual may be susceptible. This doesn't mean that in this case our individual will develop any of the above cancers. It's completely possible that our individual may develop cancers for which he doesn't appear to be at risk or he may never develop any type of cancer at all. The Layering Effect is simply an exercise designed to identify possible risks and provide individuals a tool with which they can actively participate in their own defense from those risks, through acknowledgment and action. Our third and final profile follows:

C. Profile #3

Our individual is a sixty-one-year-old female who lives in a northern European city. She began her menstrual cycle at age ten and first engaged in sexual intercourse at the age of fourteen. She practiced birth control throughout many of her reproductive years using an estrogen-based oral contraceptive at the age of fifteen for ten years before switching to the "combination" pill. She used the "combo" for an additional twelve years until her late thirties when she bore twin girls at the age of thirty-eight.

She resumed her use of the "combo" for an additional ten years until she began to experience peri-menopause at the age of forty-eight. At this time she began hormone replacement therapy, started menopause at fifty-eight, and although she's now post-menopausal, she continues to use HRT to alleviate many uncomfortable symptoms.

She's the office manager of a large legal firm and has little time for exercise. She tries to eat well, but relies on numerous supplements to provide the necessary antioxidants and nutrients she lacks in her diet. Further, she's trying to decrease her intake of fat as she's twenty-five pounds heavier than she would like to be. She smoked cigarettes heavily for fifteen years before the age of thirty-five. She began again at the age of fifty-five, although now she only smokes occasionally and only in social situations when she also drinks white wine.

Her father was diagnosed and successfully treated for colorectal cancer at the age of thirty-nine. Her younger sister also was diagnosed and successfully treated for breast cancer at the age of forty-two. Our individual has, however, been in relatively good health her entire life except for a history of the benign breast condition known as fibrosis.

Initial Risk Profile

Again, we'll begin at the top of our list with the layer of risk over which we have the least control and move through each layer, one at a time, until we reach those over which we have the most control.

1) Heredity: This layer of risk is clearly implicated in our individual's profile. First, her father had colorectal cancer, a cancer known to be genetically influenced. Additionally, her father was diagnosed with the disease at an early age, a signal that also implicates hereditary factors.

Second, her sister was diagnosed with breast cancer, which also is known to have a genetic etiology. Similarly, her sister also was diagnosed with the disease at a relatively early age, which again points to hereditary factors. And third, our individual herself has a history of benign breast disease, which also may be hereditary and in itself appears to increase a woman's risk for developing breast cancer.

In addition, women who have experienced breast cancer appear to have an increased risk for developing melanoma as well as endometrial and ovarian cancer. Further, women who develop colorectal cancer as a result of hereditary factors also appear to have a higher than average risk for developing endometrial cancer.

In summary, this woman has a family history that may put her at risk for developing either colorectal cancer or breast cancer, or both. She also may have vulnerability for melanoma, endometrial and ovarian cancer that may be linked to her possible predisposition for breast cancer and further vulnerability for endometrial cancer that may be linked to her possible genetic predisposition for colorectal cancer. As a result, heredity becomes the first layer in our risk profile.

2) Solar Radiation: From our individual's short biography, it's not clear how much time she spends outdoors. Her occupation as an office manager keeps her inside for at least five days a week and physical exercise, much of which takes place outdoors, isn't a large part of her life. We might be able to determine, therefore, that exposure to solar radiation is not a great risk for this individual. Solar radiation, however, is a constant in our environment, and the harmful free radicals it produces have the ability to penetrate many materials including glass. As a result, our skin can still be damaged even though our jobs may keep us in an office or in a car all day.

In addition, our individual also appears to have a possible genetic predisposition for breast cancer the development of which also is associated with the future development of melanoma. Solar radiation remains a risk for every individual, and although the risk in this case may not be as significant as in others, we'll add it as the second layer in our risk profile.

3) Air Pollution: As we know, this layer of risk typically will only become relevant if an individual is employed in an occupation known for harmful air pollutants and their links to cancer. Our individual is an office worker whose exposure to workplace pollutants doesn't appear to be an issue. While she lives in an industrialized part of the world where pollutants are likely to exist, the specifics of this existence are simply too difficult to substantiate. Furthermore, our individual doesn't appear to spend time in activities or outdoors in areas where specific air pollutants have been identified. As a result, this layer will not be added to our profile.

4) Water Pollution: This also is a risk the relevance of which usually will be determined by the region in which an individual lives. Unlike an individual who may live in a rural area and obtain her or his water from wells and springs, our individual lives in an industrialized city where the water supplies typically are safe and inspected regularly. In all probability this layer of risk isn't of great import to our individual and, therefore, will be omitted from her profile.

5) Pesticides/Chemicals: Again, we know these factors may exist in our environment and in our homes in the form of household cleaners and solvents. Similarly, they may exist in our food supply as the result of industrialized spraying. Our individual, however, doesn't live in a rural or agricultural region or work in an industry where this risk may be particularly relevant. As a result, we'll omit this layer from our profile as well.

6) Viruses: In our case, this particular individual has never contracted a sexually transmitted disease, has never developed herpes simplex and isn't HIV positive. She has never experienced an immunosuppression condition, EBV, hepatitis B or C or any of the other viruses that have been associated with cancer. She has no history of intravenous drug use and has never had a tattoo. This layer of risk, therefore, also will be omitted from our profile.

7) Medical Treatments/Conditions: Our individual has never been treated for cancer with chemotherapy or any of the alkylating agents. Nor is there any indication that she has ever been exposed to the additional drugs that appear to be associated with the development of certain cancers. She does, however, experience the benign breast condition known as fibrosis, which may increase her risk for developing breast cancer. Although this condition was already mentioned in our discussion of heredity, we'll include it again in this layer of risk, which becomes the third to be added to our profile.

8) Ionizing Radiation: Aside from the usual x-rays for medical and dental purposes, our individual hasn't been exposed to any damaging procedures that utilize ionizing radiation. This layer of risk, therefore, will be omitted from our profile.

9) Hormones: Unlike the several preceding risk factors, this particular layer of risk is one that has numerous implications for our individual. First, let's examine her exposure to estrogen throughout her life both in terms of exposure length, strength and intensity. She began menstruation at the age of ten and menopause at the age of fifty-eight. This means her natural production of estrogen continued for almost fifty years, which is a considerable length of time, and early menstruation and late menopause are both risk factors for breast cancer.

In addition, we know that the reproductive events in a woman's life largely influence her risk for developing breast cancer. Of these events, the most important is a woman's age at the time of her first full-term pregnancy. In this case, our individual had no children until the age of thirty-eight. Furthermore, after she bore her twins she had no additional full-term pregnancies. Her later age at the time of her pregnancy and the fact that the pregnancy was her only one are both factors that increase her risk for breast cancer. Again, these reproductive facts simply indicate that her natural production of endogenous estrogen was interrupted by pregnancy only once between the start of menstruation at the age of ten, to the start of menopause at the age of fifty-eight.

The related use of exogenous hormones – those added to the body – and the risk for breast cancer is less clear. Our individual used an estrogen based contraceptive pill for ten years beginning at the age of fifteen. She also has been on hormone replacement therapy for eleven years to relieve uncomfortable symptoms first associated with peri-menopause and now with menopause. Because it now appears that the risk for breast cancer is greater for women who are long-term users of HRT and for women who are on or have received high doses of exogenous estrogen, this information will be added to our layer of risk. The fact that our individual also began taking oral contraceptives at the relatively young age of fifteen also may increase her risk for breast cancer.

Our individual's history of estrogen exposure, however, places her in a position of increased risk for cancers other than that of the breast. The risk for both uterine cancers known as endometrial and cervical also is implicated by our individual's history. Similar to breast cancer, endometrial cancer in particular is greatly influenced by a woman's overall exposure to estrogen and the resulting hormonal imbalances. Early menstruation and late menopause, therefore, will be risk factors for this cancer as well.

Reproductive history also is important, yet in the case of endometrial cancer, a woman's age at the time of her first birth doesn't appear to be an important factor. Rather, never having children or having few children appears to be the more dominant risk factor and in our individual's case, this is relevant.

The use of exogenous estrogens in different forms is another important factor and also appears to increase a woman's risk for the disease. Our individual used an estrogen based contraceptive pill for ten years early in her life, the use of which has been linked to endometrial cancer. This contraceptive use, however, was eventually changed to use of the "combination" pill, which has been found to decrease a woman's risk for endometrial cancer. As a result, it's possible that the enduring protective effect of using the latter method may have "offset" or limited the harmful effects of using the former. Nevertheless, our individual's history of prolonged estrogen exposure and her continued use of HRT combine to raise her overall risk for developing this cancer as well.

While not directly affected by estrogen exposure or reproductive events, the second form of uterine cancer commonly known as cervical cancer does appear to be linked to a woman's sexual history. In this case, our individual first experienced sexual intercourse at the age of fourteen. While different cultures have different views regarding an acceptable age at which females may engage in sexual intercourse, the issue here is one of physical development.

Puberty is the period of time during which the female sexual characteristics develop and the sex organs mature. Typically, puberty begins in females around the age of eight or nine and continues until the age of fifteen or sixteen, or until regular menstruation is established. During this time the pituitary gland begins to secrete follicle stimulating and luteinizing hormones. The female body also begins to produce estrogen at a level approximately twenty times greater than before the onset of puberty. It's believed that the developing cervical tissues may be more vulnerable during puberty and more susceptible to damage or irritation that may occur during sexual intercourse. As a result, intercourse at an early physical age, typically before or during puberty, is one factor that appears to increase a woman's risk for cervical cancer.

Unlike other cancers, it also appears that the use of oral contraceptives, even those that combine estrogen and progesterone, may increase a woman's risk for cervical cancer. This risk, however, may be related to a decrease of folacin, a side effect of oral contraceptive use, more than to the birth control method itself. In any event, our individual's history appears to put her at an increased risk for cervical cancer as well.

Finally, our profile also must include recognition of our individual's increased risk for ovarian cancer. This cancer typically affects women who have experienced menopause and are over the age of fifty-two, factors that are relevant to our individual. Reproductive and menstrual factors also greatly influence a woman's risk for ovarian cancer. Yet, a woman's age at the time of her first full-term birth, the starts of menstruation or menopause don't appear to increase her risk. Rather, the risk is greatest for women who have difficulty conceiving or for those who have never conceived.

We know our individual conceived and bore twins at the age of thirty-eight, and we know she practiced birth control until that time. Problems conceiving, therefore, don't appear to be at issue. Her risk may be increased, however, because she only experienced one full-term pregnancy, and the risk for this cancer decreases with each complete pregnancy. On the other hand, her use of oral contraceptives over a long period of time has decreased her risk for ovarian cancer and, surprisingly, her use of estrogen through HRT is not considered a risk factor at all for this particular disease.

Even if these factors combined appear to balance one another, however, her post-menopausal age and limited pregnancies remain factors that may increase her overall risk for developing ovarian cancer. In summary, our individual's history indicates that she may be at an increased risk for breast, endometrial, cervical and ovarian cancers as a result of hormonal related factors and as such, this layer of risk will be added to our overall profile.

10) Occupation: Our individual is an office worker whose exposure to the elements is limited. It doesn't appear her position puts her at an increased risk for cancers related to solar radiation, chemicals or other significant pollutants in the atmosphere. She doesn't work in an industry in which harmful workplace elements have been studied and identified. As a result, this layer of risk will be omitted from our profile.

11) Diet: This is one layer of risk that typically plays a large role in any individual's risk profile. Here, our individual doesn't always eat properly and habitually uses antioxidant supplements to make up for this lack. Additionally, she lives in an industrialized part of the world where high fat diets are typical, and she admits to not exercising enough and being twenty-five pounds overweight.

As we know, improper diet, inadequate exercise and an overweight condition are all risk factors for colorectal cancer. We also know that consuming a high fat diet and being overweight aren't factors that are as critical to developing breast cancer as they are to developing colorectal cancer. An overweight condition, however, can make it more difficult to diagnose breast tumors in women and lack of exercise and a high fat diet contribute to this condition.

It also is true that female bodies with excess weight produce more estrogen, which in itself raises the risk for breast and other cancers. Our individual, however, is post-menopausal, which means the production of estrogen essentially has ceased and as such, won't be negatively influenced by an overweight condition. The genetic predisposition for both colorectal and breast cancers, however, may be aggravated by a high fat diet as well as cancers of the endometrium, ovaries, pancreas and possibly the kidneys. Diet, therefore, will be included as our next layer of risk in our overall profile.

12) Alcohol: This layer of risk appears to be under control. Our individual doesn't drink excessively, so the "leaching" effect of excessive alcohol consumption probably doesn't apply to her. Nor does she drink "hard" alcohols, but rather white wine and even that, only occasionally. In light of her possible genetic predisposition to cancers, including that of the breast, we will, however, add this layer to our profile although it appears to be of little, if any, impact in and of itself. Its impact is magnified, however, when combined with our next layer.

13) Tobacco: Our individual smoked cigarettes heavily for fifteen years before quitting at the approximate age of thirty-five. She began smoking again, although only occasionally, six years ago at the age of fifty-five. For former smokers, we know that their risk for developing a number of tobacco-related cancers depends upon the length of time the person smoked, the length of time since the person quit smoking, and the overall health of the person at the time she or he quit smoking.

In our case, fifteen years is a substantial amount of time to have been a heavy smoker. Yet, our individual has now been free from heavy tobacco use for almost twice that length of time, and there is no indication she suffered any health problems at the time she quit. These factors weigh positively in her profile; however, they don't negate the possibility of a continued increased risk for tobacco related cancers.

Many cancers take several years or decades to develop and irreparable damage already may have occurred during her years of smoking. We also know her risk of damage from past smoking depends upon her age at the time she began smoking with a younger age carrying more risk, the number of cigarettes she smoked each day and the number of years she smoked. Lung cancer in particular may remain a risk as we know that chemicals found in cigarette smoke "activate" certain genes within the cells of the lungs, which make them more susceptible to chemical carcinogenic harm. Our individual also may still be at risk for developing cancers of the larynx, oral cavity, esophagus, bladder, kidney, pancreas and cervix. Similarly, she may have an increased risk for stomach, liver and colorectal cancer, all of which also are believed to be linked to cigarette smoking. If we add to this information the facts that she may already have a possible increased risk for cervical cancer and a genetic predisposition for colorectal cancer, her smoking history becomes even more relevant. Moreover, her current tobacco use, although limited, continues to expose her to the harmful effects of tobacco related carcinogens.

Finally, her current tobacco use occurs with her consumption of alcohol, a combination that greatly increases the harmful effect of both, even though her use of alcohol and tobacco is in itself slight. Tobacco use, therefore, becomes our seventh and final layer of risk in our profile which includes **1) Heredity, 2) Solar Radiation, 3) Medical Treatments/ Conditions, 4) Hormones, 5) Diet, 6) Alcohol** and **7) Tobacco Use**.

Once again, we'll now examine each layer of risk in our profile and determine which can be eliminated or, at least, controlled. Beginning with **heredity**, our individual possesses a possible genetic predisposition for both breast and colorectal cancer. Her history of benign breast disease, which also may be hereditary, adds to her risk for developing breast cancer and, should this occur, she also may possess vulnerability for developing melanoma, endometrial and ovarian cancer.

Additionally, her possible genetic risk for colorectal cancer creates an indirect risk for the development of endometrial cancer as well. This layer, however, involves risks over which we have little control. As a result, this layer will remain in our profile as we look for other ways to mitigate and reduce the impact of these potential risks.

The second layer of risk involves **solar radiation** that, in our case, doesn't appear to be of major significance. Her hereditary factors for breast cancer may eventually put her at risk for developing melanoma, but this possibility isn't an issue within our current control. Our individual doesn't work outdoors, and it's not evident that she spends a great amount of leisure time outdoors. The damaging effect of free radicals, however, isn't limited to outdoor exposure or direct sunlight. While solar radiation is an environmental risk that cannot be eliminated, it can be controlled through simple means. By wearing protective clothing when necessary and using quality sunscreens on all exposed body parts every day, regardless of her location or daily activities, our individual can greatly reduce her risk for developing skin cancers.

Our next layer of risk overlaps heredity and concerns our individual's history of fibrosis. This **medical condition** is a benign breast disease that has been associated with the development of breast cancer. This isn't a condition that can be eliminated, although it can be monitored. As a result, this layer of risk will remain in our profile.

The fourth layer of risk in our profile, **hormones**, is of great significance to our individual. We've established that this individual's history as it relates to this layer of risk may put her at an increased risk for developing breast, endometrial, cervical and ovarian cancer. Her years of both endogenous and exogenous estrogen exposure, the age at which she began oral contraceptive use, her age at her first full-term pregnancy, and the fact she experienced only one full term pregnancy, are risk factors that have already occurred and cannot be altered.

She can, however, address the issue of hormone replacement therapy and the risk it may present to her in light of her background. If she can find alternative methods or treatments to combat her symptoms of menopause and post-menopause, her continued exposure to estrogen can be decreased as will her risk for breast and endometrial cancer. Knowing that, this layer of risk will remain in our profile, but its impact will be reduced.

Our next layer of risk involves **diet**, the factors of which typically are lifestyle risks that can be altered significantly when indicated. Our individual is an urban dweller who appears to be of a higher socio-economic status living in an industrialized city. High fat diets are associated with such profiles and, indeed, our individual admits to being twenty-five pounds overweight. She tries to compensate for her diet by consuming large amounts of antioxidant supplements, which indicates her diet is lacking in fruits and vegetables. Additionally, she doesn't get enough physical exercise.

First, it isn't conclusive that a high fat diet increases a woman's risk for breast cancer as current research on the subject still remains contradictory. Furthermore, as a menopausal/post-menopausal woman, our individual's excess body weight won't affect or increase her production of estrogen. Yet, she may be predisposed to developing breast cancer as indicated by her family's medical history as well as her own medical history, and her overweight condition may interfere with proper medical monitoring and the detection of the disease.

In addition, she may have a genetic predisposition for developing colorectal cancer as well, and this disease does have a strong relationship to high fat diets, an overweight condition and a lack of exercise. High fat diets also have been linked to endometrial, ovarian, kidney and pancreatic cancers. In light of these facts, therefore, it would be advisable for our individual to reduce the amount of fat in her diet.

It also would be helpful to include the recommended five or six servings of fruits and vegetables in her daily diet. Indeed, these foods and the antioxidants, vitamins and minerals they contain appear to provide a protective effect against virtually every type of cancer including that of the lungs, an issue relevant to our individual based upon her smoking history. In addition, the consumption of fruits and vegetables can replace her reliance upon antioxidant supplements, the effects of which aren't yet clearly understood.

With her physician's approval, she also may want to add the regular use of aspirin or ibuprofen to her routine as both have been found to provide a protective effect against both breast and colorectal cancer. With physician approval she also may want to increase her consumption of calcium, which appears to offer protection from colorectal cancer as well. And finally, a program of regular physical exercise will help increase her protection from these and virtually every other cancer as well. By making these changes to her daily routine, our individual can greatly reduce her risk for a number of cancers including those for which she may have a genetic predisposition.

The next layer of risk in our profile is **alcohol**. We've already established that this factor isn't significant in this case. Our individual doesn't drink excessively, so the leaching effect alcohol can produce within the body is probably not an issue. In addition, she doesn't drink hard alcohols or any type of home-brewed alcohols. Instead, she substitutes white wine. She does, however, habitually smoke cigarettes when she drinks, and we know that any harmful effect of alcohol or tobacco use is greatly increased when these two factors are combined.

Accordingly, her limited use of alcohol may still present a slight increased risk for some cancers unless she also takes steps to eliminate her continued use of tobacco. In addition, while current research remains somewhat conflicted, our individual may wish to balance her preference for white wine with an occasional red wine. By including both in her diet, she can "hedge her bet" and gain the additional antioxidant protection each beverage may offer while enjoying its culinary pleasures. While this change may be small, our individual appears to be at risk for a number of cancers, and any additional means of protection, however slight, might be welcome.

This brings us to our final layer of risk in this particular profile. Again, next to heredity, **tobacco use** is quite possibly the most significant cancer risk factor for any individual. First, as our individual smoked heavily for fifteen years, she already has been exposed to a number of chemical carcinogens and her occasional use of tobacco today increases that exposure. As a result, she runs an increased risk for eleven major cancers, including that of the lungs, colon and cervix. The latter two in particular are important as our individual appears to already have an increased risk for each of these cancers as indicated by heredity and hormonal factors.

Unfortunately, it isn't possible to eliminate damage that may have occurred to tissues years ago. Such damage, however, may be mitigated in a number of ways. First and foremost, it would be highly advisable for our individual to eliminate her current tobacco use. She also should try to avoid situations where she's exposed to environmental tobacco smoke whenever possible as she has already exposed herself to fifteen years of tobacco smoke and its related carcinogens. Second, proper diet is always important in protecting oneself against current and future carcinogenic damage.

Yet, proper diet also is essential in situations where one's goal is to reduce the effects of damage that may have occurred in the past. Foods high in antioxidants will offer our individual protection against many of the cancers for which she appears to possess an increased risk. Adequate physical exercise and the maintenance of a healthy body weight also will contribute to her overall good health and help her body fight and resist any harm it already may have sustained. In this particular case, the importance of vigilance in maintaining good health through diet and exercise cannot be overestimated.

In summary, our individual's initial profile began with seven layers of risk indicating possible vulnerabilities for the following cancers:

Heredity>

Breast Cancer
Colorectal Cancer
Melanoma (Indirectly)
Ovarian Cancer (Indirectly)
Endometrial Cancer (Twice Indirectly)

Solar Radiation>

All Skin Cancers

Medical Treatments and Conditions>

Breast Cancer (Fibrosis)

Hormones>

Breast Cancer
Cervical Cancer (Indirectly)
Endometrial Cancer
Ovarian Cancer

Diet>

(Impair Detection of Breast Cancer)
Colorectal Cancer
Endometrial Cancer
Kidney Cancer
Ovarian Cancer
Pancreatic Cancer

Alcohol>   **(Possible Slight Risk Related to Tobacco Use)**

Tobacco Use>   **Cervical Cancer**
                                      Colorectal Cancer
                                      Esophageal Cancer
                                      Kidney Cancer
                                      Laryngeal Cancer
                                      Liver Cancer
                                      Lung Cancer
                                      Oral Cavity Cancer
                                      Pancreatic Cancer
                                      Stomach Cancer
                                      Urinary (Bladder) Cancer

Adjusted Risk Profile

We can now combine these layers and analyze the types of cancers for which our profile has indicated a possible increased risk. Again, those that overlap from one layer of risk to another and appear more than once in our profile may hold more significance for our individual. We can see that the initial profile indicated possible increased risks either directly or indirectly for breast cancer four times; cervical cancer twice; colorectal cancer thrice; endometrial cancer four times; esophageal cancer once; kidney cancer twice; laryngeal cancer once; liver cancer once; lung cancer once; oral cavity cancer once; ovarian cancer thrice; pancreatic cancer twice; skin cancers, including basel and squamous cell cancer once; skin cancer including melanoma twice; stomach cancer once and urinary (bladder) once.

Overall, we have a profile that implicates seventeen different cancers that appear a total of twenty-nine times throughout our profile. In this case, those cancers suggested by heredity, those that appear more than once and those that are associated or overlap with tobacco use may be the most serious threats. Breast and colorectal cancer are certainly greater risks as the former appears four times in this profile and the latter three times, both by heredity as well as other factors.

Breast cancer also is implicated as a hormonal risk, as is cervical, endometrial and ovarian cancer all of which weigh heavily in her profile. Additional cancers that appear more than once include kidney cancer, melanoma and pancreatic cancer. Finally, those cancers associated with her tobacco use remain significant risks even though many of them, such as lung cancer, only appear once in her profile.

Although such an examination may, at first glance, appear quite overwhelming, it's important to remember that this exercise only attempts to identify possible, not certain, cancer risks. We cannot take action to reduce these possibilities until we have an understanding of what they might be. Now that we've thoroughly analyzed this initial risk profile and have accounted for the ways in which it can be altered, we're left with the following adjusted profile:

Heredity	>>>>>>>>>>>>>	**Heredity**
Solar Radiation		**{Controlled}**
Medical Condition		**Medical Condition**
Hormones		**{Modified}**
Diet		**{Controlled}**
Alcohol		**{Eliminated}**
Tobacco Use		**{Eliminated}**

Of the seven layers of risk in our initial profile only two, heredity and medical condition, remain unaltered. Our individual will continue to face the possibility that she's genetically and medically predisposed to developing breast cancer and colorectal cancer, and indirectly to melanoma, ovarian and endometrial cancers. Similarly, neither solar radiation nor her medical condition can be eliminated, yet solar radiation can be controlled in a way that greatly reduces her risk for developing skin cancers.

The hormonal factors associated with her past remain possible risks; however, a decision to eliminate or alter her current use of HRT will reduce her risks for developing breast and endometrial cancers. By changing her diet our individual will further reduce her risk for several cancers, including those already implicated in her profile, such as colorectal, endometrial and ovarian cancers. And should it occur, proper diet and body weight will facilitate early detection of breast cancer, another cancer implicated in her profile.

Overall, proper diet and good health will reduce her risk for virtually every additional type of cancer whether it's implicated in her profile or not. By adding a moderate amount of red wine to her preference for white she can maximize the antioxidant presence in her diet. And, by eliminating her tobacco use, any possible harm resulting from the combination of alcohol and cigarette smoking can be eliminated. In addition, while she cannot escape damage that may be linked to smoking in her past, she can significantly reduce her risk for many tobacco-related cancers, especially those which have already been implicated, such as cervical and colorectal cancer, by eliminating tobacco use from her current profile.

Our profile doesn't mean that our individual will or will not develop any of the cancers mentioned. We can only identify patterns, and these patterns won't account for or explain the origin, occurrence or outcome of every cancer in every situation. Based upon recognized patterns, however, this exercise can help identify some of the cancers for which she may run a higher risk. And with that knowledge, she can take pro-active steps to reduce her risk for these cancers in an informed and forthright manner, once again through acknowledgment and action.

Clearly, determining an individual's risk for developing specific cancers is far from an exact science. The factors affecting such a determination are numerous, confusing and to a large degree still misunderstood or unknown. Some factors are external such as radiation, chemicals and viruses. Others are triggered internally by inherited anomalies, hormones or immune and metabolic conditions. Some can be eliminated or controlled and, of course, some cannot.

As we know, over eleven million new cases of cancer were reported around the world in the year 2007, with nearly 1,400,000 of those occurring in the United States. In addition, approximately 560,000 Americans or 1,550 a day died of the disease in the year 2008, figures that, once calculated, are expected to be repeated in 2009.[504] Yet, it appears that approximately one third of cancer deaths result from cancers that were directly related to poor nutrition, obesity, physical inactivity and other harmful lifestyle factors.[505] These are the layers of risk within the power of most individuals to control, modify or eliminate, and these are the cancers of which literally one third can be prevented worldwide.

Such prevention, however, is a process that requires diligence and perseverance on the part of every individual. We need to understand our own potential risks for cancer and take the steps necessary to protect ourselves whenever and wherever possible. By using the Layering Effect and creating a personal Risk Profile, we're well on our way to accomplishing this crucial first step in reducing the world's overall cancer rates.

WORKSHEET

THE LAYERING EFFECT

STEP ONE: INITIAL RISK PROFILE

Begin your analysis at the top of the risk list by examining the layers over which you have the least control, progressing to those layers over which you have the most control.

With each of the thirteen layers, carefully consider any personal information that may impact your risk and write it down in the space provided. If you don't think a layer applies to you, simply cross the space out.

1) Heredity:

2) Solar Radiation:

3) Air Pollution:

4) Water Pollution:

5) Pesticides/Chemicals:

6) Viruses:

7) Medical Treatments/Conditions:

8) Ionizing Radiation:

9) Hormones:

10) Occupation:

11) Diet:

12) Alcohol:

13) Tobacco Use:

STEP TWO: RISK ANALYSIS

One by one, you've now examined each of the thirteen layers of known cancer risks and have determined which ones apply to you. Now, it's time to re-examine those layers that apply and to ask yourself if any can be eliminated, reduced or controlled. Conduct a thorough analysis as you move through each one. Use the knowledge you have of yourself, your family background and your own good common sense. Be sure to write your conclusions down in the space provided.

Again, if a particular layer of risk does not appear to impact you, simply cross it out.

1) Heredity:

2) Solar Radiation:

3) Air Pollution:

4) Water Pollution:

5) Pesticides/Chemicals:

6) Viruses:

7) Medical Treatments/Conditions:

8) Ionizing Radiation:

9) Hormones:

10) Occupation:

11) Diet:

12) Alcohol:

13) Tobacco Use:

STEP THREE: SUMMARY OF RISK

Now, it's time to cross-reference your risks with the specific cancers each may implicate. Once again, list the layers of risk that appeared in your Initial Risk Profile. Then, as we did in our hypotheticals, next to each one list all the cancers believed to be associated with that layer of risk.

The Risk: **The Cancers:**

STEP FOUR: ADJUSTED RISK PROFILE

You're almost finished. In this last step, you want to count the number of times a particular cancer shows up in step three. For example, skin cancers may be listed with heredity, solar radiation and occupation. Or, oral cancer may be listed with viruses, alcohol or tobacco use. Similarly, ovarian cancer may be listed with heredity, hormones or medical treatments and conditions.

Remember, those that appear more may carry more risk. Those that appear less may carry less risk. Also remember those layers over which you have less control, like heredity, may present greater risk simply because they may not be subject to change.

The Cancer: **Number of Times Indicated:**

Now, while the above summary may appear overwhelming, you're not finished yet. There is much you can do to change this profile.

To complete the exercise, list the layers that apply to you one more time. Summarize your analysis from Step Two and indicate if, and how, each layer may be modified. For remember, when you can reduce the risk, you can reduce the occurrence of related cancers.

The Risk: **Final Status:**

Now you're finished! So, let's review what you've accomplished.

First, you have a good picture of the known cancer risks that pertain to you. Second, you have a good picture of the cancers you may face in your lifetime based upon those risks. Third, and most importantly, you have a good picture of the steps you can take to reduce those risks and the related cancers.

The Layering Effect, of course, is only an exercise. It cannot determine with certainty what risks and related cancers you may face in your lifetime. It can identify, however, some of the risks and cancers for which you may be susceptible.

In addition, this exercise only includes the thirteen major areas of risk that pertain to **opportunity**. The second leg of cancer risk, **old age**, is not taken into account. Accordingly, readers over the age of fifty must remember that the risk for most cancers will increase as one's age increases.

Nevertheless, you've demonstrated how much power you have over your own health and well-being. You understand clearly how knowledge, common sense and lifestyle changes can reduce your cancer risks. And, you've enabled yourself to become a pro-active partici-pant in your personal battle to fight and prevent cancer. Congratulations!

Personal Note

While the Layering Effect and its Risk Profiles aren't infallible by any means, they remain help-ful in focusing an individual on her or his possible cancer risks. In my case, for instance, my Profile indicated a threat for colon cancer once based upon family history, and for breast can-cer twice based upon family history and the often inherited condition of fibrosis. My Profile also indicated a threat for skin cancers based upon my inherited light coloring and fair skin.

As we know, heredity is the layer of risk over which we have the least amount of control. As it turns out, each cancer profiled in my Risk Analysis has come to pass. The first, colon cancer, was a disease for which I was totally unprepared. I was unaware of my family history and my personal risk. As a result, I never underwent early detection procedures. I only discov-ered the cancer after symptoms presented, a situation that put me in grave danger, neces-sitated treatment with both chemotherapy and radiation and compromised my health for several years. Being more aware of my risk for the second, skin cancer, I began yearly body checks that allowed me to limit the disease to basel cell development only.

Finally, I was completely aware of my risk for the third, breast cancer, for which I underwent regular bi-annual testing. It was this awareness that kept a deadly cancer to a minimum. And, within two months I went from patient to survivor, with limited and breast-sparing treatments all conducted on an out-patient basis.

What Is An Acceptable Risk?

This question can only be answered by the individual who asks. Cancer risk itself, of course, is something that has been studied and documented for decades by medical researchers throughout the world. Yet, known risk and acceptable risk may be two different concepts—one that's determined by the medical community and another that's determined by the individual.

For example, hormone replacement therapy has been determined by researchers to be a cancer risk in some situations for some individuals. We know that excessive estrogen exposure over a woman's lifetime may increase her risk for breast cancer. If a woman experiences an early menses, a late menopause and few or no pregnancies, her natural production of estrogen has been long-term and possibly even continuous for several decades.

If she now combines her natural long-term estrogen production with HRT she may be putting herself at an increased risk for developing endometrial cancer, and if her elected use of HRT occurs in high doses or for a long period of time the accumulation of her estrogen exposure may put her at an increased risk for developing breast cancer as well. Even so, if this woman experiences severe symptoms of menopause that destroy her quality of life, and if other remedies fail to provide relief, this woman may decide that taking HRT to alleviate her symptoms, even in high doses or for a long period of time, is an acceptable risk worth taking.

Similarly, there is ample scientific evidence that links certain cancers with exposure to various products and chemicals in the workplace. As such, an individual whose occupation inherently requires her or him to work with hazardous materials may be at an increased risk for developing some form of cancer. If, however, the individual enjoys the work, takes whatever steps exist to protect her or himself, and does not believe it practical or possible to change occupations, then this individual may determine the daily exposure to these harmful materials is an acceptable risk worth taking.

Even the use of tobacco, regardless of the significant and undeniable health hazards it presents, is determined by some individuals to be an acceptable risk. Yes, urban legend would have us believe that centogenarians who smoke a pack of cigarettes a day and have never been sick a day in their lives abound. Indeed, some of these accounts may be true. Every human body is unique, and no two are exactly alike.

Just as each human face differs from every other face, the inside of each human body differs from the inside of every other human body. Physically, anomalies within the human body abound with some possessing extra or fused vertebrae, a third kidney, extra fingers, surplus ribs, or both male and female sex organs. Conversely, some human bodies lack certain parts and operate with only one kidney, or eight toes, or missing sinus passages. And just as each human body differs in its outward physical appearance and its inner construction, each develops and works somewhat differently.

For these reasons, it isn't possible to predict with certainty that what may be hazardous for one individual also will be hazardous for another. This, of course, may be one reason why some individuals choose to engage in known risky behavior. Some individuals may believe that the norm doesn't apply to them. Some believe tobacco use in particular reduces stress and anxiety. Some believe it facilitates a positive body image by helping maintain a culturally acceptable weight.

And, of course, while some simply find it too difficult to quit the habit of smoking, others may thrive on the excitement and danger of engaging in risky behavior. Some may convince themselves that they don't care about the danger, and others may ascribe to the simple bravado of youth, which often fails to recognize the fragility of life and health. Yet, tobacco use remains the most documented "cause" of cancer known to modern medicine, and the odds of staying healthy are against those individuals who engage in its use.

To borrow a phrase from American pop culture, the question one must ask is, "Do I feel lucky?" And we, of course, must respond, "Well, do you?"[506] If so, tobacco use may be an acceptable risk worth taking, and some individuals who accept this risk will beat the odds. In any event, deciding what an acceptable risk is and is not is a personal decision that each individual must make based upon her or his own lifestyle, expectations, needs and responsibilities. It must be remembered, however, that when one accepts a known cancer risk, one must accept the possible consequences of that risk as well.

Part 5:
Screening and Detection

It is not alone what we do,
but also what we do not do,
for which we are accountable.
Moliere

We've discussed the most common risks associated with cancer, and we've identified the most common cancers implicated by those risks. Moreover, in the initial step known as **primary prevention** we've outlined numerous ways in which we can protect ourselves from those risks in our daily lives. For the personal choices we make pertaining to diet, exercise, alcohol and tobacco use can play a significant role in our ability to reduce our risk for cancer.

The second step in this process is to take full advantage of all the medical procedures available today that screen for certain cancers. Known as **secondary prevention**, these screening tests are specifically designed to detect certain cancers at the earliest stage of development. Clearly, these tests are particularly important for individuals for whom Risk Profiles indicate susceptibility for a particular cancer due to older age or opportunity.

While screening tests vary greatly in their complexity and cost, they all share two common goals. The first, of course, is to monitor the health of an individual, rule out the existence of cancer and provide peace of mind. If cancer is detected, the second goal of such testing is to diagnose the disease as early as possible. For while one third of all cancers can be prevented through simple lifestyle changes, another third can be treated and cured through early detection. With this in mind, we'll discuss some of today's most common screening procedures for some of the world's most common cancers.

Chapter 24:
Breast Cancer

One of the most familiar of all screening tests is known as a **mammogram**.[507] A mammogram is a special breast x-ray designed to detect tumors in breast tissue before the tumor can be detected manually. One at a time, each breast is x-rayed while held tightly in place between two metal panels. The breast is compressed as much as possible to flatten the tissue, thereby producing the clearest picture. If a tumor is detected, it typically appears as a rounded spot or area of the breast that's grayish or dark in color.

At present, the process of mammography is the most effective tool we have in breast cancer detection. The process, however, isn't foolproof as it can fail to detect some tumors and at other times can indicate a problem when none exists. As a result, researchers continue to look for ways in which mammography can be made more reliable. For example, many mammograms are now being read by computers, which appear to increase the accuracy of the reading.

Other techniques for providing detailed pictures of the breast tissue such as **ultrasound** or **ultrasonography**[508] also are being explored. While this procedure isn't particularly useful in diagnosing the health of the breast tissue in general, it's extremely useful in diagnosing specific areas of the breast tissue. And, while it's not a replacement for mammography, ultrasound is an additional tool that may be used to clarify or confirm areas of concern that initially have been detected by mammography.

The high frequency sound waves used in ultrasound, for example, may help diagnose a shadow or obscured area of the breast that cannot be seen clearly by a mammogram alone. The procedure also can often show whether a lump in the breast tissue is a fluid filled cyst, which is non-cancerous, or a solid lump, which may be cancerous. Ultrasound use for breast cancer prevention is becoming increasingly common, especially for women who share an increased risk for developing the disease.

Indeed, the American Cancer Society has recommended that women at increased risk for the disease due to family history or a previous breast cancer diagnosis consider ultrasound in conjunction with one's scheduled mammogram. Many physicians also recommend an ultrasound for women whose mammograms may be difficult to read due to fibrosis or dense breast tissue which are, of course, conditions linked to an increased risk for the disease as well. In such cases, the combined results of mammography and ultrasonography can provide greater visual detail from which more accurate information may be derived and a more precise diagnosis may be made.

In addition, should a lump or anomaly be detected through any procedure, a **biopsy** also may be performed. This procedure, used in many medical situations, allows a physician to withdraw a small sample of cells or tissue for microscopic examination in a laboratory. If an entire tumor is removed for examination, the procedure is called an **excisional biopsy**. If only a small sample of tissue is removed, the procedure is called an **incisional,** or **core biopsy**. If a sample of tissue or fluid is removed with a needle, the procedure is referred to as a **needle biopsy,** or **fine-needle aspiration**. And, in an **en bloc biopsy,** tissue may be removed through radiofrequency waves, a procedure that proves quite effective for women with smaller breasts.[509]

Different biopsies are used in different situations, yet in the case of breast cancer the most common biopsy uses a needle, which is inserted through the breast and into the lump. If fluid is withdrawn, the tumor is in all likeliness harmless. If there's no fluid, cells from the tumor will be withdrawn and examined for cancer. At the same time, a small metal **tag** will be implanted in the suspicious tissue *just in case* the sample turns out to be cancerous. If the sample is malignant and if surgery is required to remove it, the tag will help the surgeon identify the proper area to be excised. While a biopsy is a fairly simple procedure, it's another important and necessary weapon in a woman's arsenal for screening and detecting breast cancer.

Mammography, of course, is an essential part of breast cancer detection for most women, yet there's controversy about the age at which this testing should begin. First, it should be made clear that the guidelines will vary depending upon whether or not a woman has a higher than average risk for the disease. First, if a woman's profile doesn't contain any layers of risk associated with breast cancer and she's under the age of forty, a consultation with her physician may determine mammograms are not yet necessary. If a woman's profile contains any layers of risk known to be linked with breast cancer such as a family history of the disease or fibrosis and she is under the age of forty, a personalized schedule of mammograms may be determined upon consultation with her physician.

If a woman is between the ages of forty and fifty and has no sign of an elevated risk for the disease, a personalized schedule once again may be determined after consulting with her physician. If a woman is between the ages of forty and fifty and has an elevated risk for breast cancer, a yearly mammogram is recommended. And, every woman over the age of fifty, regardless of her risk profile, should have a mammogram every year as age itself now becomes an increasingly significant breast cancer risk.

The main controversy concerning mammograms centers on whether or not an average risk woman between the ages of thirty-five and forty should have a mammogram to establish a personal **baseline**.[510] A baseline mammogram is conducted relatively early in a woman's life, at about the age of thirty-five, to clarify what is normal for her. For every woman's breast tissue is unique and what is "normal" for one woman may not be "normal" for another. It's this baseline x-ray that becomes the measure from which all a woman's future mammograms will be compared. Through this personal comparison, slight changes in her breast tissue that might otherwise go undetected may be recognized and treated if necessary. Similarly, a noncancerous anomaly in the breast tissue appearing on the baseline mammogram may be prevented from being misdiagnosed as a harmful condition in a later mammogram.

Is a baseline mammogram necessary? Perhaps not, yet this might not be the best question to ask. If we ask, "Could a baseline mammogram be helpful?" then the answer is, "Possibly, yes." The reasons for not having this baseline mammogram appear to be related to apprehensions about unnecessary radiation exposure and expense. First, while mammography twenty years ago had a relatively high radiation exposure that might have contributed to breast cancer development in some women, today's procedure exposes women to extremely small amounts of radiation. Second, mammograms often are available at free clinics or at hospitals and medical centers at reduced rates.

Additionally, mammograms, even baseline mammograms, may be covered by an individual's insurance plan. For many women, the possible increased protection provided by a baseline mammogram may be welcome and worthwhile – for others, it may be unnecessary. Whether or not a woman has a baseline mammogram is a question each woman must answer for herself after carefully evaluating her personal situation and discussing the options with her physician.

Mammography, however, is only one aspect of breast cancer protection and early detection. It also is essential for every woman to conduct a self-breast exam carefully and expertly once a month. This is a simple exam and instructions for conducting it are available from one's physician's office, hospitals, medical centers, women's clinics and a variety of health and cancer research organizations. In addition, every woman also needs to incorporate regular physician-conducted breast exams as well into her basic health routine. In fact, women of average risk who are between the ages of twenty and forty should have their breasts examined by their physician at least every three years. Women of high risk and women over the age of forty should have this examination every year.

Furthermore, for those women who have mammograms and physician-conducted breast exams annually it's advisable to schedule these procedures six months from each other, a schedule I like to refer to as the **six month split,** rather than scheduling them together. In this way, the protective effect of each is enhanced as a woman can avail herself of a professional opinion concerning the health of her breasts twice a year instead of just once.

Headline:

Schoolteachers Get More Breast Cancer[511]

Apparently, a study conducted in the United States in 2002 did, indeed, find that female schoolteachers shared a greater risk for developing breast cancer than women in other occupations. Unlike the studies conducted with airline pilots and attendants, however, these studies don't implicate the profession of teaching itself. They don't indicate, for example, that there's something inherently unhealthy with the profession or that women should avoid entering the profession for this reason. Rather, these findings most likely are linked to similarities in lifestyle associated with an increased risk for the disease. For instance, many women who teach school often postpone having children of their own until later in life. This alone is a risk factor for developing breast cancer. With the responsibilities of teaching, others may choose not to have children at all. This, of course, is another risk factor linked to the development of breast cancer.

Another possibility for the findings may have to do with the age of the sample group studied. Clearly, if the group consisted of older women the incidence rate of breast cancer might be greater than that of a younger sample group. Similarly, if the group consisted of women who live in geographic areas where a high incidence rate of breast cancer exists, or women whose dietary habits or weight contributed to the disease, the group may exhibit a higher than average rate of this cancer. Headlines can be misleading, and it's always important to analyze the facts and characteristics of the sample group to understand the study and its results.

"Can I Breathe Now?"

If there are any complaints concerning the procedure of mammography, they typically involve the discomfort that some women experience. Mammography does, after all, utilize a machine designed to compress tissue normally shaped like a balloon into a pancake. For large breasted women or for women whose breast tissue is dense due to fibrosis or other benign breast diseases the compression needed to get a clear picture of the breast may be more intense. Of course, the more pressure applied to these sensitive tissues, the more discomfort a woman may experience.

In addition, the positioning of a breast between two cold metal plates can seem at times an exercise in agility best suited to those women proficient in the arts of gymnastics or yoga. The entire breast must be placed upon one plate, the torso must be pulled back, the body must twist at an angle, the shoulders must be held out of the way and while the second plate is lowered to squeeze the breast and the corner of the lower plate is digging into the ribs, we're told to hold still, stop breathing and relax. Once the x-ray is taken, the breast is repositioned and the process is repeated from another angle. And this entire procedure, of course, must now be repeated with the second breast.

We need to note, however, that this routine of examining one breast first and then the other may be different if the pictures are taken with digital technology rather than regular film. With digital technology, the radiologist responsible for viewing the results of the mammogram may program the equipment to take digital images of the breast in any order she or he chooses. So, it may happen that the images alternate from one breast to another.

The advantage of the digital system, however, is that the radiologist can review the images from any location within the medical facility without having to come to the mammography center. This not only saves the radiologist time, but it saves the patient from having to wait for a radiologist to return to the mammography center. Furthermore, digital mammography is now believed to be fifteen to twenty-eight percent more effective than film in detecting breast tumors in women with dense breast tissue, in women under the age the age of fifty and in women entering menopause.[512]

So, yes, there may be some discomfort experienced by some women when undergoing a mammogram. Yet, this is an essential procedure that saves the lives of women the world over. No amount of discomfort should dissuade any woman from incorporating regular mammograms into her health routine. Furthermore, the technician, or the radiologic technologist depending upon the level of education, who gives the mammogram plays an important role in the amount of ease or discomfort a patient experiences with the procedure.

Less experienced technicians may have more difficulty positioning a woman properly, may take more time and may need to re-take the x-rays to get pictures with the proper clarity. On the other hand, some technicians have the ability to fly through the procedure quickly, professionally and efficiently without causing undue discomfort for their patient, and they don't forget to say when you can breathe. So, if you're a woman who dreads or dislikes having mammograms because of discomfort, find another technician.

Typically, this easily can be accomplished by making a simple request to one's physician or health care provider when making an appointment. If the facility doesn't have another technician, consider going to a facility where there's more choice. Finally, once satisfied with a technician a woman should continue to request that particular person for each mammogram she receives. If a woman's anxiety can be reduced in these small ways the probability she'll receive regular mammograms may be increased. And this, of course, is one of the important steps in reaching our goal of cancer prevention and early detection.

Special Concerns

On the day of one's mammogram it's important to refrain from using any product on the upper torso, including the arms that may interfere with the x-ray process. This means that deodorants, skin lotions and perfumes should all be avoided. In addition, women who have breast implants will face a mammogram that is somewhat more complicated and lengthy in time. Whereas the typical mammogram consists of two x-rays per breast, a top view and a side view, the procedure involves four x-rays per breast for those with implants.

First, one breast is placed upon the plate and slightly compressed for the first picture. The purpose of this is to view the implant from above to make sure that it's intact and not altered or damaged in any way. For the second picture, the implant is pushed back as far as possible against the breastbone while the nipple and the breast tissue around the nipple are compressed as tightly as possible and the x-ray is taken again from above. This picture, called the **displacement view,** strives to provide a clear picture of the major portion of the breast that lies in front of the implant.

Once these overhead views are completed, the breast is x-rayed from the side–again, without significant compression–to determine the condition of the implant. Once again, this picture is followed by a displacement view in which the implant is pushed against the breastbone and as much of the tissue as possible in front of the implant is compressed and x-rayed. Once this is accomplished, the entire process is then repeated with the other breast. The order of these pictures may, of course, differ if digital technology is used in place of film.

In either case, however, such mammograms can be more uncomfortable, even slightly painful, than those conducted on women without implants. And, it may be necessary to increase the total number of x-rays taken from eight to ten to achieve the proper result. Yet, breast implants don't compromise the quality or accuracy of the mammogram, and the final pictures should be equal to those produced in a typical procedure in which implants are not an issue.

Specific blood tests known as **tumor markers,** or **biomarkers,** also may prove valuable in preventing and detecting early breast cancers.[513] Typically, cancer in the body will produce a specific protein that can be detected within the blood. While it may be normal for these proteins to be present in small amounts within the body's blood and tissues, an excess of these proteins may indicate that cancer is present as well. Accordingly, an elevated level of these proteins can help "mark" the existence of "tumors" within the body.

The protein known as **CA 15.3**, for example, is linked to the development of breast cancer as is the protein **CA 27.29**. **Tru-Quant** is another protein that may indicate the presence of breast cancer, and the protein **CA-125** may be helpful in signaling a recurrence of breast cancer. All of these proteins have been linked in one way or another to the disease, and periodic testing for their presence, especially in high-risk women, is simply another tool one may choose to incorporate into one's regular health regimen.

What's New?

Technology is constantly advancing in the areas of breast cancer prevention and detection. In addition to the traditional mammograms, ultrasounds and physical breast exams, a new hand-held device is promising to be an effective new tool in tumor detection. This device is approximately the size of a pager and uses two infrared lights to detect specific changes in oxygen and blood flow that often indicate the presence of a tumor. When pointed at the breast, this device is programmed to emit an alarm if suspicious tissue is detected.

Furthermore, it's reported to be approximately ninety percent accurate in locating anomalies, cost effective and quite safe, as the infrared light can be used repeatedly without damaging tissues or cells. While this device may be available to the public within a few years, it's important to remember that it isn't intended to replace the traditional tools for breast cancer detection. Rather, it's intended to be used in conjunction with those forms of detection the value of which has already been scientifically proven.[514]

In addition, scientists are working on a new vaccine that holds promise for not only preventing some breast cancers, but for possibly curing others. Unlike a typical vaccine that targets viruses, this vaccine targets the human antigen a-lactalbumin. While this antigen appears in lactating women, it also appears in many breast cancer cells. The vaccine has been used on mice that have been engineered to be genetically susceptible to breast cancer. The mice that received the vaccine did not develop breast cancer when given the antigen. Mice that received a placebo did develop breast cancer when given the antigen.[515]

It also appears this vaccine is effective against tumors that have already formed. This, of course, means that the vaccine may offer curative hope as well as preventative hope. It's important to remember, however, that many cancer treatments that work in mice don't work in humans. Further, this vaccine may not work at all in breast cancers unrelated to the a-lactalbumin antigen. Nevertheless, the hope this research promises is astounding and if all goes well we could see this vaccine available to the public by the year 2020.

And, a newly developed three-dimensional mammogram may prove extremely helpful in detecting breast cancers not always found with the traditional two-dimensional mammogram. This 3D technology has the ability to find soft tissue tumors hidden behind other "over-lapping" tissue. While it does use more radiation than 2D technology, it is not believed to increase the safety risk for women who only have the procedure once a year. Although it is available in many parts of the world, as of 2010 it had yet to be approved by the Food and Drug Administration of the United States. An Advisory Panel of the FDA, however, has stated the technology is safe and actually improves tumor detection when used in combination with traditional 2D mammography.[516]

Headline:

Cell Phones Cause Cancer[517]

To date, this claim remains unsubstantiated. While the World Health Organization announced in the spring of 2011 that cell phones may be possible human carcinogens similar to lead or engine exhaust, research has yet to draw conclusive evidence that cell phone use increases one's risk for cancer, or more specifically, for brain cancer. The issue centers on the electromagnetic radiation emitted from mobile cell phones as well as all other electrical devices, including computers, televisions and alarm systems.

Cell phones, at least those used in the United States, typically operate in a frequency that ranges from about 850 megahertz, or MHZ, to about 1900. In this range, the radiation produced is known as non-ionizing radiofrequency, or RF energy. This form of energy, however, is different from ionizing radiation, which is produced by medical x-rays and similar procedures that can produce a slight health risk in certain doses.

It's true that RF energy in high levels such as that found in a microwave oven can heat living tissues to the point of biological damage. The RF energy generated by a cell phone, however, is small by comparison. Further, the main source of RF energy from a cell phone is generated from its antenna and the amount of RF energy to which one is exposed depends upon one's distance from the antenna and the frequency and duration of the cell phone use. The amount of RF energy also depends upon the age of the phone, as older analog models create a higher exposure while newer digital models create a lower exposure.

To summarize, therefore, current research has found no concrete evidence of an increased brain cancer risk related to the use of cell phones. Cell phone use, however, has only become commonplace over the last decade and, as such we lack studies on the long-term health risk their use may present. Further, some sources, including the British government, believe that children, in light of their still developing nervous systems, may be more vulnerable to potential harm from cell phone use and accordingly have issued recommendations that use by children be limited to essential calls.

It must be noted, however, that such recommendations haven't been based upon specific scientific evidence. Until further notice, therefore, those who still have concerns about cell phone safety can reduce any potential health risk by 1) placing more distance between one's body and the phone antenna by using a headset or mounting the antenna outside one's vehicle, 2) using newer digital models of cell phones, 3) limiting the number and length of cell phone calls or, 4) simply eliminating their use.

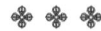

Chapter 25:
Colorectal Cancer

While colorectal cancer is one of the most common and most dangerous cancers among the world's industrialized nations, it also is one for which several early detection procedures exist. Of these, the **colonoscopy** may be the most familiar. This procedure is useful in detecting a variety of abnormal conditions or diseases of the colon and is the most accurate method of detecting cancerous or pre-cancerous intestinal polyps. It examines the entire five to six feet of colon or large intestine from the anus to the cecum, the point where the large intestine and the small intestine meet. Sometimes, the last several inches of the small intestine can be examined as well.

The procedure uses a specialized endoscope that performs two important functions. First, this flexible tube emits a puff of air that expands the sides of the colon and allows the endoscope to advance and move through the intestinal tract. Second, it contains a video chip that videotapes the intestinal walls as it moves through the colon. The video in turn is transmitted to a monitor in the examination room, which allows the examining physician to observe the procedure as it's conducted.

In this way, if an anomaly appears on the screen, such as a colon polyp, the physician can remove it immediately with an electrical loop that cuts and coagulates the tissue simultaneously. This procedure, known as a **polypectomy**, can remove suspicious or pre-cancerous tissue during the colonoscopy and in many cases, can prevent cancer from developing in the first place.[518]

A colonoscopy also can help identify problems that may have been detected in another exam by literally shedding light on the situation. If suspicious tissue is detected, a **biopsy** will be performed wherein a small sample of the tissue will be removed and examined under a microscope by a pathologist. Finally, if cancerous tissue has already developed, the colonoscopy can detect it an early stage when one's chances of a successful treatment and cure are the greatest.

As with any procedure, there's always some risk that something may go wrong. In the case of a colonoscopy, it's always possible that as the endoscope moves through the intestine it may tear or perforate the lining of the colon. This risk is very low, however, and the physicians that conduct this test are highly trained and specialized in this specific procedure.

The greater apprehension associated with this test is usually a patient's own reluctance to lie naked on an exam table, backside exposed while a stranger runs a long rubbery tube up their rear end, taking pictures no less! Granted, one is bound to feel a bit vulnerable under the circumstances yet, this is another life-saving procedure that must be utilized to prevent or detect colorectal cancer early. The best advice, therefore, for individuals who share this reluctance is simply to get over it. We're talking about matters of life and death, and concerns about modesty or misplaced embarrassment must be put aside.

Remember also that the physicians conducting these tests look at bare rear ends all day long and another one means absolutely nothing to them, for when they've seen one, they've seen 'em all. These physicians are only interested in doing their job and protecting the patient's good health. By the way, an effective sedative, such as Versaid or Propofol, is always administered intravenously before the exam unless the patient requests otherwise.

As a result, the only thing one usually remembers about the procedure is the physician saying "hello" in the exam room and a nurse saying "wake up" in the recovery room. It isn't necessary to be conscious at any time during this thirty-minute test unless one is vitally interested, for whatever reason, in viewing one's intestinal tract for her or himself. In fact, if the patient desires to be sedated and is still conscious when the procedure begins, she or he should inform the physician and request that the sedative be increased.

Perhaps surprisingly, the worst part of a colonoscopy has nothing to do with the procedure itself, but with the preparation. This begins the day before the appointment when the prospective patient exchanges normal food for clear liquids. In the afternoon, the patient will begin taking a solution that begins an hours-long period of extreme and urgent bathroom visits.

Years ago, this solution was known as "Go-Litely," a misnomer if ever there were one, and patients were required to consume a half gallon of this foul-tasting liquid the day before their procedure. Today, a four quart non-absorbable purge solution for sodium-restricted patients is often recommended. In the alternative, some patients prefer to consume an ounce and a half of soda phosphate solution or other laxative the day before the procedure. This small amount of liquid is much easier to deal with, and while the taste isn't much of an improvement, it's palatable enough when mixed with ice and a clear juice or soft drink.[519]

Similar to "Go-Litely," however, these alternatives are powerful laxatives, and the best advice here is to have the running shoes on and be prepared to move quickly. The resulting "evacuation process" will continue until late in the evening at which time most individuals will be able to sleep. In the morning, approximately five hours before the scheduled procedure one is required to take another ounce and a half dose of soda phosphate or other laxative to complete the cleansing process.

Accordingly, while many individuals prefer to schedule medical procedures early in the morning, this may not be advisable when the procedure is a colonoscopy. First, it's always helpful for one to get as much rest as possible the night before any medical procedure. Because of the required laxative needed for this particular procedure, one probably will not get to bed before midnight of the day before. If the colonoscopy is at seven the next morning the individual must wake at four to finish the remaining laxative and this leaves little time for rest. Second, one must take into account the time needed to drive to the hospital or surgical center and the fact that a bathroom may not be available.

The best time to schedule a colonoscopy, therefore, is in the late morning or early afternoon. This allows one a full night's rest and plenty of time in the morning to complete the cleansing process in the comfort of her or his home. Finally, one needs to arrange for a ride home after the procedure, and even if one elects for some reason to forego the sedative, one may still not feel up to driving.

It's recommended that individuals with no more than an average risk for colorectal cancer have their first colonoscopy between the ages of forty and fifty. If no anomalies are detected, follow-up colonoscopies may be scheduled every five years thereafter. If one's profile, however, indicates a high risk for the disease, especially if hereditary factors are implicated, the initial procedure should be conducted at an earlier age to be determined by the individual and her or his physician.

The recommended schedule of follow-up colonoscopies will then depend upon whether or not anomalies have been detected. If they have been, the procedure may have to be repeated every two or three years to monitor the individual's health and to treat additional anomalies should they develop. This is, of course, another situation in which each individual must work closely with her or his physician to design a personal schedule that offers the most protection. Finally, a colonoscopy typically is covered by insurance only if a symptom or a finding makes the procedure "medically necessary."

Personal Note

A few years ago, my husband and I, the romantics that we are, decided to have her and his colonoscopies. For me it was one of many, for my husband it was his first. We did the prep together, separate bathrooms a must, shared a cab to the clinic, filled out the paperwork and kept each other company while we waited for our respective turns. Following the procedures, we were approached by our wonderful gastroenterologist who took great delight in informing us that we were both "perfect assholes." And this, of course, was music to our ears.

"Excuse Me, But Is It Okay to Fart?"

We know that what goes up must come down, but we also need to remember that what goes in must come out. The colonoscopy is a procedure that works in part by puffing small amounts of air into the intestinal tract to expand the passage and allow the endoscope to move forward. When the procedure is over, the endoscope is removed, the air, however, remains. As a result, one may experience the normal symptoms associated with mild gastrointestinal distress. This may include cramping, bloating and yes, the need to pass gas.

These symptoms are completely normal and this is no time to stand on ceremony or typical social etiquette. Attempting to hold this gas in will only result in more cramping and bloating. So, remember that a fart here and there is totally expected and all in a day's work for every medical practitioner within the recovery room. There's no need for embarrassment; every patient is in the same boat, and the sooner the air is expelled, the better one is going to feel.

It also is quite common for one to pass a small amount of blood when having a bowel movement following the procedure. This, however, will quickly dissipate, generally within twenty-four hours, and is the result of the normal minor irritation and friction that can occur as the endoscope travels through the colon rather than an unintended injury.

Another test often used in the detection and diagnosis of colorectal cancer and other gastrointestinal anomalies is the **double contrast barium enema,** or **DCBE**.[520] The barium enema is actually a series of x-rays that permits visualization of the lining of the rectum, colon and often a part of the small intestine known as the ileum. This test is exactly what its name indicates – it's an enema that infuses material that contains barium into one's rectum instead of the water solution that typically is used. While lying on one's side on the exam table a radiologist will administer the enema. Then, to make sure the barium flows through the colon and into the small intestine, she or he will place the patient in various positions and gently palpate the abdomen.

The radiologist also may use a tube, similar to that used in a colonoscopy, to push small puffs of air into the rectum as well in an effort to move the barium into the proper position. Once the barium completely coats the lining of the colon and fills any hollow spaces, an x-ray is taken. Because an x-ray cannot pass through barium, the resulting x-ray delivers a fairly clear picture of the colon delineating the fine features of the intestinal lining as well as any anomaly.

The preparation for this procedure will require an individual to use a laxative the night before the exam and take a cleansing enema a few hours prior to the x-ray. A sedative isn't necessary for the barium enema, and the patient can drive her or himself home afterwards. Quite frankly, however, this test can be most unpleasant. As anyone who has had an enema knows, it's difficult to "hold your water" once an enema has been administered.

Yet, with a colon filled with a heavy barium material, air being pushed into the rectum and someone forcing the patient into different positions while palpitating the abdomen, "holding your water" is exactly what one has to do, and this can be difficult and uncomfortable. Additionally, after the x-ray is taken and the patient is allowed to use the bathroom to empty the colon, the radiologist may want to take another x-ray to make a "before and after" comparison.

One suggestion that may make this test less unpleasant for an individual is to meet with the radiologist before the exam to discuss any concerns. Further, as with any medical procedure, one should determine if it's important to have a radiologist of the same sex conduct the exam. If so, it's up to the individual to make this request when scheduling the procedure. As far as side effects are concerned, the test typically won't produce any except those that are clearly expected. One must remember that the barium material and the excess air must be expelled and until it is, the patient may experience moderate cramping and discomfort.

Often, one is advised to take another laxative after arriving home to insure all the barium is passed from one's system. Until it's completely passed, a process that may take several days, one should expect stool that is pink or white in color. Finally, those affected by ulcerative colitis may want to avoid this test as it has been known to aggravate this condition and even lead to perforations in the colon. As with any other procedure, the risk and benefit of a barium enema must be weighed carefully by each individual after consulting with her or his physician.

Performed in a physician's office, a **digital rectal exam, or DRE,** is a simple manual test that can help detect the presence of anomalies in the rectal area.[521] It's conducted by one's physician who gently inserts a lubricated gloved finger into the patient's rectum as the patient lies on the exam table on her or his side. Although this procedure can feel a bit uncomfortable, it's quick, easy and only needs to be performed once a year.

It's often combined with another test known as the **fecal occult blood test,** or **FOBT.** This test measures the hidden or "occult" blood that may be in an individual's stool. Determining the presence of blood is important as some cancerous and pre-cancerous tissues in the colon can bleed into the waste material carried within the intestinal tract. There are many different types of this test available most of which vary in cost and accuracy.

The most common of these, however, works by placing a small sample of stool, which can be obtained during a digital rectal exam, on a chemically treated paper card for laboratory examination. If the results of the FOBT are positive and traces of blood are found, further procedures such as a colonoscopy or a barium enema may be required to determine the cause of the bleeding. It's important to remember, however, that many positive results of this test don't indicate cancer, but rather common and noncancerous conditions such as hemorrhoids.

On the other hand, if the results are negative, the presence of harmful conditions cannot be ruled out. For while negative results might indicate a healthy colon, many cancerous tissues don't bleed and can be present without being detected by this method. To correct this problem, researchers are attempting to design stool tests that actually identify specific substances present in cancers and polyps rather than tests that detect only blood. Until such testing is available, however, it nevertheless remains helpful to incorporate the FOBT into one's annual routine of physical examinations.

Another diagnostic tool used in detecting anomalies of the colon is called a **proctoscopy**. This test utilizes a rigid hollow endoscope used to examine the rectum and the lower portion of the colon or the sigmoid. Because the instrument is inflexible, unlike the flexible tubular instrument used in a colonoscopy, this test is often called a **rigid proctoscopy**. It has the ability to not only diagnose abnormal conditions of the rectum and lower colon, it can sometimes treat them as well. This test doesn't require a sedative, takes only a few minutes and while it may be conducted as a solitary test it's often performed in conjunction with the double contrast barium enema.

Another commonly used test for preventing and detecting colorectal cancer is the **sigmoidoscopy**, also known as a **proctosigmoidoscopic exam**. This procedure is similar to a colonoscopy in that it also uses a flexible, lighted tube called a sigmoidoscope to look at the inside of the colon. It also is similar in that it can detect and remove some anomalies through a polypectomy and collect sample tissues for a later biopsy or microscopic examination as it moves through the colon.

It differs from a colonoscopy, however, in that the procedure only takes about five minutes and a sedative isn't administered. It also differs in that it only examines the rectum and the lower two feet of the colon or the sigmoid. Because the preparation only requires one or two enemas a few hours before the procedure, it's a much easier test to undergo and typically is covered by insurance. While the sigmoidoscopy does examine that portion of the colon in which approximately forty-five percent of polyps and cancers occur, it doesn't provide the same full examination or protection that the colonoscopy provides. Indeed, it must be combined with additional tests to get the same information obtained by a colonoscopy alone.

For example, the sigmoidoscopy often is used in conjunction with the barium enema. While the sigmoidoscopy examines the lower colon a barium enema confirms that information and provides additional data on the remaining part of the colon creating a complete "picture" of the intestinal tract. The guidelines for scheduling sigmoidoscopies are virtually the same as the guidelines for scheduling colonoscopies. Yet, for those in need of a complete intestinal exam and especially for those who share a high risk for colorectal cancer, it's highly advisable to forego the sigmoidoscopy and opt for the superior exam provided by the colonoscopy.[522]

Efforts to improve diagnostic testing have resulted in several new techniques one of which is known as a **virtual colonoscopy**.[523] The goal of this test was to provide a complete visualization of the colon while maintaining the comfort of the patient. This test is completely non-invasive and utilizes an x-ray that provides a computer generated three-dimensional image of the entire colon. While this test may be useful, it's important to remember that the preparation for the virtual colonoscopy is exactly the same as that for the traditional colonoscopy. That preparation cannot be escaped and, as we have discussed, it's the preparation that remains the worst part of the test.

Further, a virtual colonoscopy can only take pictures of the colon and detect anomalies. It cannot remove any anomaly in the course of the procedure as a colonoscopy does. This means that if a polyp is detected, one still must undergo a traditional colonoscopy or another procedure in order to have it removed. Accordingly, a virtual colonoscopy may be sensible only if one is affected by some chronic irritation or disease of the colon making a non-invasive test preferable as well as, perhaps, necessary. If this is the case, the same schedule of testing recommended for both the colonoscopy and sigmoidoscopy should be followed for this virtual test as well.

Chapter 26:
Lung Cancer

One of the most effective tools in the early detection of lung cancer today remains the simple **chest x-ray**. It's recommended that all individuals over the age of forty have a baseline x-ray of the chest. Follow-up x-rays should be scheduled according to an individual's risk profile at the discretion of her or his physician. For those who share a high risk of developing this disease, however, an annual chest x-ray is highly advisable. This procedure may be conducted as a part of one's yearly physical exam, and while it's simple, it's an excellent way to monitor the health of one's lungs on a regular basis.

If lung cancer is suspected, or if an individual's profile indicates a high risk for developing the disease additional tests also are available. A **sputum cytology** is a simple test that examines the cells found in the mucous obtained from a deep cough. Lung tissue provided by special biopsies also can be examined directly for evidence of cancer.

One such biopsy is a **bronchoscopy**, a test in which a thin, lighted tube is inserted through the mouth or nose and into the windpipe. This procedure allows the physician to visually inspect the air passages for anomalies and collect tissue samples for microscopic examination. Indeed, a new bronchoscopy that utilizes a fluorescent laser light now improves a physician's ability to detect the differences between cancerous and non-cancerous cells by approximately fifty percent.

Others include a **thoracentesis** in which a sample of the fluid surrounding the lungs is extracted and examined, and a **needle aspiration**, which is used to remove tissue from the inside of a tumor that has already been confirmed. Finally, in extreme cases where lung cancer is suspected yet cannot be confirmed by any of the above procedures, the physician may need to surgically open the chest in a procedure known as a **thoracotomy**, a major surgery that requires a general anesthetic and a hospital stay.[524]

What's New?

Through gene testing, physicians soon may be able to determine not only which of their patients are most likely to survive lung cancer after surgery, but also which would need the strongest additional treatments. This new research involves a panel of five genes that together assess a patient's ability to survive an initial lung cancer. Once this assessment is made, the physician is better equipped to determine the type, strength and duration of the patient's treatments such as chemotherapy and radiation. In this way, we may begin to tailor cancer treatments to fit the specific needs of each patient and increase each one's chance for survival. This, of course, would be an enormous boost in the fight against this particular form of cancer, which is the world's deadliest.

Chapter 27:
Ovarian Cancer

As we know, this disease is one of the "silent" cancers and, until recently, there was little a woman could do to monitor herself for the disease and detect it early should it arise. Regular **pelvic exams** by a woman's physician may help detect a change or abnormality in the size or shape of her reproductive organs. An occasional **barium enema** may be helpful in monitoring a high-risk woman's ovarian health. A biopsy may be used to monitor for and detect ovarian cancer. Yet, the biopsy for this cancer requires the abdomen to be opened through a procedure known as a **laparotomy** and as such, is not a practical option for regular ovarian cancer screening.

A blood test known as **CA-125 assay**, however, is an important tool that should be included in a woman's regular screening program for ovarian cancer. While CA-125 is a substance found naturally in the blood, the assay is another tumor marker test that detects excess amounts of the substance, which may indicate the presence of ovarian cancer, and may signal a recurrence of ovarian cancer as it may a recurrence of breast cancer.[525]

In addition, a new marker called **HE4** has been found to be just as effective as CA-125 in identifying approximately fifty to sixty percent of early ovarian cancer cases. Furthermore, HE4 testing also has been found to result in fewer false positives than CA-125, which is an important feature. Finally, similar to breast cancer, an excess of the proteins CA 15.3, CA 27.29 and Tru-Quant also may indicate the presence of ovarian cancer, all of which can be tested accordingly.[526]

Chapter 28:
Prostate Cancer

This cancer is extremely common among the men of the world and often deadly when not detected early. Yet, death from this cancer in almost all cases is an unnecessary result in light of the prostate cancer screening tests available today. Of the two most commonly known, the **digital rectal exam,** or **DRE,** is the first. As mentioned earlier in our discussion of colorectal cancer, this is a routine procedure in which one's physician inserts a lubricated gloved finger into the patient's rectum.

In this case, the patient typically is asked to bend forward over the exam table to allow the physician to feel the back portion of the prostate for anomalies or an abnormal enlargement of the gland. Again, the discomfort of this test is greatly outweighed by its diagnostic value. It's simple, effective and only needs to be performed once a year in men forty years of age or older.

The second important screening tool for prostate cancer is another tumor marker test called the **prostate-specific antigen blood test,** or **PSA.** The prostate produces a specific protein and it is the amount of this protein that is measured by the PSA. The PSA measures this protein in "nanograms" per milliliter of blood. While most physicians agree that four or fewer nanograms per milliliter indicate a normal PSA reading, new guidelines suggest two and a half or fewer nanograms may indicate normalcy for some men. Scores between four and ten are considered slightly elevated, while scores between ten and twenty are considered moderately elevated.

If the PSA, however, indicates a protein level higher than twenty nanograms, the score is considered highly elevated. This excessive amount of protein, or a sudden spike of protein, may indicate that cancer or another disease of the prostate exists. The PSA blood test is another simple, yet highly effective tool, used for detecting diseases of the prostate and should be performed annually in men fifty years of age or older.

Clearly, however, if an individual's profile indicates a higher than average risk for prostate cancer due to family history or other genetic predispositions, screening with both the DRE and the PSA may begin much earlier in a man's life. Again, the age at which such testing begins and the frequency of follow-up testing is an individual consideration that must be discussed thoroughly with one's physician based on one's personal and family medical history.

If any anomaly is detected as the result of either the DRE or the PSA during routine testing, one's physician will follow up with a variety of additional tests to determine the cause. These may include x-rays of the prostate that, of course, will provide a visual analysis of the problem area. Urine and blood tests also may be performed to distinguish potential prostate problems from kidney, bladder and urinary tract infections. One's physician also may perform a biopsy by extracting a small sample of tissue, which is sent to a laboratory for microscopic examination.

Such routine testing is vital as the symptoms produced by several benign conditions of the prostate mimic those produced by cancer of the prostate. For example, an enlarged prostate may only indicate a benign condition known as prostatic hyperplasia. This is a common condition that affects four out of five men by the age of eighty. Indeed, in the United States approximately thirty percent of all American men will need to have some type of procedure performed on their prostate to correct benign conditions at some point during their lifetime. Accordingly, routine DRE and PSA screening is essential for every man, not only to monitor his overall prostate health but to detect cancer at the earliest, and most treatable, stage.[527]

Chapter 29:
Skin Cancer

If we can say anything positive about cancer, we'll say it about skin cancer. For, this is the one cancer that appears on the surface of an exposed organ and often is visible to the untrained eye as well as the trained. Many skin cancers begin as obvious anomalies on the skin and, therefore, will be noticed initially through an individual's own observation. Other skin cancers, however, aren't as obvious and some begin on body parts that may be more difficult to see such as the back or the scalp.

As a result, in addition to self-examination it's advisable for every individual to schedule an annual **full body check** with her or his dermatologist. A dermatologist is highly trained to recognize any anomaly that appears on the surface of the skin. She or he also will be able to establish a baseline analysis of an individual's skin by which subsequent changes in the skin can be compared. For once again, skin tissue that may be normal for one individual may not be normal for another. Regular testing will help the dermatologist monitor the health of one's skin from one year to the next and detect possible malignancies at an early stage of development. Of course, if an area of one's skin appears suspicious, a sample of the tissue will be taken and a biopsy will be performed.[528]

Again, a full body check requires close examination of every inch of one's skin. Accordingly, one will need to determine if she or he prefers to have a dermatologist of the same sex perform the exam to feel comfortable. For the more comfortable an individual is with a cancer-screening test, the more likely she or he is to include it in a regular health care program. Once again, for individuals who share a high-risk profile for skin cancers, more than one visit each year to the dermatologist may be recommended.

Headline:

Pilots and Flight Attendants Get More Skin Cancer[529]

Apparently true. Research suggests that both females and males employed in these occupations develop more skin cancers than the general population. First, of course, these individuals spend a great deal of time in aircraft flying at high altitudes. As the altitude increases, the protective effect of the atmosphere decreases, and the harmful effects of solar radiation are intensified.

In addition, as we've already discussed, one doesn't need to be in direct sunlight to be exposed to the free radicals or harmful rays of ultraviolet light. Solar radiation permeates the atmosphere, even the atmosphere within an aircraft. The fact that pilots and flight attendants are exposed to this intensified solar radiation more than the average individual, on a continuous basis, may account for their higher incidence rate of skin cancers.

Chapter 30:
Urinary (Bladder) Cancer

As we know, this cancer strikes more men than women and typically appears in men over the age of fifty. All individuals, however, who are heavy smokers or who have histories of chronic urinary tract infections are at a greater risk for developing this cancer. A simple **urinalysis** performed during the course of an individual's annual physical exam can detect blood in the urine or hematuria. Blood can be an indication of cancer and, if this test is positive for blood, further tests will be conducted to determine its origin.

One of these tests may include a **cytoscopy,** useful in evaluating potential problems of the bladder. Similar to the colonoscopy and sigmoidoscopy, this procedure uses a narrow tube or cytoscope fitted with a special lens and fiberoptic lighting system, which allows the physician to see structures as the cytoscope passes through them. It's a technique that only takes a few minutes and can be performed in the physician's office. The cytoscope, however, must be inserted through the ureter or urethra to reach the bladder and, therefore, the procedure requires a local anesthetic. Once again, a urinalysis is one of the easiest procedures to incorporate into one's annual physical exam. It can save lives, and for those with a high risk for bladder cancer, it becomes another essential step in one's routine health care program.[530]

Chapter 31:
Uterine Cancer

A. Uterine Cervical Cancer

Cancer of the cervix, of course, is another extremely common disease that affects women around the world. Fortunately, the mortality rate for this cancer has decreased approximately seventy percent over the last fifty years thanks to the **Papanicolaou Test,** or **PAP** smear. The PAP was named for its developer Greek physician G.N. Papanicolaou and is typically administered during a woman's routine pelvic examination.[531]

It's a test that should be performed in the middle of a woman's menstrual cycle, preferably within ten to twenty days after the first day of her period. Additionally, a woman should avoid using any product that may interfere with the Pap's accuracy for approximately two days prior to the test. Such products would include spermicidal creams or foams, douching materials and the use of non-prescribed vaginal medications.

With a speculum in place to hold the vagina open, one's physician will use a cotton swab, wooden spatula or brush to gently scrape the surface of the cervix to gather sample cells. These cells, as well as cells taken from inside the cervical canal, are then "smeared" onto a glass slide and sent to a laboratory for microscopic analysis. The results will either be negative or positive, with the former indicating a normal cervix. The latter result indicates that the cervical tissue isn't normal; however, a positive PAP smear doesn't mean that cancer exists. While cancer may be the cause of the abnormal tissue, the result also may indicate a precancerous condition known as dysplasia.[532]

Dysplasia refers to the abnormal development or alteration of cells that differ in size, shape or appearance from normal cells. This condition is often the result of chronic irritation and is found most often in the respiratory tract of smokers and the cervix, a fact illustrative of our Cancer Blueprint. Cervical dysplasia may be slight or severe and may, in mild cases, simply disappear without intervention. If it doesn't disappear, it can be treated before it develops into cervical cancer. This treatment is the same as that used for severe dysplasia and may involve a **colposcopy** and a **biopsy** in which one's physician will use a magnifying lens and light to remove more cervical tissue for additional analysis.[533]

Recently, however, the use of a new diagnostic device known as an **optical wand** has become increasingly common. Specifically designed to replace the colposcope examination, the optical wand is a pencil-thin fiber optic probe that shines ultraviolet and natural light onto the cervix. It's able to detect cancerous and precancerous cells as both reflect these light waves differently than do normal cells. An optical wand also can detect the higher metabolic rate of activity associated with faster dividing cancer cells. In addition, the wand has the ability to detect an increase in red blood cells that may indicate the formation of new blood vessels needed to carry oxygen and nutrients to a developing tumor.[534]

Finally, the accuracy of this device also reduces the number of false positive readings that often occur with a colposcopy and the number of needless biopsies that follow. In some cases in which an anomaly is suspected, a physician may remove cervical tissue for further examination by using a thin wire loop and a carefully controlled electrical current. This procedure, known as a **loop electrosurgical excisional procedure,** or **LEEP,** is simply another method that aids a physician in determining whether a positive PAP smear indicates cervical cancer or some other condition that must be treated or monitored on a regular basis.[535]

Typically a PAP smear causes only slight, if any, discomfort. For many years it was recommended that every woman have her first PAP at the age of eighteen with follow-up exams annually for the rest of her life. In recent years, however, this recommendation has changed somewhat as a result of new evidence. First, it appears that cervical cancers are slow-growing and infrequent in younger and older women.

Based upon this information, some specialists believe that women may wait to be tested until the age of twenty-one or three years after they become sexually active. This reasoning also is based upon the fact that it takes three to five years for pre-cancerous cervical cells to become cancerous. Waiting until the age of twenty-one or until three years after becoming sexually active in theory, therefore, leaves plenty of time to catch any problem that may develop without "over treating" the patient.

Similarly, women who have been screened regularly throughout their life with negative results, are over the age of seventy and have the consent of their physician may decide to eliminate the PAP completely from their medical routine. For women who fall between these two categories, most medical professionals agree that all women should have annual PAP smears throughout their twenties. Women over the age of thirty who have had three normal annual tests in a row may then choose to be screened once every other year or every third year. Of course, for women who have had their cervix removed surgically through a hysterectomy PAP screening is unnecessary.[536]

It's important, however, to remember that these guidelines are just that and nothing more. Indeed, these guidelines recently have been restructured in the above way in an effort to alleviate concerns that some women are actually being harmed unnecessarily. For example, if a PAP test inaccurately indicates a problem exists, a woman may be exposed to expensive and invasive follow-up procedures. This can occur as the PAP, like any other test, is not infallible. The strength of the PAP lies in the fact that it's able to detect ninety-five percent of all cervical cancers and most importantly, detects them at an early stage before they can be seen with the naked eye.

It's at this stage that the cancer can be treated and in most cases completely cured. Testing every three years may, or may not, catch dysplasia or pre-cancerous cells before they become cancerous. On the other hand, a PAP test every year will catch any pre-cancerous cells as they develop and will allow a woman to be treated or monitored accordingly.

Furthermore, a PAP smear will occasionally detect endometrial and ovarian cancer at their earliest stage of development as well.

Additionally, the new guidelines suggesting less frequent PAP testing for women certainly don't apply to those whose profiles indicate a higher than average risk for cervical cancer. Women who began having consensual sexual intercourse at an early age or women who were sexually abused as children or teenagers may want to begin their PAP testing before the age of eighteen and then, of course, follow up with additional PAPs on an annual basis. It also is strongly advisable for women who have had multiple sexual partners, a sexually transmitted disease including HPV, a diagnosis of HIV or another immunosuppressive disease, DES mothers or any history of cervical cancer to receive PAP testing on a regular annual schedule.

Clearly, questions relating to a woman's first PAP smear and schedule of follow up testing can only be addressed on a case-by-case basis. Each woman's health history is unique, and each woman has her own level of comfort and expectation when dealing with matters of health. A thoughtful analysis, therefore, is required by every woman, in concert with her physician, to decide upon a plan of action that will provide her with the most protection as well as the greatest peace of mind.

Women should be aware of the fact that regardless of the new guidelines recommending less frequent PAP testing, the coverage supplied by many insurance companies for annual testing hasn't changed. In the alternative, a new liquid-based PAP test only requires testing every two years rather than annually. Moreover, a new HPV test can often clarify and eliminate concern when the results of a PAP test are abnormal. There are more than one hundred types of HPV, and typically each is categorized as either high risk or low risk. Several high risk HPVs appear to be responsible for the development of cervical cancer while low risk HPVs appear to be responsible for the development of genital warts.[537]

The new test, known as a **DNA HPV** test, can detect the presence of HPV in a woman's cervix. The test also can determine if these abnormal cells are high risk or low risk. If the test is positive, the abnormal cells typically are high risk, may be cancerous or may lead to cancer and must be treated. If the test is negative any abnormal cells typically are low risk and generally present no cause for alarm. In the United States, as of 2004 the combination of this DNA HPV test with a PAP wasn't readily available to all women. It remains available, however, to those women whose PAP results are uncertain or indicate an abnormality, and for all women over the age of thirty.[538]

What's New?

First, scientists in Australia have developed an important new ally in the fight against cervical cancer. Marketed today as **Gardasil**, this ally is a vaccine that will help prevent the development of this disease by protecting women against HPV type 6, 11, 16 and 18, the four most common forms of HPV associated with cervical cancer. This is extremely significant as we know that approximately seventy-five percent of sexually active women will contract some form of HPV during their lifetime.

In the Australian study, twenty-five thousand at-risk women from thirty-three countries were given either the vaccine or a placebo. The study was conducted over a two year period at the end of which only twenty-one of the test women developed cervical cancer, and all twenty-one had been given the placebo. This vaccine, which became available in late 2006, is great news for all engaged in the fight against cervical cancer and a trailblazer in the overall quest to eradicate the disease.

Second, physicians are now able to detect precancerous cervical cells, or dysplasia, in the span of an office visit. This is done by swabbing a vinegar solution onto the tissues of the cervical area. Precancerous cells will turn milky white in color in response to the solution. This, of course, allows the physician to target and treat the affected tissues before they develop into cancers.[539]

B. Uterine Endometrial Cancer

As we know, this is a cancer that typically affects women later in life. We also know that women who share a higher risk for this cancer include those with a history of infertility or failure to ovulate, those with excess body weight and those who have those who have undergone hormone replacement therapy or have experienced excessive estrogen exposure from any other cause.   When these high-risk women reach menopause it's highly advisable for them to schedule an **endometrial biopsy**. This is an office procedure conducted by one's physician and is quite similar to the Pap smear. While on the exam table with a speculum in place to hold the vagina open, the physician uses an instrument to remove a small sample of tissue from the uterine lining.[540]

This is a simple procedure that doesn't require a sedative and only takes a few minutes. The sample is then sent to a laboratory where a microscopic examination will determine if the tissue is normal. If it is, the patient is provided peace of mind and her health can continue to be monitored on a regular basis by scheduling follow-up biopsies with her physician. If the sample is abnormal, the procedure can help detect problems at an early stage of development when a successful treatment is highly likely.

Chapter 32:
Additional Screening Procedures

The acknowledgment of our weakness
is the first step toward repairing our loss.
Thomas A. Kempir

Most of us are familiar with the typical x-ray examination. It's one of the most common diagnostic procedures found in the industrialized regions of the world. Typically, x-rays have been used to view body structures such as the lungs, bones and heart. They're used in mammography to view the breasts, in dental slides to examine the teeth and other areas of the mouth and in barium contrast procedures to inspect the esophagus, stomach and intestinal tract.

These tests among others all utilize the traditional technology of an x-ray, which involves electromagnetic radiation. With the advent of new computerized scanning technologies over the last twenty years, however, the ability to examine the structures and internal organs of the human body has been virtually revolutionized. The most common of these new scanning technologies, all of which can be used in conjunction with any of the above mentioned screening procedures, include **computed tomography,** or **CT scan, magnetic resonance imaging,** or **MRI, positron emission tomography,** or **PET scan, radionuclide scanning** and **ultrasonography**.

Computed Tomography

The first, computed tomography, or CT scan, is a procedure that was first used in 1972. It requires the patient to lie flat on a movable table that slides into a chamber, or tunnel. This tunnel varies from approximately three feet long to approximately one foot long depending upon the particular scanner being used. Essentially, it forms a circle around the patient which projects ultra-thin x-ray beams from the inner walls. As these beams pass through one's body, measurements from thousands of angles are recorded by an array of special detectors. This data is then processed by a computer, which creates a composite three-dimensional picture of the body part in question. A "slice" of this three-dimensional picture can then be electronically selected and displayed as a two dimensional picture on the screen of a monitor.

With this picture, a thorough examination of the body part depicted in the slice can now be conducted, and this examination will be one hundred times more sensitive than the traditional x-ray examination. This precision is possible because different body parts absorb different amounts of the x-ray beams as they pass through the body. For example, bone is the densest structure of the body and as such it absorbs the least amount of beams. As a result, bone appears as a white representation within the image on the screen. Air, on the other hand, absorbs the greatest amount and appears black within the screen's image while all the other body structures appear as different shades of gray.

This ability to distinguish the densities of different body parts enables the CT scan to detect bone displacement, fluid accumulation, soft tissue damage and, of course, tumors. In fact, CT scanning can often tell the difference between tumors that are benign and tumors that are malignant because it's sensitive enough to detect the different densities between the two. As we know, tumors filled with liquid typically are harmless while tumors that are solid often are malignant.[541]

Moreover, in addition to its efficiency and accuracy, the CT scan is safe, painless and often eliminates the need for other high-risk invasive procedures. Although it does expose an individual to radiation, this exposure is small and equivalent to the amount of radiation exposure one would receive while on a flight from one coast of the United States to the other. The length of the procedure will vary depending upon how many body parts are to be scanned and the type of scanner being used. Most procedures, however, can be completed within fifteen minutes to half an hour.

Typically, no special preparation is necessary for the CT scan, which is usually performed on an "out-patient" basis without an overnight hospital stay. In some cases, however, the patient may be asked to drink a liquid that contains a **contrast medium** or the patient may be injected with a dye material intravenously before the procedure. Either way, these methods simply enhance the contrast of the image and neither prevents the procedure from being conducted on an out-patient basis.[542]

The intravenous dye material contains iodine, however, and as a result blood will be drawn from the patient and analyzed prior to the scan. This is done to insure that the patient doesn't suffer from any condition that would be incompatible with the use of iodine, such as diabetes or some other kidney disorder. Of course, if the patient is allergic to iodine, this portion of the procedure similarly will be eliminated. If it's used for contrast, the iodine will create a warm or "flush" feeling in the patient as it's administered, and will be easily eliminated from the body following the scan by drinking several glasses of water.

Overall, the CT scan is fairly comfortable, although the patient will be asked to hold her or his breath several times during the procedure as the images are recorded. Furthermore, there is just enough room inside the CT scan tunnel to accommodate a human body. Accordingly, when scanning the neck or head, the space between one's face and the tunnel wall only measures a few inches.

If one suffers from claustrophobia, therefore, it's advisable for the patient to discuss this with her or his physician before undergoing the procedure. Should this be the case, a mild sedative or a cool, damp cloth placed over the eyes will help alleviate the discomfort for those who experience this condition. In the alternative, a new CT scan that allows the patient to remain in a seated position while the test is conducted may be available in some facilities for specific body scanning.

Typically, CT scan screening has been a procedure used to diagnose those who have already experienced symptoms of cancer or another disease or to monitor those who run a high risk for developing such diseases or those who have been treated for such diseases. Indeed, CT scans were used initially to examine the heart and diagnose problems with cardiac function and blood flow. Recently, however, full body CT scans have become elective procedures that some individuals incorporate into their annual health care program.

The purpose of such testing is, of course, to discover potential problems of which an individual has no prior knowledge and in the alternative, to provide peace of mind if no such problems are detected. As we've discussed, the CT scan is a wonderful tool that has the ability to find many problems that other tests may miss. Similar to any other test, however, the CT scan isn't infallible. It may fail to detect a problem that exists or it may detect a "problem" that is non-existent. Indeed, the latter case is quite common as a full body scan is likely to detect multiple body sites in which the tissue appears suspicious.

If we keep in mind all the variations that exist among human bodies, it's no surprise that these suspicious areas typically prove to be harmless anomalies. Unfortunately, in many cases a "false positive" will require the patient to endure additional invasive and expensive testing to clarify the result. In addition, insurance programs in many countries, including the United States, don't cover elective CT scans at present. Yet, for individuals who believe that the additional protection and peace of mind are worth the extent and expense of the testing process, the full body CT scan may prove a practical weapon in one's personal anticancer arsenal. Of course, as with any medical procedure, the decision to include a full body scan in one's medical regimen is a choice to be made only after a thorough consultation with one's physician.

Magnetic Resonance Imaging

The second computerized scanning procedure is called **magnetic resonance imaging, or MRI**. This out-patient procedure utilizes equipment similar to the movable table and tunnel shaped chamber of the CT scan. Yet, it differs from the CT scan in that this imaging technique uses magnetic fields and radio waves to produce pictures of various body parts rather than ionizing radiation.[543]

The MRI works by creating a strong magnetic field around the patient's body. This field causes the nucleus of a body cell that contains an odd number of protons to align and rotate around the axis of the field. The application of a radiofrequency pulse then causes the protons to resonate and the removal of the pulse allows the protons to relax. As they do so, the protons release energy detected as a radio signal. An analysis of the amplitude and frequency of this signal provides information about the nuclei in the tissue and this information is computed into an image.[544]

The MRI is especially useful when examining the central nervous system, the spinal cord and areas of the head where soft and hard tissues meet. It also is effective for imaging the pelvic area and organs, including the kidneys, pancreas, liver and urinary tract. The procedure typically doesn't require a contrast medium, although an intravenous injection of **gadolinium**, a rare metallic earth element, may be administered to intensify the image.[545] As it's necessary for the patient to lie completely still to insure the clearest MRI images, a sedative for children and an anti-anxiety drug for individuals who suffer from claustrophobia may be advised.

Further, because the procedure is quite noisy, resembling the sound of loud metal tumblers falling into place, earplugs should be provided. Finally, because imaging rooms often are quite cold, a blanket also will be offered. While those individuals with metallic devices within their bodies such as pacemakers, clips or foreign objects cannot take advantage of the MRI, this procedure remains an effective, safe and painless diagnostic tool for many other individuals around the world.

Positron Emission Tomography

Positron emission tomography, or PET scan, is a computerized imaging technique that uses radioactive substances to examine the metabolic state of various body parts and organs. This scan is similar to the CT scan in that the patient once again is instructed to lie flat upon a moveable table that slides into a round chamber. Unlike the CT scan, however, which provides anatomical information including the size, shape and location of various body structures, the PET scan determines the actual biological functioning of the body structures.

While the PET scan itself is a non-invasive procedure, the patient is required to inhale or to be injected with a metabolically significant substance prior to scanning. Such substances, such as glucose, carry a radioactive element that emits positively charged particles known as **positrons**. When these positrons combine with the electrons normally found in the cells of the body, gamma rays are created. The PET has the ability not only to detect and map these gamma rays, but also to construct color-coded images based upon their location and intensity. These color images indicate the amount of metabolic activity taking place within the body part being scanned.[546]

Now, if the activity taking place within the body part appears to be abnormal in any way, the presence of a tumor or another physical anomaly may be indicated. Similar to the CT scan, the PET does expose the patient to radiation, however, the radioactive isotopes used are short lived and the patient's exposure is minimal. Furthermore, the PET is a relatively comfortable procedure that may take from thirty to sixty minutes to perform and typically is conducted on an out-patient basis.

Radionuclide Scanning

This imaging process uses nuclear technology to detect anomalies in the soft tissues and organs of the body as well as the bones. This process uses small amounts of radioactive particles, or **radioisotopes**, attached to various substances known as **radiopharmaceuticals**.

Once the particles and the substance are combined, the preparation is administered to the patient by injection, ingestion or inhalation.[547]

Similar to other scanning procedures, the patient must lie still on a table while a special detector called a **gamma camera** takes pictures of the targeted body area. In essence, this procedure is the reverse of a traditional x-ray in that the radiation source is coming from inside the body rather than from the outside. The pictures measure the level of radioactivity in the tissue and if an uneven distribution of the radiopharmaceutical is found within the tissue, an anomaly may exist. For example, an accumulation of the substance or a "hot spot" may indicate the presence of disease such as cancer, or the presence of non-threatening conditions such as a benign cyst, arthritis or an old bone fracture.

Like all body scans, therefore, the results of the radionuclide scan may produce several false positives that may be misleading and may require further testing for clarification. It remains, however, a tool especially useful in monitoring and detecting disease such as cancer in the bone, liver and lung. Further, no special care is needed following the procedure, and the radioactive substance typically will be cleared from the body within one to two days.

Ultrasonography

The fifth computerized scanning technique is known as **ultrasonography,** or **ultrasound**. This technique utilizes high frequency sound waves to produce moving pictures of the body's internal structures. A device called a transducer is placed upon and gently moved over a specific part of the body. As the transducer moves over the body, it sends high frequency sound waves through the body's tissues. As these waves are reflected back to the transducer, a computer translates the information into a moving image that, in turn, is displayed on a monitor for examination.[548]

Ultrasound has become useful in many medical applications, including fetal monitoring and the imaging of internal organs. It's particularly useful when a thorough and noninvasive examination is required of the abdominal organs, such as the pancreas, kidneys, uterus, ovaries and prostate. Not only does ultrasound have the ability to detect tumors and other anomalies of the internal organs, it can help guide the biopsy procedure should a tumor be found. It's a simple and effective test that requires no special preparation and is performed typically on an out-patient basis. Additionally, similar to the MRI, ultrasound doesn't use x-ray beams and doesn't expose the patient to even the smallest amount of ionizing radiation.[549]

At present, the above screening procedures, both specific and general, are the most effective and most common screening measures found throughout the world. Research continues on a daily basis, however, to improve these procedures and provide new and even more effective ones. It's, therefore, the responsibility of each individual to maintain an open dialogue with her or his physician to make sure one's knowledge is current and up to date. Each individual must know which screening tests pertain to her or him, when the screening should begin and how often the screening should be repeated.

For those at high risk for developing certain cancers due to personal and family histories, this knowledge becomes even more important. If one's risk for breast cancer is greater than average, that woman must avail herself of regular self and physician-conducted breast exams and the appropriate schedule of mammograms at a relatively early age. If one's risk for colorectal cancer is greater than average, that individual must undergo one or a series of the recommended screening procedures and also must do so at an earlier than average age.

The importance of these measures in the prevention and early detection of cancer cannot be overstated. Such testing will provide great reassurance when the results are normal and will provide the greatest chance for a complete cure if cancer, or another disease, is detected. These procedures, combined with one's knowledge of her or his body, as well as regular self-examination and observation, create powerful tools that literally can make the difference between life and death.

Part 6:
A Quick Review

We now have a fundamental understanding of what cancer is and how it develops. Our Cancer Blueprint provides us with a simplified explanation of why cancer begins in some cells and not others. We know that weak or damaged cells provide the perfect environment for a cancer to begin, and we know that such cells typically are the result of old age and opportunity. Although we have little control over the process of aging, we have more control over the opportunities that contribute to cancer growth such as diet and the environment.

Furthermore, we have a solid understanding of the relationship between these opportunities, or risk factors, and the cancers most commonly associated with them. Through our Layering Effect we can examine each risk independently and determine which impact our personal life. This, of course, provides us with an individual Risk Profile that helps pinpoint the cancers for which we may have an increased risk of developing. And, with this knowledge we can begin to modify, control or even eliminate some of our risk for developing these cancers by making specific lifestyle changes.

We know the scientific and medical communities of the world estimate that one third of all cancers expected to affect humankind over the next few decades can be prevented through the dedication to a healthy lifestyle or primary prevention. Proper diet and adequate exercise are essential components of primary prevention as is the avoidance of harmful activities such as alcohol abuse and tobacco use. Continued efforts to protect oneself from known carcinogens such as ultraviolet radiation or chemical exposure help complete the elements of this first step in cancer prevention.

In addition, secondary prevention refers to the dedication and commitment one must make to undergo the recommended cancer screening procedures available today. It's the combination of a healthy lifestyle and regular screening that removes or reduces some of the opportunities that allow cancers to develop in the first place. In this way, primary and secondary prevention work together to prevent one third of the world's cancers by maintaining and monitoring healthy body tissues, and by detecting and removing unhealthy tissues before they become cancerous.

In spite of all the precautions that an individual may take, cancer still may strike. If we have an individual, for example, who has adopted a healthy lifestyle and has regular cancer screening tests performed based upon her or his risk profile, who nevertheless is diagnosed with cancer, two things are likely. First, this individual, regardless of the diagnosis, typically will have a generally healthy body that will be better equipped to handle the cancer that has developed and recover from the disease more quickly.

In fact, proper diet and exercise and the avoidance of harmful substances and situations will result in a body the overall health of which may slow the growth of the cancer, limit the growth and spread of the cancer and withstand many of the harmful effects of the cancer. It's a simple fact that the healthier one is going into an illness, the more likely one is to emerge from it.

Second, as a result of the individual's commitment to regular cancer screening, the cancer most likely will have been detected at an early stage of development. And, when most cancers are detected early, the chances for a complete recovery are very good. Clearly, it's fallacy to believe that one's dedication to a healthy lifestyle has failed if one still develops cancer. Furthermore, general good health will help an individual to not only withstand the harmful effects of the cancer, but to withstand the harmful effects of the treatments as well. For many cancer treatments can be debilitating and even lethal in and of themselves.

So, let's suppose for a moment that an individual has just undergone her or his annual physical exam replete with the appropriate cancer screening tests. The results are examined, the physician arranges a conference with the individual and the findings, which in spite of one's best efforts, indicate a problem may exist.

Never give up, for that is just the place and time that the tide will turn.
Harriet Beecher Stowe

END OF VOLUME 1

REFERENCES

[1] NATIONAL CANCER INSTITUTE, CLOSING IN ON CANCER 3-35 (1998).

[2] Benjamin F. Miller, M.D., Lawrence Galton, The Complete Medical Guide 430 (5th ed. 1978).

[3] www.cancer.org/downloads/STT/CAFF2006PWSecured.pdf; www.cdc.gov/nchs/data/nvsr/nvsr57/nvsr57_14.pdf

[4] www.who.int/cancer/en/; www.cancer.org/downloads/STT/CAFF2006PWSecured.pdf; www.theheart.org/article/749039.do; www.cdc.gov/nchs/data/nvsr/nvsr57/nvsr57_14.pdf.

[5] Mario F. Triola, Elementary Statistics 3 (3rd ed. 1986).

[6] Random House Webster's Dictionary 702 (4th ed. 2001).

[7] Mario F. Triola, Elementary Statistics 4 (3rd ed. 1986).

[8] Id. at 5.

[9] Id.

[10] Id. at 7.

[11] Id. at 8.

[12] Mario F. Triola, Elementary Statistics 8 (3rd ed. 1986).

[13] Id. at 11.

[14] Id.

[15] Id. at 9.

[16] Mario F. Triola, Elementary Statistics 8 (3rd ed. 1986).

[17] Id. at 10.

[18] Id.

[19] Id.

[20] *SEER Cancer Statistics Review* (CSR); http://www.seer.cancer.gov; http://cis.nci.gov/fact/1_10.htm.

[21] NATIONAL CANCER INSTITUTE, CANCER RATES AND RISKS 9 (4th ed. 1996).

[22] AMERICAN CANCER SOCIETY, CANCER FACTS & FIGURES (2009).

[23] Id.

[24] http://www.who.int/mediacentre/releases/2003/pr27/en.

[25] Cancer.org/downloads/STT/CAFF2006PWSecured.pdf.

[26] WORLD HEALTH ORGANIZATION, GLOBAL CANCER RATES COULD INCREASE BY 50% TO 15 MILLION BY 2020 (2003).

[27] REUTERS LIMITED, CANCER DEATHS TO DOUBLE BY THE YEAR 2030 (2010).

[28] Id.

[29] Id. The most recent data also confirms that one third of all cancer deaths in 2009 could have been prevented by adhering to proper diets and nutrition, increasing physical

exercise, taking sun-safe precautions and eliminating tobacco use. AMERICAN CANCER SOCIETY, CANCER FACTS AND FIGURES 1 (2009).

[30] Boyce Rensberger, Instant Biology 30 (1996).

[31] Id. at 91-93.

[32] Mayo Clinic Family Health Book 1291 (2nd ed. 1991).

[33] Id.

[34] Joel Achenbach, *The skinny on aging*, NATIONAL GEOGRAPHIC, March 2003.

[35] Mosby's Medical, Nursing & Allied Health Dictionary 707 (6th ed. 2002).

[36] http://www.healingdaily.com/conditions/free-radicals.htm.

[37] Benjamin F. Miller, M.D., Lawrence Galton, The Complete Medical Guide 430-431 (5th ed. 1978).

[38] Mayo Clinic Family Health Book 419 (4th ed. 2009).

[39] Id. at 964.

[40] David M. Prescott, The Cancer Reference Book 5 (1978).

[41] Mayo Clinic Family Health Book 418 (4th ed. 2009).

[42] Id. at 1053-1055.

[43] NATIONAL CANCER INSTITUTE, CANCER RATES AND RISKS 22 (4th ed. 1996).

[44] Random House Webster's Dictionary 14 (4th ed. 2001).

[45] longevity.about.com/od/longevity101/a/why_we_age.htm.

[46] American Medical Association Encyclopedia of Medicine 78 (1989).

[47] Id.

[48] Richard A. Goldsby et al, Immunology (5th ed. 2002).

[49] Joel Achenbach, *The skinny on aging*, NATIONAL GEOGRAPHIC, March 2003.

[50] It's true that aging creates a greater risk of developing cancer. Some cancers, however, require a co-factor such as hormones. For example, if women ovulated until the age of seventy, the rates of breast, endometrial and ovarian cancer would rise dramatically. On the other hand, if women began menopause at the age of thirty it's believed that none of these cancers would occur. Lori Oliwenstein, *The age of cancer*, USC HEALTH, Spring 2005, at 5-9.

[51] David M. Prescott, The Cancer Reference Book 8 (1978).

[52] Mayo Clinic Family Health Book 820 (4th ed. 2009).

[53] Random House Webster's Dictionary 337 (4th ed. 2001).

[54] NATIONAL CANCER INSTITUTE, CANCER RATES AND RISKS 133 (4th ed. 1996).

[55] Li FP: Molecular epidemiology studies of cancer in families. *Brit J Cancer* 68:217-219, 1993.

[56] John L. Ziegler, MD, MSc, *Hereditary susceptibility to cancer*, UCSF CANCER RISK PROGRAM Oct. 23, 2000.

[57] NATIONAL CANCER INSTITUTE, CANCER RATES AND RISKS 107 (4th ed. 1996).

[58] Id. at 108-109.

[59] Kinlen LJ: Immunosuppressive therapy and acquired immunological disorders. *Cancer Res* [suppl] 52:5474s-5476s, 1992.

[60] NATIONAL CANCER INSTITUTE, CANCER RATES AND RISKS 90 (4th ed. 1996).

[61] Id. at 90-92.

[62] Id. at 84-85.

[63] Id. at 61-62.

[64] Id. at 67; AMERICAN CANCER SOCIETY, CANCER FACTS AND FIGURES 47-50 (2009).

[65] NATIONAL CANCER INSTITUTE, CANCER RATES AND RISKS 120 (4th ed. 1996).

[66] Id. at 77; Mayo Clinic Family Health Book 424 (4th ed. 2009).

[67] http://www.cancer.gov/dictionary/?CdrID=460150.

[68] Sarah Huoh, *A cluster of cancers: a cancer atlas of Los Angeles area communities chronicles cancer patterns,* USC HEALTH, Winter 2005.

[69] NATIONAL CANCER INSTITUTE, CANCER RATES AND RISKS 77 (4th ed. 1996); Li FP: Familial cancer syndromes and clusters. *Curr Prob Cancer* 14:73-114, 1990; Valerie Ulene, *Cancer clusters or pure chance?,* LOS ANGELES TIMES, April 7, 2003.

[70] NATIONAL CANCER INSTITUTE, CANCER RATES AND RISKS 77 (4th ed. 1996).

[71] Friend SH et al: Oncogenes and tumor-suppressing genes. *N Engl J Med* 318:618-622, 1988.

[72] NATIONAL CANCER INSTITUTE, CANCER RATES AND RISKS 77 (4th ed. 1996).

[73] Id. at 148.

[74] Id. at 77, 126.

[75] NATIONAL CANCER INSTITUTE, CLOSING IN ON CANCER 43 (1998).

[76] Loescher LJ: Genetics in cancer prediction, screening, and counseling: Part 1, genetics in cancer prediction and screening. *Oncol Nurs Forum* 22:10-15, 1995.

[77] As of 2009, states that had not enacted laws prohibiting the use of genetic information in health insurance include Mississippi, North Dakota, Pennsylvania and Washington. Hsien-Hsien, L. State Laws Governing Genetic Discrimination. *DNA and the Law*. Jan. 7, 2009.

[78] Alissa Johnson, *Plunging into the gene pool,* STATE LEGISLATURES MAGAZINE, March 2007.

[79] NATIONAL CANCER INSTITUTE, CANCER RATES AND RISKS 163-165, 188-189 (4th ed. 1996).

[80] Unna PG: Die Histopathologie der Hauptkrankheiten. Berlin: August Hirschwald, 1894.

[81] NATIONAL CANCER INSTITUTE, CANCER RATES AND RISKS 103-4 (4th ed. 1996); Jane E. Allen, *Next in skin cancer fight: protection from UVA rays,* LOS ANGELES TIMES, May 20, 2002, at S6.

[82] ALTRUIS BIOMEDICAL NETWORK, SUNBURNS (2005).

[83] NATIONAL CANCER INSTITUTE, CANCER RATES AND RISKS 103 (4th ed. 1996).

[84] Fears TR et al: Mathematical models of age and ultraviolet effects on the incidence of skin cancer among whites in the United States. *Am J Epidemiol* 105:420-427, 1977.

[85] Farman JC et al: Large losses of total ozone in Antarctica reveal seasonal ClOxNOx interaction, *Nature* 315:207-210, 1985.

[86] Id.

[87] NATIONAL CANCER INSTITUTE, CANCER RATES AND RISKS 104 (4th ed. 1996).

[88] Id. at 105.

[89] SID KIRCHHEIMER, WEBMD, INC., FLIGHT CREWS HAVE HIGHER CANCER RISK (2003).

[90] NATIONAL CANCER INSTITUTE, CANCER RATES AND RISKS 56 (4th ed. 1996).

[91] Id.

[92] Mumford JL et al: Lung cancer and indoor air pollution in Xuan Wei, China. *Science* 232:217-220, 1987.

[93] Wu-Williams AH et al: Lung cancer among women in northeast China. *Br J Cancer* 62:982-987, 1990.

[94] Xu ZY et al: Smoking, air pollution, and the high rates of lung cancer in Shenyang, China. *J Natl Cancer Inst* 81:1800-1806, 1989.

[95] Id.

[96] NATIONAL CANCER INSTITUTE, CANCER RATES AND RISKS 57 (4th ed. 1996).

[97] Lubin JH et al: Estimating Rn-induced lung cancer in the United States. *Health Phys* 57:417-427, 1989.

[98] NATIONAL CANCER INSTITUTE, CANCER RATES AND RISKS 57 (4th ed. 1996).

[99] Id.

[100] Lee Snodgrass, *What you need to know about asbestos*, THIS OLD HOUSE (Magazine).

[101] Environmental Protection Agency: Respiratory Health Effects of Passive Smoking: Lung cancer and other disorders. Washington, DC: EPA, 1992.

[102] http://www.scientificamerican.com/article.cfm?id=what-is-third-hand-smoke.

[103] NATIONAL CANCER INSTITUTE, CANCER RATES AND RISKS 56 (4th ed. 1996).

[104] Id. at 57-59.

[105] Id. at 57-58.

[106] Lee Snodgrass, *What you need to know about asbestos*, THIS OLD HOUSE (Magazine).

[107] NATIONAL CANCER INSTITUTE, CANCER RATES AND RISKS 57-58 (4th ed. 1996).

[108] Chen CJ and Wang CJ: ecological correlation between arsenic level in well water and age-adjusted mortality from malignant neoplasms. *Cancer Res* 50:5470-5474, 1990.

[109] Chromium 3 also known as trivalent and chromium 6 also known as hexavalent: NATIONAL CANCER INSTITUTE, RATES AND RISKS 58 (4th ed.1996); http://www.oehha.ca.gov/public_info/facts/chrom6facts.html.

[110] NATIONAL CANCER INSTITUTE, RATES AND RISKS 58 (4th ed. 1996).

[111] http://www.chemicool.com/elements/radium.html.

[112] NATIONAL CANCER INSTITUTE, RATES AND RISKS 90 (4th ed. 1996).

[113] Samet J M: Radon and lung cancer. *J Natl Cancer Inst* 81:745-757, 1989.

[114] NATIONAL CANCER INSTITUTE, CANCER RATES AND RISKS 59 (4th ed. 1996).

[115] Id.

[116] Id. at 58-59.

[117] Id. at 59.

[118] NATIONAL CANCER INSTITUTE, CANCER RATES AND RISKS 99 (4th ed. 1996).

[119] Blair A., et al: Clues to cancer etiology from studies of farmers, *Scand J. Work Environ Health,* 18:209-215, 1992.

[120] Id.; International Agency for Research on Cancer (1987, 1991).

[121] UNITED STATES ENVIRONMENTAL PROTECTION AGENCY, http://www.epa.gov/history/topics/ddt/01.htm.

[122] NATIONAL CANCER INSTITUTE, CANCER RATES AND RISKS 99-100 (4th ed. 1996).

[123] Id. at 100; Hayes et al: Case-control of canine malignant lymphoma, *J National Cancer Institute* 83:1226-1231, 1991.

[124] LORIE RITCHIE, WHAT IS AGENT ORANGE? (2004).

[125] Id.

[126] Donna A. et al: Triazine herbicides and ovarian neoplasms. *Scand J Work Environ Health* 15:203-209, 1989.

[127] Mayo Clinic Family Health Book 444 (4th ed. 2009).

[128] NATIONAL CANCER INSTITUTE, CANCER RATES AND RISKS 107 (4th ed. 1996); Mayo Clinic Family Health Book 444 (4th ed. 2009).

[129] NATIONAL CANCER INSTITUTE, CLOSING IN ON CANCER 20 (1998); NATIONAL CANCER INSTITUTE, CANCER RATES AND RISKS 107 (4th ed. 1996).

[130] NATIONAL CANCER INSTITUTE, CANCER RATES AND RISKS 107 (4th ed. 1996); Boyce Rensberger, Instant Biology 44 (1996).

[131] NATIONAL CANCER INSTITUTE, RATES AND RISKS 107-108 (4th ed. 1996).

[132] Id.

[133] Mayo Clinic Family Health Book 1057 (2nd 1991).

[134] NATIONAL CANCER INSTITUTE, CANCER RATES AND RISKS 107 (4th ed. 1996).

[135] Id.

[136] Blattner W: HIV epidemiology: past, present, and future. *FASEB J* 5:2340-2348, 1991.

[137] Mayo Clinic Family Health Book 475-477 (4th ed. 2009).

[138] NATIONAL CANCER INSTITUTE, CANCER RATES AND RISKS 108 (4th ed. 1996).

[139] Gail MH et al: Projections of the incidence of non-Hodgkin's lymphoma related to acquired immunodeficiency syndrome. *J Natl Cancer Inst* 83(10):695-701, 1991.

[140] NATIONAL CANCER INSTITUTE, CANCER RATES AND RISKS 109 (4th ed. 1996); http://www.cdc.gov/ncidod/EID/vol5no3//campadelli.htm.

[141] NATIONAL CANCER INSTITUTE, CANCER RATES AND RISKS 80 (4th ed. 1996); http://www.cdc.gov/std/herpes/STDFact-herpes.htm.

[142] NATIONAL CANCER INSTITUTE, CANCER RATES AND RISKS 80-81 (4th ed. 1996); http://www.STD/HPV/STDFact-HPV.htm.

[143] Thomas H. Maugh II, *Rectal cancer rates increase in people under 40, researchers say,* August 23, 2010.

[144] Mayo Clinic Family Health Book 478-479, 876 (4th ed. 2009).

[145] Id. at 876-877.

[146] Id. at 215-216.

[147] Herbst H et al: Epstein-Barr virus latent membrane protein expression in Hodgkin and Reed-Sternberg cells. *Proc Natl Acad Sci USA* 88:4766-4770, 1991; Litter E et al: Diagnosis of nasopharyngeal carcinoma by means of recombinant Epstein-Barr virus proteins. *Lancet* 337 (8743):685-689, 1991.

[148] LARRY AXMAKER, EDD, PHD AND LYNNE HASSELMAN, MPH, WELLSOURCE, INC., SAFE SEX REDUCES CANCER RISK (2004).

[149] NATIONAL CANCER INSTITUTE, CANCER RATES AND RISKS 64-65 (4th ed. 1996).

[150] Id.

[151] Id.

[152] Id. at 64.

[153] NATIONAL CANCER INSTITUTE, CANCER RATES AND RISKS 87-88 (4th ed. 1996).

[154] Hoover R: Effects of drugs: immunosuppression. In Origins of Human Cancer. Cold Spring Harbor Lab. Press 369-379, 1977; Kinlen LJ: Immunosuppressive therapy and acquired immunological disorders. *Cancer Res* [suppl] 52:5474s-5476s, 1992.

[155] PSLGROUP.COM, ADA MEETING: ORGAN TRANSPLANT PATIENTS AT HIGH RISK FOR DEVELOPING SKIN CANCER (1999).

[156] Hoover R and Fraumeni JF Jr: Drug-induced cancer. *Cancer* 47:1071-1080, 1981.

[157] Id.

[158] DANIEL DENOON, NEW BREAST CANCER DRUGS MAY BEAT TAMOXIFEN (March 15, 2004).

[159] Fisher B et al: Endometrial cancer in tamoxifen-treated breast cancer patients: Findings from the National Surgical Adjuvant Breast and Bowel Project (NSABP) b-14. *J Natl Cancer Inst* 86:527-537, 1994.

[160] Dr. Isadore Rosenfeld, *Good news—a better treatment for breast cancer*, PARADE, March 6, 2005, at 10.

[161] ELI LILLY AND COMPANY, UNDERSTANDING EVISTA (2006); AMERICAN CANCER SOCIETY, INS., RALOXIFENE AS GOOD AS TAMOXIFEN TO PREVENT BREAST CANCER (2006).

[162] NATIONAL CANCER INSTITUTE, CANCER RATES AND RISKS 87 (4th ed. 1996).

[163] Id. at 88.

[164] Id. at 87.

[165] Id. at 88.

[166] NATIONAL CANCER INSTITUTE, CANCER RATES AND RISKS 88 (4th ed. 1996).

[167] Id.

[168] Id.

[169] NAS: Health Effects of Exposure to Low Levels of Ionizing Radiation (BEIR 4). Washington, DC: Natl Acad. Press, 1990.

[170] NATIONAL CANCER INSTITUTE, CANCER RATES AND RISKS 88 (4th ed. 1996).

[171] Id. at 90.

[172] Id.

[173] Darby SC et al: Long term mortality after a single treatment course with x-rays in patients treated for ankylosing spondylitis. *Br J Cancer* 55:179-190, 1987.

[174] Boice JD Jr. et al: Frequent chest x-ray fluoroscopy and breast cancer incidence among tuberculosis patients in Massachusetts. *Radiat Res*, 125:214-222, 1991.

[175] Shore RE et al: Thyroid tumors following thymus irradiation. *J Natl Cancer Inst*, 74:1177-1184, 1985.

[176] Ron E et al: Thyroid neoplasia following low-dose radiation in childhood. *Radial Res*, 120:516-531, 1989.

[177] NATIONAL CANCER INSTITUTE, CANCER RATES AND RISKS 91 (4th ed. 1996).

[178] NAS: Health Effects of Exposure to Low Levels of Ionizing Radiation (BEIR 4). Washington, DC: Natl Acad Press, 1990.

[179] Bithell JF, Stewart AM: Pre-natal irradiation and childhood malignancy: a review of the British data from the Oxford Survey. *Br J Cancer* 31:271-287, 1975.

[180] NAS: Health Effects of Exposure to Low Levels of Ionizing Radiation (BEIR 4). Washington, DC: Natl Acad Press, 1990.

[181] Lubin JH et al: Radon and lung cancer risk: a joint analysis of 11 underground miners studies. National Cancer Institute. NIH Publ. No. 94-3644, Bethesda, Md, 1994.

[182] NATIONAL CANCER INSTITUTE, CANCER RATES AND RISKS 92, 159 (4th ed. 1996); Cold Spring Harbor Laboratory Press, Origins of Human Cancer 187-188 (1991).

[183] NATIONAL CANCER INSTITUTE, CANCER RATES AND RISKS 92 (4th ed. 1996).

[184] Judy Foreman, *Hormone therapy is all in the timing*, LOS ANGELES TIMES, Feb. 27, 2006, at F8; Mayo Clinic Family Health Book 1204-1205 (4th ed. 2009).

[185] Id.; Jane E. Allen, *Bone study gives estrogen therapy another chance*, LOS ANGELES TIMES, Sept. 1, 2003, at F5.

[186] Thomas DB: Steroid hormones and medications that alter cancer risks. *Cancer* 62:1755-1767, 1988.

[187] Brinton LA: Estrogen replacement therapy and endometrial cancer: Unresolved issues. *Obstet Gynecol* 81:265-271, 1993.

[188] Brinton LA: The relationship of exogenous estrogens to cancer risk. *Cancer Detect Prevent* 7:159-171, 1984.

[189] Stanford JL et al: Oral contraceptives and endometrial cancer risk: Do other risk factors modify the association? *Intl J Cancer* 54:243-248, 1993.

[190] Van Leeuwen FE and Rookus MA: The role of exogenous hormones in the epidemiology of breast, ovarian and endometrial cancer. *Eur J Cancer Clin Oncol* 25:1961-1972, 1989.

[191] Stanford JL et al: Oral contraceptives and endometrial cancer risk: Do other risk factors modify the association? *Int J Cancer* 54:243-248, 1993.

[192] Id.

[193] Id.; Susan Pierres, *The hormone replacement dilemma, so what's a woman to do?*, HEALTH, at 134.

[194] NATIONAL CANCER INSTITUTE, CANCER RATES AND RISKS 84 (4th ed. 1996).

[195] Id. at 85.

[196] Id.

[197] Sally Lehman, *Concerns rise as more men use hormone therapy*, LOS ANGELES TIMES, Nov. 3, 2003, at F-1.

[198] NATIONAL INSTITUTE OF DRUG ABUSE, NIDA INFOFACTS: STEROIDS (ANABOLIC-ANDROGENIC) (2005).

[199] Id.

[200] NATIONAL CANCER INSTITUTE, CANCER RATES AND RISKS 94, 159 (4th ed. 1996); Cold Spring Harbor Laboratory Press, Origins of Human Cancer 186 (1991).

[201] NATIONAL CANCER INSTITUTE, CANCER RATES AND RISKS 94 (4th ed. 1996).

[202] Id.; Cold Spring Harbor Laboratory Press, Origins of Human Cancer 171 (1991).

[203] NATIONAL CANCER INSTITUTE, CANCER RATES AND RISKS 94 (4th ed. 1996).

[204] Id.; Cold Spring Harbor Laboratory Press, Origins of Human Cancer 177 (1991).

[205] NATIONAL CANCER INSTITUTE, CANCER RATES AND RISKS 98 (4th ed. 1996); Cold Spring Harbor Laboratory Press, Origins of Human Cancer 177 (1991).

[206] NATIONAL CANCER INSTITUTE, CANCER RATES AND RISKS 97-98 (4th ed. 1996).

[207] Id. at 73.

[208] http://www.americanheart.org/presenter.jhtml?identifier=3045792.

[209] Id.

[210] Americanheart.org/presenter.jhtml?identifier=3045792.

[211] Howe GR et al: Dietary factors and risk of breast cancer: Combined analysis of 12 case-control studies. *J Natl Cancer Inst* 82-561-569, 1990.

[212] Willett WC et at: Dietary fat and fiber in relation to risk of breast cancer. *JAMA* 268:2037-2081, 1992.

[213] NATIONAL CANCER INSTITUTE, CANCER RATES AND RISKS 73 (4th ed. 1996).

[214] Id.

[215] Id.

[216] Id. at 74.

[217] NATIONAL CANCER INSTITUTE, CANCER RATES AND RISKS 74 (4th ed. 1996).

[218] Id.

[219] Block G et al: Fruit, vegetables, and cancer prevention: A review of the epidemiologic evidence. *Nutr Cancer* 18:1-29, 1992.

[220] NATIONAL CANCER INSTITUTE, CANCER RATES AND RISKS 74-75 (4th ed. 1996).

[221] Id. at 74.

[222] Elena Conis, *Antioxidants: have they been hyped?*, LOS ANGELES TIMES, Oct. 27, 2003, at F1, F10.

[223] Id.

[224] NATIONAL CANCER INSTITUTE, CANCER RATES AND RISKS 75 (4th ed. 1996).

[225] Id.

[226] Thomas H. Maugh II, *Aspirin might reduce recurrence risk for breast cancer survivors, study finds,* LOS ANGELES TIMES, Feb. 17, 2010.

[227] NATIONAL CANCER INSTITUTE, CANCER RATES AND RISKS 61 (4th ed. 1996).

[228] Id. at 62.

[229] Id.

[230] Id. at 61.

[231] Lester Haines, *Beer fights cancer: official*, THE REGISTER, Jan. 20, 2005.

[232] NATIONAL CANCER INSTITUTE, CANCER RATES AND RISKS 62 (1996).

[233] Id.

234 Id. at 62, 175-176.

235 Id. at 67-68; AMERICAN CANCER SOCIETY, CANCER FACTS AND FIGURES 47-51 (2009).

236 NATIONAL CANCER INSTITUTE, CANCER RATES AND RISKS 67 (4th ed. 1996).

237 Id. at 70.

238 Mosby's Medical, Nursing, & Allied Health Dictionary 280 (6th ed. 2002).

239 Id. at 385.

240 http://medical-dictionary.thefreedictionary.com/tumor+promoter.

241 NATIONAL CANCER INSTITUTE, CANCER RATES AND RISKS 67-68 (4th ed. 1996).

242 U.S. Environmental Protection Agency. Respiratory health effects of passive smoking: Lung cancer and other disorders. The Report of the U.S. Environmental Protection Agency. Smoking and Tobacco Control Monograph no. 4. NIH Pub. No. 93-3605. Bethesda, MD, 1993.

243 NATIONAL CANCER INSTITUTE, CANCER RATES AND RISKS 68 (4th ed. 1996).

244 REUTERS, Lung cancer disparity, LOS ANGELES TIMES, June 27, 2005, at F3.

245 NATIONAL CANCER INSTITUTE, CANCER RATES AND RISKS 68 (4th ed. 1996).

246 Cold Spring Harbor Laboratory Press, Origins of Human Cancer 173 (1991).

247 NATIONAL CANCER INSTITUTE, CANCER RATES AND RISKS 58 (4th ed. 1996).

248 Id. at 68.

249 Id. at 70.

250 Most recent available at time of printing U.S. figures for most common and most deadly cancers for men and women, amcancersoc.org/cgi/content/full/58/2/71.

251 Most recent available at time of printing worldwide figures for most common and most deadly cancers for men and women, cancer.org/downloads/STT/Global_Cancer_Facts_ and_Figures_2007_rev.pdf; who.int/mediacentre/factsheets/fs297/en/index.html.

252 AMERICAN CANCER SOCIETY, CANCER FACTS AND FIGURES (2009).

253 NATIONAL CANCER INSTITUTE, CANCER RATES AND RISKS 26 (1996).

254 Timothy Gower, *A diagnosis that takes men by surprise*, LOS ANGELES TIMES, July 12, 2004, at F3.

255 Mayo Clinic Family Health Book 796-797 (6th ed. 2009).

256 http://www.mayoclinic.com/health/breast-cancer/WO00095.

257 NATIONAL CANCER INSTITUTE, CANCER RATES AND RISKS 120 (4th ed. 1996).

258 Id.

259 Id. at 121.

260 Daniel Costell, *An enduring battle: cancer and abortion*, LOS ANGELES TIMES, March 10, 2003, at F1, F7.

261 NATIONAL CANCER INSTITUTE, CANCER RATES AND RISKS 121 (4th ed. 1996).

262 Id.; Geoffrey Cowley and Karen Springen, *The end of the age of estrogen*, NEWSWEEK, July 22, 2002, at 41-45.

263 NATIONAL CANCER INSTITUTE, CANCER RATES AND RISKS 120-121 (4th ed. 1996).

264 Kelsey JL et al: Reproductive and hormonal risk factors: reproductive factors and breast cancer. *Epidemiol Rev* 15:36-47, 1993.

[265] Id. While fat intake alone has been found to increase a woman's risk for breast cancer in some studies, other studies have failed to show an association. Hunter DJ and Willett WC: Diet, body size, and breast cancer. *Epidemiol Rev* 15:110-132, 1993.

[266] Kelsey JL and Gammon MD: Epidemiology of breast cancer. *Epidemiol Rev* 12:228-240, 1990.

[267] NATIONAL CANCER INSTITUTE, CANCER RATES AND RISKS 120 (4th ed. 1996); Mayo Clinic Family Health Book 1225 (4th ed. 2009).

[268] NATIONAL CANCER INSTITUTE, CANCER RATES AND RISKS 120 (4th ed. 1996).

[269] Nicole Fawcett, *Study finds black women more likely than white women to have more aggressive, less treatable form of breast cancer*, UNIVERSITY OF MICHIGAN COMPREHENSIVE CANCER CENTER REPORT, Sept. 7, 2007.

[270] In particular, this information pertains to women who have atypical hyperplasia as well as women with Dy and P2 patterns. Bodian CA: Benign breast diseases, carcinoma in situ, and breast cancer risk. *Epidemial Rev* 15:177-187, 1993; Oza AM, Boyd NF: Mammographic parenchymal patterns: a marker of breast cancer risk. *Epidemial Rev* 15:196-208, 1993.

[271] NATIONAL CANCER INSTITUTE, CANCER RATES AND RISKS 122 (4th ed. 1996).

[272] Kelsey JL and Gammon MD: Epidemiology of breast cancer. *Epidemiol Rev* 12: 228-240, 1990.

[273] Hunter DJ and Willett WC: Diet, body size, and breast cancer. *Epidemiol Rev* 15: 110-132, 1993.

[274] NATIONAL CANCER INSTITUTE, CANCER RATES AND RISKS 120-121 (4th ed. 1996); AMERICAN CANCER SOCIETY, BREAST CANCER RATES ON THE RISE AMONG ASIAN AMERICANS: JAPANESE-AMERICAN WOMEN MAY BE HARDEST HIT, August 1, 2002.

[275] SCIENCEDAILY,COM, JAPANESE WOMEN FOUND TO HAVE LOWER RECURRENCE OF BREAST CANCER (2005).

[276] Coyle YM: Physical activity as a negative modulator of estrogen-induced breast cancer. *Cancer Causes Control* 19(10):1021-1029, 2008.

[277] Longnecker MP et al: A meta-analysis of alcohol consumption in relation to risk of breast cancer. *JAMA* 260:62-656, 1988.

[278] http:/www.nutritionbox.com/index.php/article/articleview/10/.

[279] NCERX LLC, DRINKING RED WINE MAY HAVE A PREVENTIVE EFFECT IN CERTAIN CANCERS (2005).

[280] Daniel J. DeNoon, *Vitamin D fights colon cancer but colon cancer protection limited to the lean and active, researchers say*, July 10, 2007.

[281] Id.

[282] Pharma Marketletter, Review study suggests NSAIDs, including aspirin, may cut risk of developing breast cancer 20%, March 17, 2008.

[283] Kelsey JL and Gammon MD: Epidemiology of breast cancer. *Epidemiol Rev* 12:228-240, 1990.

[284] NATIONAL CANCER INSTITUTE, MOLECULAR TEST CAN PREDICT BOTH THE RISK OF BREAST CANCER RECURRENCE AND WHO WILL BENEFIT FROM CHEMOTHERAPY (2004).

[285] Dr. Philip Norrie, MBBS, MSc, MSocSc, ALCOHOL IN MODERATION, RED WINE VERSUS WHITE WINE—IS THERE A DIFFERENCE IN HEALTH BENEFIT? (2003).

[286] Mohammed Abbas, *Red wine slows lung cancer, white raises risk*, REUTERS, Oct. 27, 2004.

[287] NCERX LLC, DRINKING RED WINE MAY HAVE A PREVENTIVE EFFECT IN CERTAIN CANCERS (2005).

[288] NATIONAL CANCER INSTITUTE, CANCER RATES AND RISKS 129 (4th ed. 1996).

[289] Mayo Clinic Family Health Book 787 (2nd ed. 1996); Mayo Clinic Family Health Book 856 (4th ed. 2009).

[290] Id.

[291] NATIONAL CANCER INSTITUTE, CANCER RATES AND RISKS 129 (4th ed. 1996); AMERICAN CANCER SOCIETY, CANCER FACTS AND FIGURES 12 (2009).

[292] Whelan SL et al: Patterns of cancer in five continents. Lyon, France: International Agency for Research on Cancer. IARC Scientific Publication No. 102, 1990.

[293] Spiegelman D, Wegman DH: Occupation-related risks for colorectal cancer. *J Natl Cancer Inst*, 75:813-21, 1985; Lashner BA and Epstein SS: Industrial risk factors for colorectal cancer. *Int J Health Serv* 20:459-83, 1990.

[294] Lashner BA and Epstein SS: Industrial risk factors for colorectal cancer: *Int J Health Serv* 20:459-83, 1990.

[295] Ziegler RG et al: Epidemiologic patterns of colorectal cancer. 209-32. In Important Advances in Oncology. Philadelphia: J.P. Lippincott, 1985; McMichael AJ and Giles GG: Cancer in migrants to Australia: Extending the descriptive epidemiological data. *Cancer Res* 48:751-56, 1988.

[296] NATIONAL CANCER INSTITUTE, CANCER RATES AND RISKS 131-32 (4th ed. 1996).

[297] Bruce WR: Recent hypotheses for the origin of colon cancer. *Cancer Res* 47:4237-42, 1987.

[298] NATIONAL CANCER INSTITUTE, CANCER RATES AND RISKS 131 (4th ed. 1996).

[299] Id.

[300] Aaron Brown, FOOD CHANNEL, June 29, 2005, (Television).

[301] REUTERS LIMITED, RED MEAT, WHITE MEAT (2005); BERGEN MEATS, THE COLOR OF MEAT AND POULTRY (2005).

[302] ICBS, Inc., Holisticonline.com. Fat Content of Foods (2009).

[303] KAREN COLLINS, MS, RD, CDN, MICROSOFT CORPORATION, THE GRILLING QUESTION (2005); Sugimura T: Past, present, and future of mutagens in cooked foods. *Environ Health Perspect* 67:5-10, 1986.

[304] Id.

[305] Reddy BS: Diet and excretion of bile acids. *Cancer Res* 41:3766, 1981.

[306] Potter JD et al: Colon cancer: A review of the epidemiology. *Epidem Rev* 15:499-544, 1993.

[307] Slattery ML et al: Diet and colon cancer: Assessment of risk by fiber type and food source. *J Natl Cancer Inst* 80:1474-1480, 1988.

[308] Willett WC et al: The search for the causes of breast and colon cancer. *Nature* 338:389, 1989.

[309] Giovannucci E et al: Intake of fat, meat, and fiber in relation to risk of colon cancer in men. *Cancer Res* 54:2390-97, 1994.

[310] Garland C et al: Dietary vitamin D and calcium and risk of colorectal cancer: A 19-year prospective study in men. *Lancet* 1:307-09, 1985; Glynn SA and Albanes D: Folate and cancer: A review of the literature. *Nutr and Cancer* 22:101-19, 1994 .

[311] Bostick RM et al: Relation of calcium, vitamin D, and dairy food intake to incidence of colon cancer among older women: The Iowa Women's Health Study. *Am J Epidemiol* 137:1302-17, 1993.

[312] NATIONAL CANCER INSTITUTE, CANCER RATES AND RISKS 132 (4th ed. 1996).

[313] NATIONAL CANCER INSTITUTE, ASPIRIN MAY REDUCE RISK OF COLON POLYPS (2005); CBSNEWS, ASPIRIN NO COLON CANCER PANACEA (2005).

[314] Wu AH et al: Alcohol, physical activity and other risk factors for colorectal cancer. A prospective study. *Brit J Cancer* 55:687-94, 1987.

[315] Lee IM et al: Physical activity and risk of developing colorectal cancer among college alumni. *J Natl Cancer Inst* 83:1324-9, 1991.

[316] Cannon-Albright LA et al: Common inheritance of susceptibility to colonic adenomatous polyps and associated colorectal cancers. *N Engl J Med* 319:533-37, 1988.

[317] Grodon J et al: Identification and characterization of the familial adenomatous polyposis coli gene. *Cell* 66:589-600, 1991; Mayo Clinic Family Health Book 857 (4th ed. 2009). Similarly, Gardner's syndrome is a variant of FAP causing polyps to develop throughout one's colon and small intestine.

[318] Leach FS et al: Mutations of a mutS homolog in hereditary nonpolyposis colorectal cancer. *Cell* 75:1215-25, 1993; Mayo Clinic Family Health Book 857 (4th ed. 2009). HNPCC includes Lynch I and Lynch II syndromes. The former causes a small number of polyps to develop in the colon that quickly become malignant. The latter causes tumors in other body organs as well as the colon to develop.

[319] In women, an early diagnosis of colon cancer typically indicates a hereditary factor is responsible. If this hereditary factor is HNPCC, Lynch Syndrome I or II also is indicated. Women with this genetic anomaly who develop colon cancer have a thirty to fifty percent chance of developing endometrial cancer as well. Lynch HT and Lynch JF: Familial factors and genetic predisposition to cancer: Population studies. *Cancer Detection and Prevention* 15(1):49-57, 1993; Lynch HT et al: Hereditary factors in cancer. Study of two large midwestern kindreds. *Arch Intern Med* 117(2): 206-12, 1966.

[320] Random House Webster's Dictionary 535 (4th ed. 2001).

[321] Mayo Clinic Family Health Book 826 (4th ed. 2009).

[322] NATIONAL CANCER INSTITUTE, CANCER RATES AND RISKS 136 (4th ed. 1996).

[323] Brown LM et al: Environmental factors and high risk of esophageal cancer among men in coastal South Carolina. *J Natl CancerInst* 80:1620-1625, 1988.

[324] Blot WJ et al: Smoking and drinking in relation to oral and pharyngeal cancer. *Cancer Res* 48:3282-3287, 1988.

[325] NATIONAL CANCER INSTITUTE, CANCER RATES AND RISKS 61 (4th ed. 1996).

[326] Brown LM et al: Environmental factors and high risk of esophageal cancer among men in coastal South Carolina. *J Natl Cancer Inst* 80:1620-1625, 1988.

[327] Kallner AB et al: On the requirements of ascorbic acid in man: Steady-state turnover and body pool in smokers. *Am J Clin Nutr* 34:1347-1355, 1981; Broitman SA et al: Ethanolic beverage consumption, cigarette smoking, nutritional status, and digestive tract cancers. *Semin Oncol* 10:322-329, 1983.

[328] NATIONAL CANCER INSTITUTE, CANCER RATES AND RISKS 137 (4th ed. 1996); Cold Spring Harbor Laboratory Press, Origins of Human Cancer 192 (1991).

[329] Graham GM et al: Nutritional epidemiology of cancer of the esophagus. *Am J Epidemiol* 131:454-467, 1990.

[330] Ghadirian P: Thermal irritation and oesophageal cancer in Northern Iran. *Cancer* 60:1909-1914, 1987.

[331] Brown LM et al: Adenocarcinoma of the esophagus and esophagastric junction in white men in the United States: Alcohol, tobacco and socioeconomic factors. *Cancer Causes Control* 5:333-340, 1994.

[332] Mayo Clinic Family Health Book 886-887 (4th ed. 2009).

[333] Devesa SS et al: Comparison of the descriptive epidemiology of urinary tract cancers. *Cancer Causes and Control* 1:133-141, 1990.

[334] Id.

[335] McLaughlin JK et al: Cigarette smoking and cancers of the renal pelvis and ureter. *Cancer Res* 52: 254-257, 1992.

[336] NATIONAL CANCER INSTITUTE, CANCER RATES AND RISKS 146 (4th ed. 1996).

[337] Id. at 145-146.

[338] Id. at 146.

[339] William G. Kaelin, Jr.: The von Hippel-Lindau Gene, Kidney cancer, and Oxygen Sensing. *J Am Soc Nephrol* 14:2703-2711, 2003.

[340] Coppes MJ at al: Genetic events in the development of Wilms' tumor. *N Engl J Med* 331(9):586-90, 1994.

[341] Alison Levitt, MD, *Baked or fried: acrylamide*, EXPERIENCE LIFE, March 2004, at 22-24;

[342] Mayo Clinic Family Health Book 1048-1053 (4th ed. 2009).

[343] This form of acute leukemia also is called monocytic or myelogenic leukemia as well as nonlymphocytic leukemia, which distinguishes it from leukemias that affect the lympho-cytes. Monocytic and myelogenic are interchangeable terms for leukemias. Mayo Clinic Family Health Book 1048-1053 (4th ed. 2009); RUSH UNIVERSITY MEDICAL CENTER RUSH BONE MARROW TRANSPLANT CENTER, WHAT IS BONE MARROW TRANSPLANT? (2005).

[344] Mayo Clinic Family Health Book 1048-1053 (4th ed. 2009).

[345] Id.

[346] Id.

[347] Id.

[348] Id.

[349] NATIONAL CANCER INSTITUTE, GLEEVEC (ST1571) (2005).

350 NATIONAL CANCER INSTITUTE, CANCER RATES AND RISKS 107, 151 (4th ed. 1996); TULANE UNIVERSITY, HTLV-1 (2005).

351 Blattner WA: Human T-cell lymphotrophic viruses and cancer causation. In Cancer: Principles and Practice of Oncology Philadelphia: J.B. Lippincott, 1993.

352 International Agency for Research on Cancer: Monographs on the Evaluation of the Carcinogenic Risk of Chemicals to Man. Wood, Leather, and Some Associated Industries, vol 25. Lyon, IARC, 1981, 1-97.

353 Blair A et al: Clues to cancer etiology from studies of farmers. *Scand J Work Environ Health* 18:209-215, 1992.

354 Savitz DA and Chen J: Parental occupation and childhood cancer: A review of epide-miologic studies. *Environ Health Perspect* 88:325-337, 1990; MIRANDA HITTI, WEBMD, BENZENE LINKED TO CHILDHOOD LEUKEMIA (2004).

355 Id.; NATIONAL CANCER INSTITUTE, CANCER RATES AND RISKS 150-51 (4th ed. 1996).

356 http://www.oehha.ca.gov/public_info/facts/chrom6facts.html.

357 NATIONAL CANCER INSTITUTE, CANCER RATES AND RISKS 149-150 (4th ed. 1996).

358 Kinlen LJ et al: Rural population mixing and childhood leukaemia. Effects of the North Sea oil industry in Scotland, including the area near Dounreay nuclear site. *BMJ* 306:743-748, 1993; Roman E et al: Case-control study of leukaemia and non-Hodgkin's lymphoma among children aged 0-4 years living in West Berkshire and North Hampshire health dis-tricts. *BMJ* 306:615-621, 1993.

359 Jablon S et al: Cancer in populations living near nuclear facilities. *JAMA Assoc* 265: 1403-1408, 1991; Hjalmars U et al: Risk of acute childhood leukaemia Group: Risk of acute child-hood leukaemia in Sweden after the Chernobyl reactor accident. *BMJ* 309:154-157, 1994.

360 NAS: Health Effects of Exposure to Low Levels of Ionizing Radiation (BEIR 4). Washington DC: Natl Acad Press, 1990.

361 MacMahon B: Prenatal X-ray exposure and childhood cancer. *J Natl Cancer Inst* 28:1173-1191, 1962; Boice JD Jr. et al: Diagnostic X-rays and risk of leukemia, lymphoma, and mul-tiple myeloma. *JAMA Assoc* 265:1290-1294, 1991.

362 Darby et al: Long-term mortality after a single treatment course with X-rays in patients treated for ankylosing spondylitis. *Br J Cancer* 55:179-190, 1987.

363 NATIONAL CANCER INSTITUTE, CANCER RATES AND RISKS 150 (4th ed. 1996).

364 Sandler DP and Collman GW: Cytogenetic and environmental factors in the etiology of the acute leukemias in adults. *Am J Epidemiol* 126:1017-1032, 1987.

365 Id.

366 Blattner WA: Human T-cell lymphotrophic viruses and cancer causation. In Cancer: Principles and Practice of Oncology Philadelphia: J.B. Lippincott, 1993.

367 http://www.answers.com/topic/retrovirus.

368 TULANE UNIVERSITY, HTLV-1 (2005).

369 Blattner WA: Human T-cell lymphotropic viruses and cancer causation. In Cancer: Principles and Practice of Oncology. Philadelphia: J.B Lippincott, 1993.

370 Id.

371 NATIONAL CANCER INSTITUTE, CANCER RATES AND RISKS 64-65, 148-149 (4th ed. 1996).

372 Id.; http://www.medterms.com/script/main/art.asp?articlekey=32631.

373 NATIONAL CANCER INSTITUTE, CANCER RATES AND RISKS 151 (4th ed. 1996); Clinical Reference Systems, *Diethylstilbestrol (DES). (Women's Health Advisor 2002.1)* Jan. 1, 2002.

374 Theriault G et al: Cancer risks associated with occupational exposure to magnetic fields among electric utility workers in Ontario and Quebec, 139:550-572, 1994; National Radiological Protection Board: Electromagnetic Fields and the Risk of Cancer. Report of an Advisory Group on Non-Ionising Radiation, vol 1, no. 1. Chilton, Didcot, Oxon, United Kingdom: National Radiological Protection Board, 1992.

375 Evidence does suggest that a mother's diet may help protect her fetus from developing leukemia as a child. SCIENCEDAILY, NEW STUDY SUGGESTS LINK BETWEEN MATERNAL DIET AND CHILDHOOD LEUKEMIA RISK, August 24, 2004.

376 Peggy Peck, *Paternal smoking before conception increases risk of childhood leukemia in off-spring: presented at AACR*, DGDISPATCH, July 17, 2003.

377 Mayo Clinic Family Health Book 783-787 (4th ed. 2009).

378 Id.

379 Id.

380 Id.

381 U.S. Department of Health and Human Services: A Report of the Surgeon General: The Health Benefits of Smoking Cessation. DHHS Publ. No. (CDC) 90-8416, 1990.

382 Id.

383 NATIONAL CANCER INSTITUTE, CANCER RATES AND RISKS 159 (4th ed. 1996).

384 Id.

385 Blot WJ and Fraumeni JF Jr: Lung and pleura. In Cancer Epidemiology and Prevention, 2nd ed. Philadelphia: WB Saunders, 1992.

386 Blot WJ at al: Lung cancer after employment in shipyards during World War II. *N Engl J Med* 299:620, 1978; NATIONAL CANCER INSTITUTE, CANCER RATES AND RISKS 160 (4th ed. 1996).

387 Xu ZY et al: Smoking, air pollution, and the high rates of lung cancer in Shenyang, China. *J Natl Cancer Inst* 81:1800-1806, 1989.

388 Id.

389 NATIONAL CANCER INSTITUTE, CANCER RATES AND RISKS 90-91, 160 (4th ed. 1996).

390 Id. at 77.

391 Id. at 74, 151.

392 Id. at 161.

393 Bonnie Liebman, *B-C: no magic bullet*, NUTRITION ACTION HEALTHLETTER, Nov. 1, 1996; Lyn Patrick, *Beta-C: the controversy continues*, ALTERNATIVE MEDICINE REVIEW, Dec. 1, 2000.

394 Mayo Clinic Family Health Book 1035-1036 (4th ed. 2009).

395 Id.

396 Beral V et al: AIDS-associated non-Hodgkin lymphoma. *Lancet* 337:805-809, 1991.

[397] Kinlen L et al: Collaborative United Kingdom-Australasian study of cancer in patients treated with immunosuppressive drugs. *BMJ* 2:1461-1466, 1979.

[398] NATIONAL CANCER INSTITUTE, CANCER RATES AND RISKS 170-171 (4th ed. 1996).

[399] Hoar SK et al: Agricultural herbicide use and risk of lymphoma and soft-tissue sarcoma. *JAMA* 256:1141-1147, 1986.

[400] NATIONAL CANCER INSTITUTE, CANCER RATES AND RISKS 171 (4th ed. 1996).

[401] Id.

[402] Id. at 172.

[403] Id.

[404] WEBMD, INC., HAIR DYE LINKED TO BLOOD CANCER (2003).

[405] CANCER WEEKLY, MORE STUDY NEEDED TO ASSESS DERMAL ABSORPTION OF RISKY AMINES FOUND IN HAIR DYE, March 16, 2004.

[406] Mayo Clinic Family Health Book 1225-1226 (4th ed. 2009); Johannes CB et al: Site of origin of epithelial ovarian cancer. *BMJ* 304(6818):27-28, 1992.

[407] NATIONAL CANCER INSTITUTE, CANCER RATES AND RISKS 179 (4th ed. 1996).

[408] Id.

[409] Id. at 83, 179.

[410] AMERICAN CANCER SOCIETY, CANCER FACTS AND FIGURES 16 (2005).

[411] HNPCC not only is implicated in the development of colorectal, it is implicated in the development of ovarian, stomach and uterine endometrial cancer. Mayo Clinic Family Health Book 1225 (4th ed. 2009).

[412] Amos CI and Struewing JP: Genetic epidemiology of epithelial ovarian cancer. *Cancer* 71 (2suppl):566-572, 1993.

[413] Parazzini F et al: The epidemiology of ovarian cancer. *Gynecol Oncol* 43:9-23, 1991.

[414] NATIONAL CANCER INSTITUTE, CANCER RATES AND RISKS 179 (4th ed. 1996).

[415] Weiss NS and Harlow BL: Why does hysterectomy without bilateral oophorectomy influence the subsequent incidence of ovarian cancer? *AM J Epidermiol* 124:856-858, 1986.

[416] Id.

[417] Harlow BL et al: Perineal exposure to talc and ovarian cancer risk. *Obstet Gynecol* 80(1): 19-26, 1992.

[418] Id.

[419] Mayo Clinic Family Health Book 1225-1227 (4th ed. 2009).

[420] Id. at 870-872.

[421] Id. at 871-873.

[422] Lauran Neergaard, AP ONLINE NEWS WIRES, FEW GET SURGERY FOR GRIM PANCREATIC CANCER, Feb. 5, 2009.

[423] NATIONAL CANCER INSTITUTE, CANCER RATES AND RISKS 183 (4th ed. 1996).

[424] Parkin DM et al: Cancer Incidence in Five Continents, vol VI. IARC Scientific Publication No. 120. World Health Organization, IARC, Lyon, 1992.

[425] NATIONAL CANCER INSTITUTE, CANCER RATES AND RISKS 182-183 (4th ed. 1996).

[426] Id.

[427] AMERICAN CANCER SOCIETY, CANCER FACTS AND FIGURES 16 (2009).

[428] Mack TM et al: Pancreas cancer and smoking, beverage consumption, and past medical history. *J Natl Cancer Inst* 76:49-60, 1986.

[429] *Pancreatic cancer likelier in diabetics*, LOS ANGELES TIMES, Aug. 8, 2005, at F5.

[430] AMERICAN CANCER SOCIETY, CANCER FACTS AND FIGURES 18 (2009); Mayo Clinic Family Health Book 871-872 (4th ed. 2009).

[431] Id.; NATIONAL CANCER INSTITUTE, CANCER FACTS AND FIGURES 182 (4th ed. 1996).

[432] NATIONAL CANCER INSTITUTE, CANCER FACTS AND FIGURES 182 (4th ed. 1996).

[433] Dr. Isadore Rosenfeld, *Protect your prostate*, PARADE MAGAZINE, June 15, 2003, at 6-7; Mayo Clinic Family Health Book 1245-1246 (4th ed. 2009).

[434] Males with a mutation in the BRCA 1 and 2 genes have an increased risk for male breast cancer, prostate and testicular cancer. These cancers, however, appear to be more strongly associated with a mutation in the BRCA 2 gene. Thompson D and Easton DF: The Breast Cancer Linkage Consortium. Cancer incidence in BRCA 1 mutation carriers. *J Natl Cancer Inst* 94(18):1358-1365, 2002; The Breast Cancer Linkage Consortium. Cancer risk in BRCA 2 mutation carriers. *J Natl Cancer Inst* 91(15): 1310-1316, 1999.

[435] AMERICAN CANCER SOCIETY, CANCER FACTS AND FIGURES 19 (2009).

[436] Dr. Isadore Rosenfeld, *Protect your prostate,* PARADE MAGAZINE, June 15, 2003, at 6-7; AMERICAN CANCER SOCIETY, CANCER FACTS AND FIGURES 17 (2005).

[437] Bosland M: The etiopathogenesis of prostate cancer with special reference to environmental factors. *Adv Cancer Res* 51:1-106, 1988.

[438] Id.

[439] NATIONAL CANCER INSTITUTE, CANCER RATES AND RISKS 185 (4th ed. 1996).

[440] Foods rich in lycopene such as tomatoes, apricots and watermelon appear to have a protective effect for this cancer. http://www.cancer.org/docroot/ETO/content/ETO_5_3X_Lycopene.asp.

[441] Kolonel LN et al: Diet and prostatic cancer: A case-control study in Hawaii. *Am J Epidemiol* 127:999-1012, 1988.

[442] Id. at 185; CLINICAL ADVISOR, SOY MAY PREVENT PROSTATE CANCER, May 1, 2007.

[443] Ross RK et al: Case-control studies of prostate cancer in blacks and whites in Southern California. *J Natl Cancer Inst* 78:869-874, 1987.

[444] NATIONAL CANCER INSTITUTE, CANCER RATES AND RISKS 186 (4th ed. 1996).

[445] Id.

[446] AMERICAN CANCER SOCIETY, CANCER FACTS AND FIGURES 19 (2009).

[447] Kurihara M et al: Cancer mortality statistics in the world 1950-1985, Nagoya: University of Nagoya Press, 1989.

[448] AMERICAN CANCER SOCIETY, CANCER FACTS AND FIGURES 19 (2009).

[449] Timothy Gower, *A man's tough choice*, LOS ANGELES TIMES, Nov. 8, 2004, at F1, F8.

[450] Lindsey Tanner, *Study disputes sex-prostate cancer link*, LOS ANGELES TIMES, April 7, 2004.

[451] SKIN CANCER FOUNDATION: http://www.skincancer.org/skincancer-facts.php.

[452] Mayo Clinic Family Health Book 1066-1067 (4th ed. 2009).

453 Id.

454 Id. at 1104-1109.

455 Id.

456 Mayo Clinic Family Health Book 1109 (4th ed. 2009).

457 Id.

458 Tucker MA: Individuals at high risk of melanoma. In Pigment Cell, vol 9 (Makie RM, ed.). Basel, Switzerland: S. Karger, 1988, 95-109.

459 NATIONAL CANCER INSTITUTE, CANCER RATES AND RISKS 165 (4th ed. 1996).

460 Mayo Clinic Family Health Book 1109-1110 (4th ed. 2009).

461 Timothy F. Kim, SKIN AND ALLERGY NEWS, STUDIES SHED NEW LIGHT ON MELANOMA SUN RISK, Dec. 1, 2005.

462 NATIONAL CANCER INSTITUTE, CANCER RATES AND RISKS 164 (4th ed. 1996).

463 Id. at 163.

464 Id. at 164-165.

465 Id.

466 Rhodes AR et al: Risk factors for cutaneous melanoma. A practical method for recognizing predisposed individuals. *JAMA* 258:3146-3154, 1987.

467 NATIONAL CANCER INSTITUTE, CANCER RATES AND RISKS 189 (4th ed. 1996).

468 Tucker MA: Individuals at high risk of melanoma. In Pigment Cell, vol 9 (Makie RM, ed.). Basel, Switzerland: S. Karger, 1988, 95-109.

469 Id.

470 NATIONAL CANCER INSTITUTE, CANCER RATES AND RISKS 197 (4th ed. 1996).

471 Id.

472 Id.

473 Id.

474 Li FP: Cancer families: Human models of susceptibility to neoplasia – The Richard and Hinda Rosenthal Foundation Award lecture. *Cancer Res.* 48:5381-5386, 1988.

475 NATIONAL CANCER INSTITUTE, CANCER RATES AND RISKS 197-198 (4th ed. 1996).

476 Silverman DT et al: Epidemiology of bladder cancer. *Hematol Oncol* 6:1-30, 1992a.

477 NATIONAL CANCER INSTITUTE, CANCER RATES AND RISKS 197-198 (4th ed. 1996).

478 Id.

479 Id. at 200-201.

480 Brinton LA and Fraumeni JF Jr: Epidemiology of uterine cervical cancer. *J Chron Dis* 39:1051-1065, 1986.

481 DR. JOE GLICKMAN, JRL, M.D., CONTRACTING HPV, HPV IN WOMAN (2005).

482 Brinton LA et al: The male factor in the aetiology of cervical cancer among sexually monogamous women. *Int J Cancer* 44:199-203, 1989b.

483 Schiffman MH et al: Epidemiologic evidence showing that human papillomavirus infection causes most cervical intraepithelial neoplasia. *J Natl Cancer Inst* 85:958-964, 1993.

484 Brinton LA: Oral contraceptives and cervical neoplasia. *Contraception* 43:581-595, 1991.

485 Id.

[486] Slattery ML et al: Dietary vitamins A, C, and E and selenium as risk factors for cervical cancer. *Epidemiology* 1:8-15, 1990; Zeigler RG et al: Diet and the risk of invasive cervical cancer among white women in the United States. *Am J Epidemiol* 132:432-445, 1990.

[487] NATIONAL CANCER INSTITUTE, CANCER RATES AND RISKS 201 (4th ed. 1996).

[488] Winkelstein W Jr: Smoking and cervical cancer—Current status: a review. *Am J Epidemiol* 131:945-957, 1990.

[489] AMERICAN CANCER SOCIETY, SMOKING MAY DOUBLE CERVICAL CANCER RISK, Jan. 19, 2004.

[490] NATIONAL CANCER INSTITUTE, WHAT YOU NEED TO KNOW ABOUT CANCER OF THE CERVIX, NIH PUBLICATION NO. 08-2047 (2008); Mayo Clinic Family Health Book 1177 (2nd ed. 1991).

[491] REPORT OF THE SURGEON GENERAL, THE HEALTH CONSEQUENCES OF SMOKING: 2004; http://www.cdc.gov/tobacco/sqr/sqr2004/; http://info.cancerresearchuk.org/cancerstats/types/cervix/riskfactors/.

[492] Mayo Clinic Family Health Book 1183 (2nd ed. 1991).

[493] Weiss NS et al: Increasing incidence of endometrial cancer in the United States. *N Eng J Med* 294:1259-1262, 1976.

[494] Fisher B et al: Endometrial cancer in tamoxifen-treated breast cancer patients: (NSABP) b-14. *J Natl Cancer Inst* 86:527-537, 1994.

[495] NATIONAL CANCER INSTITUTE, CANCER RATES AND RISKS 203 (4th ed. 1996).

[496] Brinton LA et al: Estrogen replacement therapy and endometrial cancer risk: Unresolved issues. *Obstet Gynecol* 81:265-271, 1993.

[497] Cancer and Steroid Hormone Study of the Centers for Disease Control and the National Institute of Child Health and Human Development; Combination oral contraceptive use and the risk of endometrial cancer. *JAMA* 257:796-800, 1987.

[498] Id.

[499] Weiss NS et al: Increasing incidence of endometrial cancer in the United States. *N Engl J Med* 294:1259-1262, 1976.

[500] Potischman N et al: Dietary associations in a case-control study of endometrial cancer. *Cancer Causes Control* 4:239-250, 1993.

[501] Id.; Swanson CA et al: Relation of endometrial cancer risk to past and contemporary body size and body fat distribution. *Cancer Epidemiol Biomarker Prev* 2:321-327, 1993.

[502] NATIONAL CANCER INSTITUTE, CANCER RATES AND RISKS 203 (4th ed. 1996).

[503] SID KIRCHHEIMER, WEBMD INC., TANNING SALONS BOOST SKIN CANCER RISK (2003); Jane E. Allen, *Next in skin cancer fight: protection from UVA rays*, LOS ANGELES TIMES, May 20, 2002, at S6.

[504] http://www.who.int/features/qa/15/en/; http://www.cancer.org/docroot/PRO/content/PRO_1_1_Cancer Statistics 2008 Presentation.asp.

[505] AMERICAN CANCER SOCIETY, CANCER FACTS AND FIGURES 1 (2009).

[506] DIRTY HARRY, Warner Bros. Productions, Release date Dec. 22, 1971.

[507] Mayo Clinic Family Health Book 330, 806-807 (4th ed. 2009).

[508] Id. at 1268.

[509] NATIONAL CANCER INSTITUTE, WHAT YOU NEED TO KNOW ABOUT BREAST CANCER, NIH PUBLICATION NO. 03-1556 (2009).

[510] http://www.medicinenet.com/mammogram/article.htm.

[511] Leslie Bernstein et al: High breast cancer incidence rates among California teachers: results from the California Teachers Study (United States), Kluwer Academic Publishers, *Cancer Causes and Control* 13:625-635, 2002.

[512] Shawn Farley, Women with dense breasts, women younger than 50, and those who are premenopausal or perimenopausal may benefit from digital mammograms, American College of Radiology Imaging Network (ACRIN) Digital Mammography (DMIST) Trial, Sept. 19, 2005.

[513] Mosby's Medical, Nursing & Allied Health Dictionary 1763 (6th ed. 2002); DANA DELANY, BREASTCANCER.ORG, TUMOR MARKERS (ALSO CALLED BIOMARKERS) (2004); BREASTCANCER.ORG, BLOOD TESTS (2004).

[514] ABC NEWS INTERNET VENTURES, HAND-HELD DEVICE SHOWS PROMISE IN BREAST CANCER DETECTION (2005).

[515] Doug Stanglin, *Cleveland clinic doctor reports a possible vaccine to prevent breast cancer*, USA TODAY, June 1, 2010; Dana Blankenhorn, *A breast cancer vaccine is still far away*, SMARTPLANET, June 1, 2010.

[516] http://www.bloomberg.com/news/2010-09-24/hologic-3d-mammogram-s-benefits-outweigh.

[517] TAMAR NORENBERG, U.S. FOOD AND DRUG ADMINISTRATION, CELL PHONES AND CANCER: NO CLEAR CONNECTION (2000); VIRTUAL HEALTH, CELL PHONES AND CANCER RESEARCH (2004); JOSHUA LEVIN, DO CELL PHONES CAUSE CANCER? (2005).

[518] NATIONAL CANCER INSTITUTE, WHAT YOU NEED TO KNOW ABOUT CANCER OF THE COLON AND RECTUM, NIH PUBLICATION NO. 06-1552 (2006).

[519] Soda phosphate has been known to cause kidney failure in some patients and as a result it is not available for sale in some areas. When it is available, physicians often ask patients to sign a release form. In the alternative, patients may choose to take a tablet preparation known as Visicol. The correct preparation will be determined by the health of the patient.

[520] NATIONAL CANCER INSTITUTE, WHAT YOU NEED TO KNOW ABOUT CANCER OF THE COLON AND RECTUM, NIH PUBLICATION NO. 06-1552 (2006).

[521] Id.

[522] Id.; Mayo Clinic Family Health Book 857-860 (4th ed. 2009).

[523] http://www.bing.com/health/article/mayo-119674/Virtual-colonoscopy?q+virtual+colonoscopy.

[524] NATIONAL CANCER INSTITUTE, WHAT YOU NEED TO KNOW ABOUT LUNG CANCER, NIH PUBLICATION NO. 07-1553 (2007).

[525] NATIONAL CANCER INSTITUTE, WHAT YOU NEED TO KNOW ABOUT OVARIAN CANCER, NIH PUBLICATION NO. 06-1561 (2006).

[526] http://www.researchherpathways.com/researchherpath/her4/index.

[527] NATIONAL CANCER INSTITUTE, WHAT YOU NEED TO KNOW ABOUT PROSTATE CANCER, NIH PUBLICATION NO. 08-1576 (2008); Mayo Clinic Family Health Book 1250-1254 (4th ed. 2009); Thomas H. Maugh II, *Researchers open several new fronts on prostate cancer*, LOS ANGELES TIMES, June 14, 2004.

[528] http://www.betterhealthandliving.com/articles/whos_afraid_of_a_full_body_skin_check/.

[529] Sid Kirchheimer, *Flight crews have higher cancer risk*, WEBMD HEALTH NEWS, Oct. 21, 2003; BBC NEWS, PILOTS 'HAVE HIGHER SKIN CANCER RISK', Feb. 17, 2000.

[530] Mayo Clinic Family Health Book 903-906 (4th ed. 2009).

[531] Id. at 1223-1224.

[532] Id. at 1222.

[533] NATIONAL CANCER INSTITUTE, WHAT YOU NEED TO KNOW ABOUT CANCER OF THE CERVIX, NIH PUBLICATION NO. 08-2047 (2008).

[534] Linda Marsa, *Optical wand used to detect cervical cancer*, LOS ANGELES TIMES, May 24, 2004, at F3.

[535] NATIONAL CANCER INSTITUTE, WHAT YOU NEED TO KNOW ABOUT CANCER OF THE CERVIX, NIH PUBLICATION NO. 08-2047 (2008).

[536] Jane E. Allen, *A change in routine for Pap testing*, LOS ANGELES TIMES.

[537] Dr. Isadore Rosenfeld, *Do you know about HPV?*, PARADE, Oct. 10, 2004, at 15.

[538] Id.; Mayo Clinic Family Health Book 1224 (4th ed. 2009).

[539] http://www.gardasil.com/what-is-gardasil/information-or-gardasil.

[540] Mayo Clinic Family Health Book 1220-1221 (4th ed. 2009); NATIONAL CANCER INSTITUTE, WHAT YOU SHOULD KNOW ABOUT CANCER OF THE UTERUS, NIH PUBLICATION NO. 01-1562 (2002).

[541] Mayo Clinic Family Health Book 1269-1270 (4th ed. 2009).

[542] Id.

[543] Id.

[544] Id.

[545] Mosby's Medical, Nursing & Allied Health Dictionary 716 (6th ed. 2002).

[546] PETSCANINFO.COM, WHAT IS PET? (2005).

[547] Mayo Clinic Family Health Book 1270-1271 (4th ed. 2009).

[548] Id. at 1268.

[549] Id.

INDEX

About the Author

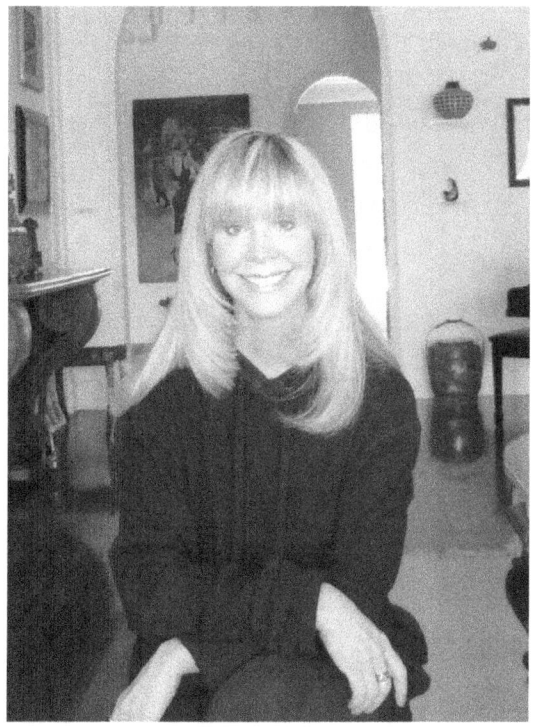

For more information, visit www.swilkinghoran.com

Ms. Horan received her Bachelor's Degree in Psychology from California State University, Northridge and her Juris Doctor Degree from Loyola Law School, Los Angeles. She has been an author, an attorney and an advocate for patient rights over the last twenty years. At present, she is living quietly and cancer free, with her attorney husband and Labrador Retriever in Los Angeles, California.